ADOLESCENT MEDICINE: STATE OF THE ART REVIEWS

Advances in the Treatment of Endocrine Disorders in Adolescents

GUEST EDITORS

Irene N. Sills, MD

Martin M. Fisher, MD

August 2015 • Volume 26 • Number 2

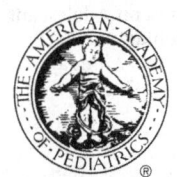

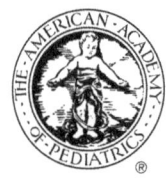

ADOLESCENT MEDICINE:
STATE OF THE ART REVIEWS
August 2015
Editor: Carrie Peters
Marketing Manager: Linda Smessaert
Production Manager: Shannan Martin
eBook Developer: Houston Adams

Volume 26, Number 2
ISBN 978-1-58110-887-3
ISSN 1934-4287
MA0730
SUB1006

The recommendations in this publication do not indicate an exclusive course of treatment or serve as a standard of medical care. Variations, taking into account individual circumstances, may be appropriate.

Statements and opinions expressed are those of the author and not necessarily those of the American Academy of Pediatrics.

Products and Web sites are mentioned for informational purposes only. Inclusion in this publication does not imply endorsement by the American Academy of Pediatrics. The American Academy of Pediatrics is not responsible for the content of the resources mentioned in this publication. Web site addresses are as current as possible but may change at any time.

Every effort has been made to ensure that the drug selection and dosage set forth in this text are in accordance with the current recommendations and practice at the time of publication. It is the responsibility of the health care provider to check the package insert of each drug for any change in indications and dosage and for added warnings and precautions.

Copyright © 2015 American Academy of Pediatrics. All rights reserved. No part of this publication may be reproduced or transmitted in any form or by any means, electronic or mechanical, including photocopying, recording, or any information retrieval system, without written permission from the Publisher (fax the permissions editor at 847/434-8780).

Adolescent Medicine: State of the Art Reviews is published three times per year by the American Academy of Pediatrics, 141 Northwest Point Blvd, Elk Grove Village, IL 60007-1019. Periodicals postage paid at Arlington Heights, IL.

POSTMASTER: Send address changes to American Academy of Pediatrics, Department of Marketing and Publications, Attn: AM:STARs, 141 Northwest Point Blvd, Elk Grove Village, IL 60007-1019.

Subscriptions: Subscriptions to *Adolescent Medicine: State of the Art Reviews* (AM:STARs) are provided to members of the American Academy of Pediatrics' Section on Adolescent Health as part of annual section membership dues. All others, please contact the AAP Customer Service Center at 866/843-2271 (7:00 am–5:30 pm Central Time, Monday–Friday) for pricing and information.

Adolescent Medicine: State of the Art Reviews

Official Journal of the American Academy of Pediatrics
Section on Adolescent Health

EDITORS-IN-CHIEF

Victor C. Strasburger, MD
Distinguished Professor Emeritus
of Pediatrics
Founding Chief, Division of Adolescent
Medicine
University of New Mexico
School of Medicine
Albuquerque, New Mexico

Donald E. Greydanus, MD, Dr HC
(ATHENS)
Professor & Founding Chair
Department of Pediatric &
Adolescent Medicine
Western Michigan University
Homer Stryker M.D. School of
Medicine
Kalamazoo, Michigan

ASSOCIATE EDITORS

Robert T. Brown, MD
Camden, New Jersey

Paula K. Braverman, MD
Cincinnati, Ohio

Megan A. Moreno, MD, MSED, MPH
Seattle, Washington

Sheryl Ryan, MD
New Haven, Connecticut

Martin M. Fisher, MD
Manhasset, New York

Alain Joffe, MD, MPH
Baltimore, Maryland

ADVANCES IN THE TREATMENT OF ENDOCRINE DISORDERS IN ADOLESCENTS

EDITORS-IN-CHIEF

VICTOR C. STRASBURGER, MD, Distinguished Professor Emeritus of Pediatrics, Founding Chief, Division of Adolescent Medicine, University of New Mexico, School of Medicine, Albuquerque, New Mexico

DONALD E. GREYDANUS, MD, Dr HC (ATHENS), Professor & Founding Chair, Department of Pediatric & Adolescent Medicine, Western Michigan University Homer Stryker M.D. School of Medicine, Kalamazoo, Michigan

GUEST EDITORS

MARTIN M. FISHER, MD, Chief, Division of Adolescent Medicine, Cohen Children's Medical Center, North Shore–Long Island Jewish Health System, Professor of Pediatrics, Hofstra–North Shore LIJ School of Medicine, New Hyde Park, New York

IRENE N. SILLS, MD, Professor of Pediatrics, Pediatric Endocrinologist, SUNY Upstate Medical University, Syracuse, New York

CONTRIBUTORS

SHARA R. BIALO, MD, Division of Pediatric Endocrinology, Rhode Island Hospital and Alpert Medical School of Brown University, Providence, Rhode Island

CLIFFORD A. BLOCH, MD, Clinical Professor of Pediatrics, University of Colorado School of Medicine, Pediatric Endocrine Associates, P.C., Greenwood Village, Colorado

CHARLOTTE M. BONEY, MD, MS, Division of Pediatric Endocrinology, Baystate Medical Center and Tufts University School of Medicine, Springfield, Massachusetts

DENNIS E. CAREY, MD, Division of Pediatric Endocrinology, Cohen Children's Medical Center of New York, Associate Professor of Pediatrics, Hofstra–North Shore LIJ School of Medicine, New Hyde Park, New York

LINDA CARMINE, MD, Division of Adolescent Medicine, Cohen Children's Medical Center, North Shore–Long Island Jewish Health System, Hofstra–North Shore LIJ School of Medicine, Hempstead, New York

MEGHAN CRAVEN, MD, Division of Pediatric Endocrinology, Cohen Children's Medical Center of New York, North Shore–Long Island Jewish Health System, New Hyde Park, New York; Hofstra–North Shore LIJ School of Medicine, Hempstead, New York

NEVILLE H. GOLDEN, MD, Chief, Division of Adolescent Medicine, The Marion and Mary Elizabeth Kendrick Professor of Pediatrics, Stanford University School of Medicine, Palo Alto, California

PAULA J. ADAMS HILLARD, MD, Professor of Obstetrics and Gynecology, Stanford University Medical Center, Stanford University School of Medicine, Palo Alto, California

YEOUCHING HSU, MD, Division of Pediatric Endocrinology, Cohen Children's Medical Center of New York, Assistant Professor of Pediatrics, Hofstra–North Shore LIJ School of Medicine, Lake Success, New York

SUZANNE E. KINGERY, MD, Division of Pediatric Endocrinology, Department of Pediatrics, University of Louisville School of Medicine, Louisville, Kentucky

JASON KLEIN, MD, Division of Pediatric Endocrinology, Cohen Children's Medical Center of New York, North Shore–Long Island Jewish Health System, New Hyde Park, New York; Hofstra–North Shore LIJ School of Medicine, Hempstead, New York

AMIT LAHOTI, MD, Division of Pediatric Endocrinology, Le Bonheur Children's Hospital, University of Tennessee Health Science Center, Memphis, Tennessee

SUNIL NAYAK, MD, Assistant Clinical Professor of Pediatrics, University of Colorado School of Medicine, Pediatric Endocrine Associates, P.C., Greenwood Village, Colorado

NADIA SALDANHA, MD, Division of Adolescent Medicine, Cohen Children's Medical Center, North Shore–Long Island Jewish Health System, Hofstra–North Shore LIJ School of Medicine, Hempstead, New York

DAVID E. SANDBERG, PhD, University of Michigan, Pediatrics & Communicable Diseases and Child Health Evaluation & Research (CHEAR) Unit, Ann Arbor, Michigan

IRENE N. SILLS, MD, Professor of Pediatrics, Pediatric Endocrinologist, SUNY Upstate Medical University, Syracuse, New York

PHYLLIS W. SPEISER, MD, Chief, Division of Pediatric Endocrinology, Cohen Children's Medical Center of New York, Professor of Pediatrics, North Shore-Long Island Jewish Health System, Hofstra–North Shore LIJ School of Medicine, Hempstead, New York

SUSAN E. STRED, MD, Clinical Professor of Pediatrics, Pediatric Endocrinology Center, SUNY Upstate Medical University, Syracuse, New York

PATRICIA M. VUGUIN, MD, MSc, Division of Pediatric Endocrinology, Cohen Children's Medical Center of New York, North Shore–Long Island Jewish Health System, New Hyde Park, New York; Hofstra–North Shore LIJ School of Medicine, Hempstead, New York

KUPPER A. WINTERGERST, MD, Division of Pediatric Endocrinology, Department of Pediatrics, University of Louisville School of Medicine, Louisville, Kentucky

ADVANCES IN THE TREATMENT OF ENDOCRINE DISORDERS IN ADOLESCENTS

CONTENTS

Preface xiii

Thyroid Disorders in Adolescents 233
YeouChing Hsu

> Adolescence is a critical period for management of congenital hypothyroidism as well as other newly diagnosed thyroid disorders. Disorders seen more frequently in adults are on the rise in children and adolescents, particularly autoimmune thyroid disorders. This article summarizes the evaluation process for common causes of thyroid disorders and thyroid malignancy, discusses the prognosis for these disorders, and presents appropriate management in view of recent clinical updates.

Update on Diabetes in Children and Adolescents 256
Clifford A. Bloch, Sunil Nayak

> There has been an increased incidence of type 1 and type 2 diabetes mellitus in adolescents during the past 3 to 4 decades. The reasons for the increased incidence of type 1 diabetes mellitus remain unclear. The increases in type 2 diabetes mellitus have not reached epidemic populations, as had been predicted by some experts. In this article, we review new information on the etiology and management of diabetes mellitus, with a focus on the newer technologies available for treatment, especially continuous glucose monitoring systems (CGMS) and CGMS sensor-augmented insulin pump therapy with automated insulin suspension. The roles of diabetes education and a complete diabetes management team are emphasized.

Update on Puberty and Its Disorders in Adolescents 269
Amit Lahoti, Irene N. Sills

> Puberty, the process of transformation of a child into a young adult, involves both physical and psychosocial maturation. It is characterized by secretion of gonadal hormones, development of secondary sexual

characteristics, and maturation of gametogenesis and reproductive functions. This developmental stage is also characterized by a period of rapid growth, the pubertal growth spurt. Pubertal onset and progression are important because they are closely linked to optimum and timely growth during this phase and an adolescent's ability to fit in among his peers. It is also associated with long-term health outcomes not immediately apparent to the adolescent and the physician. This article focuses on developments over the past few years which have allowed us to better understand the genetic and epigenetic determinants of pubertal development and its underlying processes, the pathophysiology of deviations from normal, and the management of patients with these deviations. Epidemiologic studies evaluating a change in the timing of puberty are reviewed.

Bone Health in Adolescence 291
Dennis E. Carey, Neville H. Golden

As the understanding of osteoporosis in adults expands, there is increasing awareness that the antecedents of adult osteoporosis exist in children and adolescents, as do various forms of childhood bone disease and osteoporosis. In this article, we review the current state of knowledge on bone development, assessment of bone health, conditions associated with low bone mass, and the prevention and treatment of low bone mass in adolescents.

Polycystic Ovarian Syndrome 326
Jason Klein, Meghan Craven, Patricia M. Vuguin

Polycystic ovarian syndrome (PCOS), the most common endocrine disorder in women of reproductive age, is a process with polygenic and epigenetic origins. An adverse intrauterine environment, premature adrenarche, or childhood obesity may precede the typical presentation of chronic anovulation, hyperandrogenism, or abnormal uterine bleeding (AUB). As a diagnosis of exclusion, other causes of hyperandrogenism and AUB must be ruled out before a diagnosis of PCOS is made. Metabolic dysfunction, including insulin resistance, obesity, and dyslipidemia, are often seen in association with PCOS and increase the risk of early cardiovascular disease. Hormonal contraception, insulin sensitizers, antiandrogens, and lifestyle modifications have roles in improving the symptoms of PCOS and are reviewed in this article.

Adrenal Dysfunction 343
Phyllis W. Speiser

> Adrenal cortical disease, especially adrenal insufficiency, is more common than adrenal medullary disease and often goes unrecognized for extended periods. Physicians should consider the diagnosis of adrenal insufficiency in any patient with nonspecific unexplained signs or symptoms, including hypoglycemia, growth failure, weight loss, vomiting, or lethargy. The clinical features may be mistaken for, and should be differentiated from, infection, malnutrition, gastrointestinal disease, inborn errors of metabolism, anorexia nervosa, chronic fatigue syndrome, and depression. The spectrum of diseases causing adrenal dysfunction is more limited compared with those causing hypofunction.

Screening and Treatment of Common Lipid Disorders in Adolescents 364
Shara R. Bialo, Charlotte M. Boney

> Among adolescents aged 12 to 19 years, the prevalence of abnormal lipid levels is as high as 20.3%. This statistic comprises genetic and secondary dyslipidemias. Familial hypercholesterolemia has a prevalence of 1 in 500 individuals in western populations, causes increased low-density lipoprotein cholesterol from birth, and leads to early cardiovascular events. The most common cause of secondary dyslipidemia is obesity, and the incidence continues to increase in the setting of the current obesity epidemic. In this article we will review basic lipid metabolism, describe common dyslipidemias affecting children and adolescents, and discuss the 2011 screening and treatment guidelines for childhood lipid disorders. Based on our own evidence-based practice in a multidisciplinary lipid clinic, we have included "clinical tips" as useful principles for the physician.

Prevention and Management of Pregnancy in Adolescents with Endocrine Disorders 382
Paula J. Adams Hillard

> Most adolescent pregnancies are unintended, and adolescents with chronic medical conditions are as likely as healthy teens to be sexually involved. Preventing unintended pregnancies among teens with chronic endocrine conditions, including diabetes mellitus (both types 1 and 2), polycystic ovary syndrome (PCOS), and thyroid dysfunction, is critically important.

Evidence-based guidelines are available to assist with assessment of the risks versus the benefits of specific options for contraception in teens with these and other medical conditions. In most adolescents, the top-tier contraceptive methods—implants and intrauterine devices—represent the most effective, safest, and most successful contraceptive options. Prepregnancy counseling is an important tool for managing chronic endocrine conditions and lowering the risks for both mother and fetus, but it is underutilized among all women, particularly adolescents. The management of pregnancies complicated by diabetes mellitus, PCOS, and thyroid conditions is facilitated by a coordinated effort among obstetricians, endocrinologists, dietitians, and nurse educators. Primary physicians should be aware of their potential role in preventing unplanned pregnancies among all adolescents, but particularly among those with chronic medical conditions. Special care should be taken during the transition of care from pediatric subspecialists to those caring for adults.

Endocrine Abnormalities in Patients with Eating Disorders 393
Nadia Saldanha, Linda Carmine

The endocrine consequences of eating disorders are among the most severe and potentially longest lasting of any of the medical complications associated with anorexia nervosa, bulimia nervosa, and binge eating disorder. Endocrine complications include alterations in levels of cortisol, growth hormone, insulinlike growth factor-1, estradiol, testosterone, gut neuropeptides (leptin, ghrelin, peptide YY), and thyroid hormone, which lead to delayed puberty and amenorrhea and have an effect on both bone density and bone growth. Depending on the duration and degree of illness, most of the endocrine consequences can be reversed, with the exception of decreased bone density. Most of the endocrine changes are due primarily to the energy deficit created by malnutrition and thus are seen most commonly in anorexia nervosa. However, some neuroendocrine manifestations are seen in both bulimia nervosa and binge eating disorder as well. This review will highlight what has been well established in the literature with regard to endocrine abnormalities in the eating disorders as well as discuss more recent findings.

Turner Syndrome and Klinefelter Syndrome 411
Suzanne E. Kingery, Kupper A. Wintergerst

Two of the most common sex chromosome disorders are Turner syndrome and Klinefelter syndrome. Turner syndrome is caused by the complete or partial absence of the second X chromosome in females, whereas

Klinefelter syndrome is characterized by an additional X chromosome to the typical male XY karyotype. Each of these disorders has typical features and disease associations, some of which warrant close monitoring by medical specialists. Recent investigations regarding conditions associated with these sex chromosome disorders, as well as advances in treatment and updated clinical guidelines, are reviewed, as early identification of these disorders can improve patient outcomes.

Disorders of Sex Development: Why Adolescent Medicine Specialists Should Care   428

David E. Sandberg

Disorders of sex development (DSD) is an umbrella term covering congenital conditions in which chromosomal, gonadal, or anatomic sex development are atypical. Disorders of sex development exhibit a wide range of gonadal phenotypes, such as partial or complete gonadal dysgenesis and ovotestis; external genital phenotypes, such as hypospadias, clitoromegaly, and ambiguous genitalia; or fully masculinized or feminized genitalia discordant with karyotype or gonadal histology. This review focuses on clinical management challenges which remain in a state of flux and controversy. The case is made for increasing the involvement of the adolescent medicine specialist in multidisciplinary teams caring for youth affected by these conditions and their families.

Endocrine Consequences of Treatment for Childhood Cancer   448

Susan E. Stred

More than 80% of children and adolescents diagnosed with cancer during childhood will become long-term survivors. Of these survivors, at least half will develop 1 or more endocrine disorders. Chemotherapy with alkylating agents represents a major risk factor for gonadal failure. Radiation therapy accounts for most of the remaining disorders. Although short stature, pubertal disorders, and thyroid disorders are well-established sequelae of antineoplastic treatment, there are newly emerging data on increased risk of development of diabetes mellitus and the metabolic syndrome in adolescent and young adult survivors. This article outlines the guidelines for surveillance by primary care physicians and adolescent specialists for endocrine disorders during adolescence.

Index   461

Advances in the Treatment of Endocrine Disorders in Adolescents

Providing state-of-the-art medical care to adolescents always requires updated endocrinology knowledge. Whether one is monitoring the pubertal growth spurt, looking for those long-awaited pubertal changes, including the establishment of fertility, or asking questions about optimal ways to ensure health as an adult, expertise in endocrinology is always needed.

This issue of *AM:STARs* discusses advances in basic endocrinology, including evaluation and treatment of thyroid disorders in adolescents with congenital hypothyroidism who are now in their teen years, as well as thyroid disorders that are acquired in later childhood as a result of autoimmune etiologies and medications. The prevalence of thyroid malignancy is increasing, and a complete discussion of this important topic is offered in the article on thyroid disorders.

New information on disorders of growth and diagnostic evaluation for adolescents who have not achieved puberty at the expected time is discussed in the article on growth and puberty. Because of the frequent occurrence of the 2 most common sex chromosome disorders that are associated with delayed puberty (ie, Turner syndrome and Klinefelter syndrome), an article to update the adolescent medicine specialist about the diagnosis, treatment, and long-term follow-up of these disorders is included. Adrenal disorders are less commonly well understood by many medical professionals despite the need for prompt evaluation and treatment when they do occur; therefore, we thought a thorough review of this topic would be helpful.

As adolescent medicine physicians, it is important that we be concerned about decreasing the risk factors for poor health as adults. We recognize the importance of good bone health and healthful lipid profiles and therefore have included 2 articles to update these issues. In addition, new information on polycystic ovarian syndrome and a review of endocrine disorders in patients with eating disorders are presented because both of these conditions are commonly diagnosed in adolescent girls. Although teen pregnancy is currently less prevalent, a discussion of pregnancy in those with endocrine disorders is still a worthy topic to review and update.

Diabetes mellitus is one of the most common chronic diseases of childhood and adolescence. Although many adolescent patients will receive care from pediatric endocrine specialists, it remains important that adolescent medicine physicians understand the recent advances in treatment so that patients can access primary care from well-informed medical professionals.

Increasing expertise in the successful treatment of childhood cancer has given us an expanding number of patients who are at risk for long-term endocrine disorders. Not all of these patients return to their cancer treatment teams for long-term follow-up, and it is increasingly important that all medical professionals who care for these children and adolescents know how and when to screen for potential endocrinologic disease.

Finally, it is quite likely that most adolescent medicine physicians will encounter some patients with disorders of sexual differentiation. The adolescent years bring special challenges to this group of patients, and physicians who are caring for these patients should have updated information on the recent approaches to their psychosocial management.

We thank all of the authors for their efforts in adhering to tight timelines and for providing such excellent manuscripts. We also thank Carrie Peters and the American Academy of Pediatrics for giving us the opportunity to share with you the excitement that new knowledge brings to our abilities to provide the best care we can for our patients.

Irene N. Sills, MD, FAAP
Professor of Pediatrics
Pediatric Endocrinologist
SUNY Upstate Medical University
Syracuse, New York

Martin M. Fisher, MD, FAAP
Chief, Division of Adolescent Medicine
Cohen Children's Medical Center
North Shore–Long Island Jewish
Health System
Professor of Pediatrics
Hofstra–North Shore LIJ School of Medicine
New Hyde Park, New York

Thyroid Disorders in Adolescents

YeouChing Hsu, MD

Division of Pediatric Endocrinology, Cohen Children's Medical Center of New York, Assistant Professor of Pediatrics, Hofstra-North Shore LIJ School of Medicine, Lake Success, New York

APPROACH TO SUSPECTED THYROID DISORDER

Within the adolescent population, weight-related complaints are sometimes believed to be caused by a thyroid disorder. Although the incidence and prevalence of obesity have been a major concern, endocrinopathy remains a negligible cause of the obesity epidemic.[1] Obese adolescents without signs or symptoms of hypothyroidism are unlikely to have thyroid dysfunction. Prepuberal or peripubertal adolescents with hypothyroidism are unlikely to have isolated obesity without symptoms of growth failure, as growth is highly affected by thyroid dysfunction.[2] Similarly, poor weight gain or significant weight loss without symptoms consistent with thyrotoxicosis (eg, tachycardia, goiter, changes in behavior) is unlikely to be secondary to thyroid dysfunction but likely is secondary to gastroenterologic or nutritional disorders. Figures 1 and 2 show brief algorithms of evaluation for hypo- and hyperthyroidism.

Yearly screening of children and adolescents for thyroid disorders is not recommended unless specific risk factors are present. Adolescents who are at risk for a thyroid disorder and who are recommended to have routine thyroid testing include patients with type 1 diabetes mellitus, who have a reported risk of autoimmune thyroiditis of approximately 15% to 20%.[3] Patients with syndromes known to be associated with acquired thyroid dysfunction include Down syndrome,[4] Turner syndrome,[5] and Klinefelter syndrome.[6] For all of these syndromes, autoimmune thyroid disease is the most likely cause of the thyroid dysfunction.

Thyroid disorders as a result of abnormalities at the level of the pituitary gland are rare; therefore, tests for thyroid disorders, when indicated, should be focused

---

E-mail address: yhsu@nshs.edu

Copyright © 2015 American Academy of Pediatrics. All rights reserved. ISSN 1934-4287

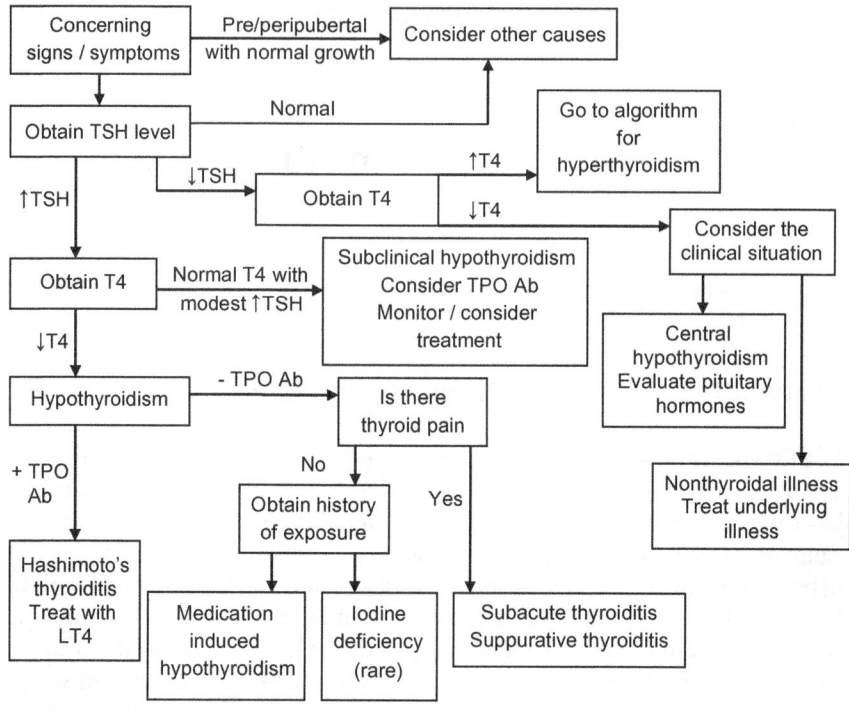

Fig 1. Algorithm for a patient with the concern of hypothyroidism. TSH, thyroid stimulating hormone; T4, thyroxine

on checking for primary thyroid disorders. Primary thyroid disorders can be evaluated with a thyroid-stimulating hormone (TSH) test first. If an abnormality is noted on the TSH level, then a thyroxine (T4) level can be obtained. If and only if TSH is suppressed and thyrotoxicosis is suspected should triiodothyronine (T3) level be obtained. T3 toxicosis can be the presenting picture for primary hyperthyroidism. Otherwise, the T3 test has low sensitivity and specificity for hypothyroidism, as levels can remain normal with increased peripheral conversion. The most common cause of primary thyroid disorder in an iodine-sufficient country such as the United States is autoimmune thyroid disease; therefore, based on the results of the TSH, T4, and T3 tests, thyroid antibody levels may be obtained to elucidate the cause of the thyroid disorder, as summarized in Figures 1 and 2.

In the evaluation of the adolescent with a thyroid concern, a detailed history of exposures is essential, including a detailed medication history to check for goitrogens. Lithium, best known for its use in treating bipolar disorder, is a known goitrogen, with complex effects on the thyroid gland. Lithium concentrates in the thyroid cells, where it may initially induce iodine retention and then subsequently decrease thyroid iodine uptake. As treatment is continued it may cause

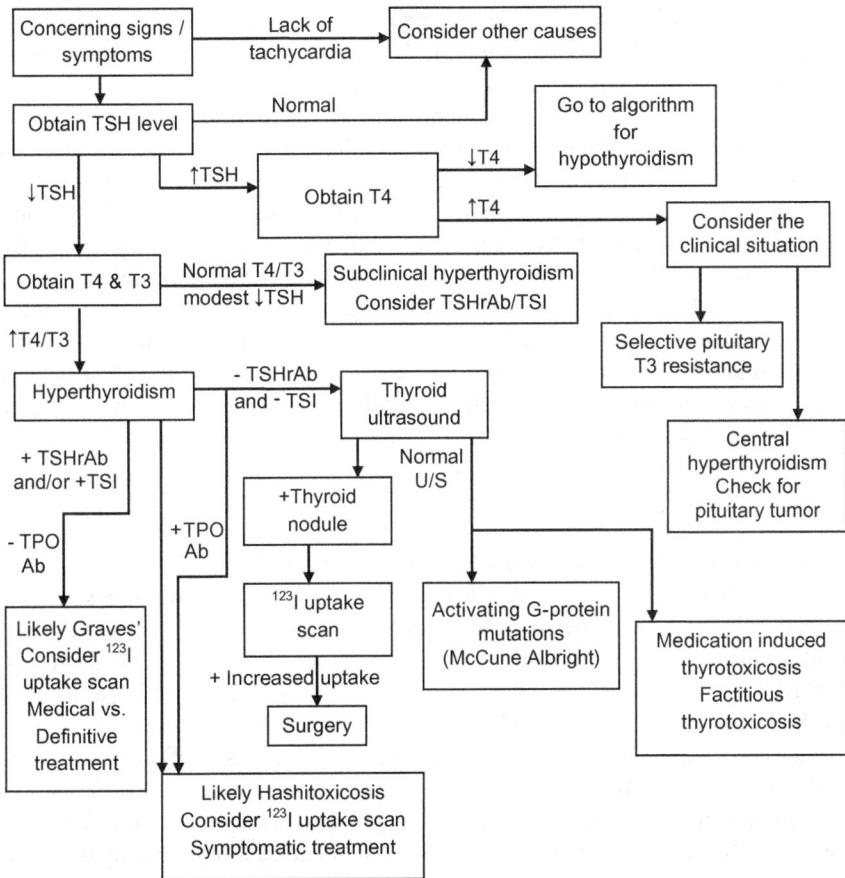

Fig 2. Algorithm for a patient with the concern of hyperthyroidism. T3, triiodothyronine; T4, thyroxine; TSH, thyroid-stimulating hormone.

increased uptake of iodine as a result of increased secretion of TSH. Lithium also inhibits the synthesis and release of thyroid hormone through alteration of the structure of thyroglobulin, which in turn leads to an associated reduction in hepatic deiodination and clearance of free T4. Hypothyroidism and subclinical hypothyroidism, with or without goiter, are seen in up to 50% of those receiving lithium treatment. Female gender and those with positive thyroid antibodies are at an increased risk for development of hypothyroidism.[7,8] A high percentage of lithium-induced hyperthyroidism is thought to be secondary to transient thyroiditis, but, as in hypothyroidism, most cases are believed to be autoimmune in origin.[9] Studies have shown that those at highest risk for lithium-induced thyroid dysfunction have preexisting thyroid autoimmunity; thus, some physicians recommend checking thyroid antibodies before starting lithium treatment.

Amiodarone, a benzofuranic iodine-rich antiarrhythmic drug, is well documented to cause thyroid dysfunction. Adult data show that most patients on treatment for amiodarone have at least mild abnormalities in thyroid hormone test results, and 5% to 20% of patients have frank thyroid dysfunction.[10] The incidence appears to be less common in children and adolescents.[11,12] Much of the thyroid dysfunction results from the large iodine load in amiodarone, which at typical treatment dosage is many hundreds times greater than the recommended daily iodine intake. This leads to hypothyroidism as a result of the Wolff-Chaikoff effect (see next paragraph).[13] Amiodarone-induced thyrotoxicosis (AIT) occurs via 2 main mechanisms. Type 1 AIT occurs as a result of the Jöd-Basedow effect (discussed later) from excessive iodine exposure, and type 2 is secondary to destructive thyroiditis caused by amiodarone itself. The 2 types may occur together and potentially can be discerned by an iodine uptake scan, which has implications for treatment.[10] Table 1 summarizes additional medications that can cause abnormalities in thyroid hormone test results or cause frank thyroid dysfunction.[14]

Iodine is the mineral that is most important in thyroid hormone regulation. It is a main substrate for the production of thyroid hormone. Hormone synthesis is enhanced by administration of iodine; however, at a critical level of intrathyroidal iodide, iodine organification and hormone synthesis are blocked, the so-called *Wolff-Chaikoff effect*. Chronic repeated administration of large doses of iodine then causes a decrease in iodide transport and thus a decrease in intrathyroidal concentration.[15,16] Conversely, thyrotoxicosis as a result of excessive iodine intake, termed the *Jöd-Basedow phenomenon*, is more common in patients with a history of nontoxic diffuse or nodular goiters and is more common in areas of iodine deficiency.[17] Withdrawal of the source of excess iodine usually is associated with normalization of thyroid function.

The use of supplements is important because many minerals and anions can interfere with the concentration of iodine, including bromide, fluoride, cobalt, and cadmium.[18-20] Environmental toxins such as nitrates, thiocyanate, perchlorates, and bisphenyls, each of which has been shown to cause thyroid dysfunction, have been found to be measurable in water and processed foods.[21-23] Although the levels detected in most over-the-counter supplements and in the environment have not been shown to be clinically significant, the consequences of exposure to these toxins may be significant in patients with a history of unusual amounts of exposure. In patients already undergoing thyroid hormone replacement therapy, ingestion of minerals along with levothyroxine is known to cause decreased absorption; therefore, multivitamins with minerals should not be taken with levothyroxine.[24]

Table 1
Drugs that cause thyroid dysfunction

Decrease TSH secretion/cause TSH suppression
    Glucocorticoids
    Dopamine agonists
    Somatostatin analogues
    Rexinoids
    Carbamazepine/oxcarbamazepine?*
    Metformin?*

TSH elevation
    Metyrapone

Decrease thyroid hormone secretion
    Iodide
    Amiodarone
    Lithium

Increase thyroid hormone secretion
    Iodide
    Amiodarone

Increase T4 and T3 metabolism
    Phenobarbital
    Rifampin

Increase hepatic metabolism
    Phenytoin
    Carbamazepine

Inhibition of T4/T3 synthesis
    Lithium
    Thioamides (carbimazole and methimazole)
    Propylthiouracil

Increase serum TBG
    Estrogens
    Heroin
    Methadone
    Mitotane
    Fluorouracil

Decrease serum TBG
    Androgens
    Anabolic steroids

Displacement from TBG (laboratory abnormality)
    Furosemide
    Phenytoin
    Salicylates
    Heparin
    Nonsteroidal anti-inflammatory drug

TBG, thyroxine-binding globulin; TSH, thyroid stimulating hormone.
?*, conflicting reports of whether these drugs cause thyroid dysfunction.
Adapted with permission from Kundra P, Burman K. The effects of medication on thyroid function. *Med Clin North Am.* 2012;96:283-295.

PHYSICAL EXAMINATION OF THE THYROID

The orthotopic thyroid gland is just caudal to the thyroid cartilage in the anterior neck. For good visualization, the patient's head is held in slight hyperextension with good cross light. The thyroid can be palpated through the anterior or posterior approach. Attempts should be made to first palpate the centrally located isthmus and then slide the fingers laterally. The opposite lobe can be palpated with the other hand from the opposite direction, and the patient should be directed to swallow to determine the movement of the gland. The texture, symmetry, and any concerning masses should be noted while the size of each lobe is being estimated.[25] In addition, it is important to palpate for any cervical lymphadenopathy and any features of the lymph nodes that can increase the likelihood of malignancy, such as adherence of the lymph nodes to adjacent structures.[26]

HYPOTHYROIDISM

To detect primary hypothyroidism, the best test is a measurement of TSH level with reflex to T4 (ie, the laboratory automatically performs a T4 test if the TSH is elevated). Age-appropriate norms should be used to ascertain whether true thyroid dysfunction exists. The more common forms of hypothyroidism are discussed here; a full listing of the differential diagnoses and an algorithm to evaluate the causes of hypothyroidism are given in Table 2 and Figure 1. If pharmacologic treatment is the cause of the hypothyroidism, the risks versus benefits should be discussed with the prescribing physician to determine whether thyroid hormone replacement or removal of the medication causing the hypothyroidism is preferable. In those who have only a mild laboratory test abnormality consistent with subclinical hypothyroidism, ongoing monitoring is an option.

Iodine deficiency as a cause of goiter and acquired hypothyroidism is rare in the United States given the iodinization of salt. However, recently there have been concerns of increasing cases of marginal iodine deficiency secondary to high intake of processed foods that often are made with non-iodized salt, increasing

Table 2
Differential diagnosis of hypothyroidism

Exposure to goitrogens (including medications)
Thyroid dysgenesis
Thyroid dyshormonogenesis
Hashimoto thyroiditis
Iodine deficiency
Nonthyroidal illness
Consumptive hypothyroidism
Subacute thyroiditis
Suppurative thyroiditis
Central hypothyroidism

exposure to nitrates, increasing popularity of non-iodized salt, and avoidance of salt because of health concerns.[19] If the clinical suspicion is high, a good dietary history may be important, and a urinary iodine level can be obtained to rule out iodine deficiency.[27] This is important information when evaluating children who come from the many countries around the world where iodine deficiency still is epidemic.

Clinical features of hypothyroidism include bradycardia, cold intolerance, dry skin, fatigue, menstrual irregularities, and alopecia.[28] Normocytic to macrocytic anemia that is refractory to iodine treatment can occur because thyroid hormone is an important stimulator of erythropoietin production. Hyperlipidemia, with a significant increase in low-density lipoprotein (LDL) and triglycerides and a decrease in high-density lipoprotein (HDL), occurs because thyroxine is important in the regulation of proteins necessary for biosynthesis and clearance of lipids and for upregulation of cholesterol receptors.[29] In the adolescent who has not yet completed growth, growth failure is a cardinal feature of hypothyroidism because of the direct effect on cartilage as well as its permissive effect on growth hormone.[2]

Hashimoto Thyroiditis

The most common cause of acquired hypothyroidism in iodine-sufficient countries is Hashimoto thyroiditis, also known as chronic lymphocytic thyroiditis. It was first described in 1912 by Hakaru Hashimoto, a thyroid surgeon. In this condition, the thyroid gland has a characteristic diffuse infiltration of plasma cells and lymphocytes, fibrosis, and parenchymal atrophy with eosinophilic degeneration.[30] The cause of acquired hypothyroidism in Hashimoto thyroiditis is lymphocytic infiltration, not antibody-mediated destruction. High levels of antithyroperoxidase (anti-TPO) antibodies have a good predictive value for long-term thyroid failure and are correlated with the histopathologic findings of chronic lymphocytic thyroiditis, whereas antithyroglobulin antibody levels have been shown to have a poor predictive value.[31]

The incidence and prevalence of Hashimoto thyroiditis increase with advancing age. Prevalence is estimated to be approximately 3 to 5 per 100 in adults,[32] compared to 3.0 to 8.2 per 1000 children and adolescents.[33]

On physical examination, the thyroid gland usually is enlarged and firm, and the lobular structures are more pronounced on palpation.[34] Ultrasound of the thyroid gland is not recommended in those with diffuse enlargement of the thyroid gland; it is indicated only when physical examination indicates a possible thyroid nodule or asymmetry, for evaluation of possible thyroid cancer. Ultrasound findings in Hashimoto thyroiditis include a heterogeneous echotexture of the thyroid gland and the appearance of lobulations (pseudo-nodules). Calcification can be present without concern of malignancy.[35,36]

Autoimmune thyroid disease, both Hashimoto thyroiditis and Graves disease, has a strong genetic susceptibility. The risk of autoimmune thyroid disease is noted to be as high as 20% to 30% in siblings, and the prevalence of antibodies is up to 50%. There is a concordance rate of 30% to 60% in monozygotic twins.[37] Genes identified to be associated with thyroid autoimmunity include the human leukocyte antigen on chromosome 6p, the cytotoxic T lymphocyte antigen-4 gene on chromosome 2q33, and the PTPN22 gene on chromosome 1p13. Other potential genes include the CD40 molecule, the tumor necrosis factor (TNF) receptor superfamily member 5 on 20q11, IL2RA (CD25), and Fc receptor-like 3.[38]

Treatment of patients with an elevated TSH level and a low T4 consistent with hypothyroidism is thyroid hormone replacement with levothyroxine with the goal of achieving normal TSH without causing thyrotoxicosis. The signs and symptoms, if they are secondary to hypothyroidism, improve with thyroid hormone replacement, and the prognosis is excellent. In the adolescent with significant growth failure, however, height may not completely normalize at the end of treatment, particularly in the adolescent who is diagnosed at a peripubertal age. Commencement of treatment may cause rapid progression through puberty and closure of the growth plates, which subsequently may stunt final adult height. There are case reports of success with use of gonadotropin-releasing (GnRH) agonists, with or without growth hormone, to delay pubertal progression and to allow for optimal catch-up growth.[39,40] However, a small retrospective review by Nebesio et al[41] was unable to show that growth-promoting treatments significantly improve adult height. It should be noted that, albeit small, autoimmune thyroid disorders do modestly increase the risk for thyroid cancer.[37] Thus, regular examination of the thyroid gland and cervical lymph nodes should be performed in all patients with autoimmune thyroid disorders.

Subclinical Hypothyroidism

Subclinical hypothyroidism is defined as a condition of normal T4 accompanied by modestly elevated TSH, and although definitions vary, most quote a TSH level of up to 10 µIU/mL.[42] As the term suggests, adolescents with subclinical hypothyroidism are asymptomatic. There has long been concern that even mild thyroid dysfunction can cause low bone mineral density and an increase in cardiovascular risk in adults, although the data are conflicting.[43,44] Data in adolescents are limited. In a study by DiMase et al,[45] children and adolescents with subclinical hypothyroidism with TSH values between 4.2 and 10 µIU/mL were not found to have any difference in dual-energy X-ray absorptiometry and quantitative ultrasound determinations of bone mineral density.[45] Similarly, no large-scale studies in children have suggested that treatment improves the lipid profile, which is a marker of cardiovascular risk.[46] Currently there is no consensus on treatment of subclinical hypothyroidism because of its unclear benefit.[47]

Congenital Hypothyroidism and Thyroid Dysgenesis

The most common cause of congenital hypothyroidism (90%-95%) is thyroid dysgenesis (ie, ectopic glands or abnormally formed glands); second (5%-10%) is thyroid dyshormonogenesis (ie, abnormalities in hormone synthesis and release); and small percentages (0%-5%) are the result of maternal antibodies causing transient thyroid dysfunction and central hypothyroidism.[48,49] Expansion of universal newborn screening has been instrumental in detecting congenital hypothyroidism early to facilitate early thyroid hormone replacement with levothyroxine. Early treatment has virtually eliminated the significant intellectual disabilities, ranging from severe learning disorders to frank mental retardation, previously seen in children and adolescents. Previous data have suggested that the incidence of congenital hypothyroidism is 1 in 4000; however, with a lowering of the upper limit of TSH on the newborn screen, more recent US data suggest an incidence as high as 1 in 1714.[49] With this high incidence rate, it would not be uncommon for physicians who treat adolescents to see patients with congenital hypothyroidism. With faster normalization of TSH as a result of thyroid hormone replacement, the prognoses for both intelligent quotient and growth have been excellent.[50] But despite these results, follow-up data have suggested a concern for decreased quality of life and self-worth.[51] There is ongoing concern that those with athyreosis (ie, total absence of the thyroid gland) have a slightly higher TRH set point that requires increased thyroid hormone replacement to achieve normalization of TSH, but without further data the current goal of treatment is normalization of TSH and T4.[52]

A variety of mild thyroid dysgeneses may not be detected until adolescence. One example is a lingual thyroid, in which remnant hypertrophy occurs, causing signs consistent with a retropharyngeal mass. A thyroglossal duct cyst that becomes infected can be another cause of a thyroid disorder that presents during the adolescent years. Management of a frequently infected thyroglossal duct cyst is removal, but care should be taken to determine whether the adolescent has a normal, orthotopic thyroid gland before the lesion is removed; otherwise surgery will render the adolescent hypothyroid.[53] Although removal of the lesion still may be necessary, this alerts the physician and the family that thyroid hormone replacement will be necessary after surgery.

There also is concern that ectopic thyroid tissue should be monitored for signs of malignancy. Thyroid cancer in the adolescent age group generally has an excellent prognosis, and at this point there is no recommendation for radiologic screening of ectopic thyroid tissue that is not palpable (see section on Evaluation of a Thyroid Mass/Thyroid Nodule). If thyroid cancer is noted, however, the current recommendation is removal of the ectopic thyroid tissue along with a total thyroidectomy of the orthotopic thyroid gland if one is present.[54] Treatment of thyroid malignancy should be performed at a center that has expertise in its management.

HYPERTHYROIDISM (THYROTOXICOSIS)

As with hypothyroidism, hyperthyroidism may be detected on incidental testing. Signs include tachycardia, weight loss, heat intolerance, tremor, hypertension (systolic with increased pulse pressure), and polyuria with polydipsia. Symptoms include hyperactivity, often present with poor school performance, or, conversely, fatigue, because of sleep disturbance, along with palpitations, emotional lability and irritability, increased stool frequency, and increased appetite.[55] Figure 2 shows an algorithm for evaluation of hyperthyroidism, and Table 3 lists the full differential diagnosis of thyrotoxicosis.

Pharmacologic causes of hyperthyroidism are rare but, as noted previously, well documented in amiodarone and lithium treatment.[9,10] A dialogue should occur with the physician who prescribed these treatments to determine whether the thyrotoxicosis should be separately treated or the primary medication discontinued or given a trial of cessation.

Graves Disease

Graves disease is the most common cause of hyperthyroidism in adolescents. It is an autoimmune disorder resulting from thyrotropin receptor stimulation by autoantibodies. Children account for about 1% to 5% of all cases of Graves disease. The incidence rate in adolescents in the United States is approximated to be about 3 per 100,000 person-years, with a prevalence rate of 1 in 10,000 to 1 in 100,000.[56]

Laboratory findings of thyrotoxicosis show undetectable or suppressed TSH levels. Patients with Graves disease usually have significantly elevated T4 and T3 levels, but some may have isolated T3 toxicosis, which is observed more frequently with early diagnosis or during relapse.[57] T3 toxicosis is more commonly present in prepubertal than pubertal children.[58] In patients with suspected hyperthyroidism with a low TSH level, T3 and T4 levels should be obtained.

Two tests can be obtained to check for the cause of Graves disease: TSH receptor immunoglobulin (TSHrAb, also known as TSH-binding inhibitory immunoglobulin [TBII]) and thyroid-stimulating immunoglobulin (TSI). The former test detects antibody binding to the TSH receptor; the latter is a functional study that measures adenosine monophosphate (AMP) production using in vitro thyroid cells.[55] Frequently, thyroid peroxidase antibodies as well as thyroid globulin antibodies are also detected at high levels, which places hashitoxicosis in the differential diagnosis (discussed in the section on Hashitoxicosis). In most cases, clinical findings, duration of symptoms, and presence of autoantibodies can distinguish Graves disease from other causes of thyrotoxicosis. A thyroid uptake scan with radioactive iodine showing diffusely increased uptake of the thyroid gland would definitively establish the diagnosis.[56]

Table 3
Differential diagnosis of hyperthyroidism

Graves disease
Autonomously functioning thyroid nodule
Activating G-protein mutations (McCune-Albright)
Central hyperthyroidism
  Pituitary tumor
  Selective pituitary T3 resistance
Factitious hyperthyroidism

The goiter in Graves disease usually is uniformly large and firm, but it is softer than the gland in Hashimoto thyroiditis and is smooth to palpation. Graves ophthalmopathy is much less severe in adolescents than in adults, generally characterized by lid lag and proptosis. True exophthalmos, which is secondary to increased retro-orbital deposition of mucopolysaccharides, is rare. Malignant Graves ophthalmopathy is virtually unheard of, and surgery is rarely needed.[59,60]

Graves disease can be treated with antithyroid medications, surgery, or radioactive iodine. In children and adolescents, many practitioners start with antithyroid medication in an attempt to achieve medical remission and avoid definitive therapy, which is generally associated with lifelong thyroid hormone replacement.[61] The commonly used medications are thioamides, which include carbimazole and its active metabolite methimazole (MMI), and propylthiouracil (PTU). The mechanism of action of these medications is interference with thyroid peroxidase-mediated iodination of tyrosine residues in thyroglobulin. Because of a recent black box warning of fulminant hepatic failure that has been seen with use of PTU, the first-line treatment is now methimazole. Propylthiouracil also has the disadvantage of requiring 3 doses daily, but it has the advantage of preventing peripheral conversion of T4 to T3. Methimazole has adverse reactions, including mild hepatitis and hyperlipidemia, which resolve with cessation of therapy; however, no cases of hepatic failure have been reported. Frequent, yet minor, reactions occur in 5% to 25% of patients taking methimazole; these include rash, urticaria, arthralgia, and gastrointestinal complaints. Antineutrophil cytoplasmic antibody (ANCA)-associated vasculitis has been described in long-term treatment.[62] Female patients should be counseled regarding the risk of carbimazole embryopathy, which is limited to the first trimester.[63,64] The current recommendations for pregnant women are use of PTU during the first trimester and then a switch to methimazole for the second and third trimesters.[65]

Clinical judgment is used for dosage adjustments; this includes primarily the rate at which T3 and T4 decrease and ultimately the normalization of these values. Thyroid-stimulating hormone can take longer to normalize, so whether it continues to be suppressed is of less importance when adjusting medication dosage.[66] Previously, the "block and replace" method, in which a reasonable dosage of methimazole is used to suppress thyroid hormone synthesis and release with concomitant thyroid hormone replacement, was thought to be advantageous in improving rates of remission. However, recent studies have refuted this advantage; thus, most practitioners use the lowest dosage of antithyroid medication possible to achieve a euthyroid state.[67]

Evidence from available data shows that the chances of long-term remission are low if medical remission cannot be achieved with 24 to 36 months of antithyroid medication treatment.[68] Although long-term treatment with antithyroid medication is a possibility, there is ongoing concern of adverse reactions, including a higher risk for the development of agranulocytosis and an increased risk of ANCA-associated vasculitis with longer treatment.[62] Recent studies have suggested that the medical remission rate likely is less than 30% in children and adolescents compared to 40% to 60% in adults, thus increasing the push for earlier definitive therapy.[68]

Radioactive iodine treatment is generally well tolerated, with short-term adverse reactions of nausea, salivary gland dysfunction, altered taste, and increased caries. Despite the concern for an increased risk of malignancy, many studies have shown a low risk of malignancy with this modality for the treatment of children, adolescents, and adults. Another concern, given the age of the children and adolescents, is fertility. Many practitioners avoid radioactive iodine until after puberty, but no evidence has shown prepubertal use of radioactive iodine to be detrimental.[69]

Surgical total thyroidectomy as a method of definitive treatment has the risk of recurrent laryngeal or superior laryngeal nerve injury, which has been reported to occur in up to 1% of cases. There is a risk of hypocalcemia from hypoparathyroidism as a result of damage to the parathyroid gland or release of calcitonin during surgery, but the hypocalcemia usually is transient and responds well to calcium and calcitriol. The appearance of a neck scar can be minimized in the hands of a well-experienced surgeon. Because pediatric ear, nose, and throat (ENT) surgeons may be presented with fewer total thyroidectomy cases, the best surgeon for this procedure usually is an adult thyroid surgeon who performs a high number of cases, with appropriate pediatric anesthesiology and surgical team support.[70] Currently in the United States, the preferred definitive treatment is radioactive iodine ablation because of its much lower long-term risks, but which treatment is used more frequently varies based on location.[66]

Autonomously Functioning Nodules

Autonomously functioning nodules often are palpable. In a patient who has laboratory and clinical evidence of thyrotoxicosis but does not have a diffusely enlarged thyroid and has negative antibodies, a careful physical examination is necessary. Most autonomously functioning thyroid nodules are palpable if they are larger than 1 cm, and an ultrasound examination can be performed to confirm the presence of a nodule. An iodine-123 (^{123}I) uptake and scan then can be performed to confirm that the nodule is functioning autonomously.[71] Although autonomously functioning thyroid nodules carry a much lower risk of malignancy, children and adolescents have a higher risk of malignant nodules than adults (see section on Evaluation of a Thyroid Mass/Thyroid Nodule); thus, the preferred treatment is surgery for removal of the nodules rather than use of radioactive iodine or ethanol injection.

Hashitoxicosis

Hashitoxicosis is an acute inflammatory stage of Hashimoto thyroiditis. Diagnosis is supported by the presence of thyroperoxidase antibodies with negative TSHrAb and TSI. This is confirmed by ^{123}I uptake and scan, which shows a low uptake.[72] Generally, treatment beyond supportive care and monitoring is rarely needed. Glucocorticoids can potentially be used to decrease the destructive thyrotoxicosis, but the length of treatment should be limited, and symptoms can be managed with beta-blockers. In long-term follow-up, most patients become euthyroid or hypothyroid.[73]

EVALUATION OF A THYROID MASS/THYROID NODULE

When an adolescent presents with an isolated complaint of a neck mass, the first step in evaluation is to ascertain whether the mass is associated with the thyroid gland. During the examination of the thyroid, it is important to pay special attention to asymmetry and texture of the thyroid, and the presence of any lymphadenopathy. A diffusely enlarged, smooth thyroid gland likely is secondary to chronic lymphocytic thyroiditis or Graves disease, and ultrasonographic evaluation is not recommended. Cervical lymphadenopathy is common in children, but a concerning quality of the lymphadenopathy should also be noted. Figure 3 shows an algorithm for evaluation of thyroid mass.

A thyroid nodule in a patient without risk factors is most commonly detected on physical examination or is noted by the family. Gupta et al[74] evaluated 141 children who presented with thyroid nodules that were larger than 1 cm. Forty-one percent of nodules were noted on physical examination in the office, 40% were detected by the patient, family, or friends, and only 18% were radiographic "incidentalomas."[74] There is no evidence in either the adult or pediatric literature suggesting that nodules have a different risk for malignancy based on whether they were palpated or incidentally noted; thus, all lesions should be evaluated based on their ultrasound characteristics.

It has long been shown that the risk for thyroid nodules being malignant is higher in children than in adults.[75] The reported range of risk for malignancy in the pediatric population is 15% to 50%, compared to 5% to 15% in adults,[76] or

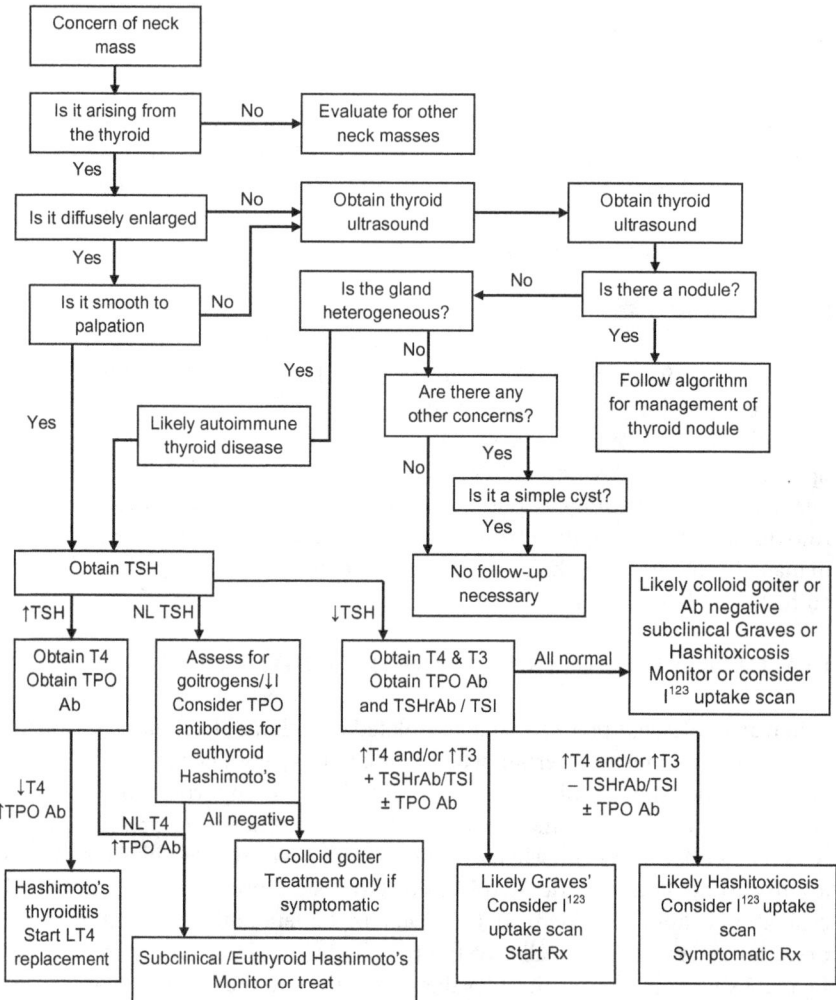

Fig 3. Algorithm for evaluation of thyroid enlargement or mass. ↓I, iodine deficiency; T3, triiodothyronine; T4, thyroxine; TG Ab, thyroglobulin antibody; TPO Ab, thyroperoxidase antibody; TSH, thyroid-stimulating hormone; TSHrAb, thyroid-stimulating hormone receptor antibody; TSI, thyroid-stimulating immunoglobulin.

about a 3- to 5-fold increase in risk compared to adults.[77] This finding continues to hold true, with one study of patients seen at the Children's Hospital Boston showing that the cancer rate in children with nodules larger than 1 cm was 22%, which is higher than the adult rate of 14%.[78]

Previously, the American Thyroid Association[79] and the American Association of Clinical Endocrinologists[80] had guidelines for the evaluation and management of thyroid nodules that were recommended for use in children and adolescents. Pediatric thyroid nodules and thyroid cancers behave differently from adult thyroid nodules, and in April 2015 the American Thyroid Association Guidelines Task Force on Pediatric Thyroid Cancer published management guidelines for children with thyroid nodules and differentiated thyroid cancer (Figure 4).[81] Although the recommendation still stands that thyroid nodules larger than 1 cm be evaluated with ultrasound-guided fine needle aspiration (FNA), because thyroid volume is different in children than adults, the recommendation is to base the decision for biopsy more heavily on suspicious clinical features on ultrasound findings and clinical context, such as suspicious lymphadenopathy, a history of head and neck irradiation, and a history of thyroid cancer in a first-degree relative.[79-81]

Obtaining a TSH level and performing a detailed ultrasound examination are the first steps in evaluation upon discovery of a thyroid nodule. If the TSH level is suppressed, a radioactive iodine uptake scan can be performed to evaluate

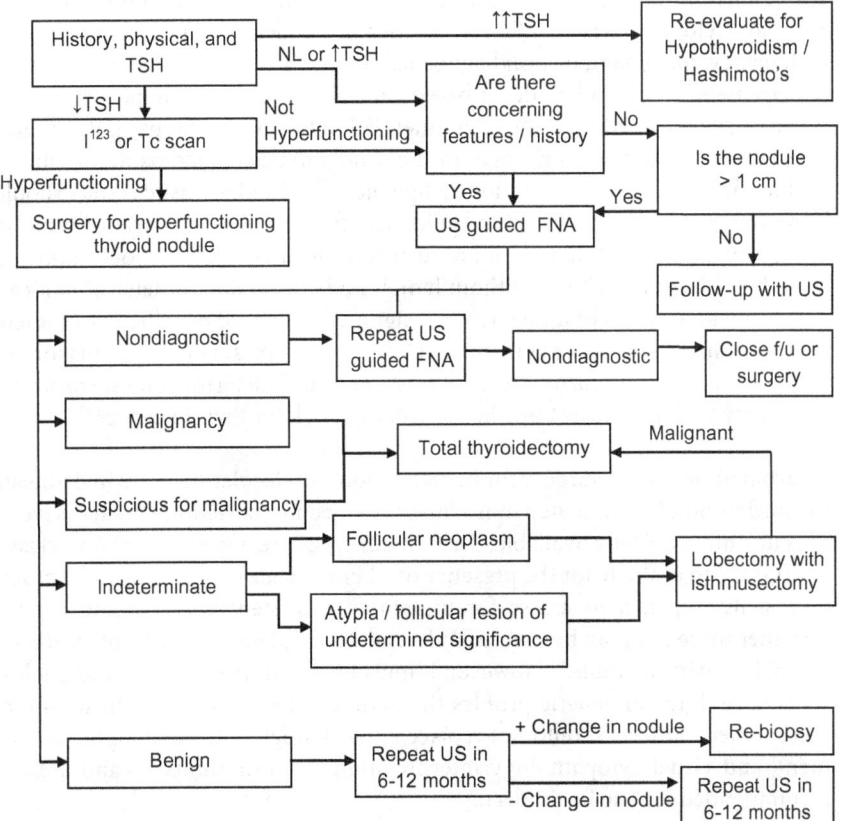

Fig 4. Algorithm for management of an ultrasound (US)-confirmed solid/mixed thyroid nodule. FNA, fine needle aspiration biopsy; TSH, thyroid-stimulating hormone.

whether the thyroid nodule is hyperfunctioning, isofunctioning, or nonfunctioning. In adults, a thyroid nodule that is hyperfunctioning is rarely malignant. In adolescents, however, given the increased risk for malignancy even in hot nodules, the recommendation is for surgical removal, and no FNA is needed prior to surgery.[80,81]

Ultrasound findings that may increase suspicion of malignancy of the thyroid nodule include nodule hypoechogenicity, increased intranodular vascularity, irregular infiltrative margins, presence of microcalcifications, an absent halo, and greater nodule height than width. Suspicious cervical lymphadenopathy is a specific but not sensitive finding for the higher likelihood of a malignant nodule. One feature of a thyroid nodule that is much less concerning for malignancy is a purely cystic appearance. A spongiform appearance, from an aggregation of multiple microcystic components in more than 50% of the nodule volume, is 99.7% specific for identification of a benign thyroid nodule.[80]

The results of the FNA are categorized into The Bethesda System for Reporting Thyroid Cytopathology (TBSRTC) as benign, indeterminate, suspicious for malignancy, malignant, or nondiagnostic.[82] Figure 4 shows an algorithm for the management of thyroid nodules based on FNA results. A completely benign lesion can be followed, with the recommendation for another biopsy if the nodule enlarges significantly or if changes in the sonographic characteristics or clinical findings increase the suspicion for malignancy.[79,80] Nondiagnostic results should be repeated with careful ultrasound guidance after a minimum delay of 3 months. Malignant lesions and those that are suspicious for malignancy should undergo total thyroidectomy, with or without lymph node dissection. Indeterminant categories include atypia of undetermined significance (AUS) or follicular lesion of undetermined significance (FLUS), and follicular neoplasm or suspicious for follicular neoplasm. The current recommendations for indeterminant categories are lobectomy with isthmusectomy because of high risk for thyroid cancer.[81]

To avoid unnecessary surgery for benign lesions, molecular markers to delineate the likelihood of malignancy in nodules have been in development, and several are currently clinically available. The 2 main types are a gene expression classifier (GEC), to evaluate for the presence of a benign gene expression, and a mutation analysis panel, to assess for mutations consistent with thyroid cancer. Together these tests can be used to differentiate about 60% of well-differentiated thyroid cancers in adults.[83] However, it must be noted that children and adolescents have different genetic profiles than adults. The current consensus is that these molecular tests should not replace clinical judgment, sonographic assessment, and visual cytopathology interpretation, even in adults,[79,83] and are not recommended for use in children.[82,84]

Surgery is not recommended for a diffusely enlarged but euthyroid goiter or for a thyroid nodule that is deemed benign, unless there are compressive symptoms including neck pressure, dysphagia, shortness of breath, hoarseness, or pain. An exception is thyroid nodules that are larger than 4 cm in size because FNA has decreased sensitivity for the diagnosis of malignancy in large nodules. Therefore, surgery should be considered especially if the nodule is solid and lobectomy is preferred.[81] Treatment with levothyroxine has not been shown to decrease thyroid nodule size and is not recommended.[79,80]

DIFFERENTIATED THYROID CANCER

Pediatric cancer rates overall have been on the rise, and thyroid cancer rates, although still rare, have also been on the rise. The rate of increase is reportedly highest among female adolescents.[85] Differentiated thyroid cancer (DTC) is the most common, with 90% to 95% being papillary thyroid carcinoma (PTC) and 5% to 10% being follicular thyroid cancer (FTC). Medullary thyroid cancer is rare, often associated with familial medullary cancer syndromes, and anaplastic and undifferentiated thyroid cancers are exceedingly rare. The age standardized rates of DTC are reported to be 3.51 cases per million for 10- to 15-year-olds and 15.2 cases per million for 15- to 19-year-olds.[86] The increased rate does not seem to be linked to increased incidental findings.[74] Speculation is that the increase may be the result of increased ionizing radiation from environmental sources and radiologic studies, increasing rates of obesity, or the presence of perchlorate or polybrominated diphenyl ethers in the environment.[79] Radiation exposure is particularly concerning, as evidenced by the infamous Chernobyl nuclear power plant accident that caused a large amount of ^{131}I to spread over hundreds of square kilometers, resulting in a significant subsequent increase in the rate of childhood thyroid cancer in the area.[87] Radiation from radiologic studies is of greater concern in children than adults because they probably will undergo more studies within their lifetimes, and there is a suggestion that the exposure dose may be higher in children than adults because of failure to optimize radiologic parameters relative to body size.[88]

Syndromes that are associated with an increased risk of differentiated thyroid cancer include McCune-Albright syndrome, PTEN hamartoma syndrome, Carney complex, familial adenomatous polyposis, and DICER1PPB familial tumor predisposition syndrome.[83] In families without syndromic causes of cancer, first-degree female relatives of a patient with papillary thyroid carcinoma have a 2% risk of developing thyroid cancer, which is 3 times that of the general population. In those with more than 2 relatives with thyroid cancer, the risk is 10% for females and 24% for males.[89]

The prognosis for well-differentiated thyroid cancer in children and adolescents is excellent, with overall survival of 100% at 20 years and 94.4% at 30 years.[90] Previously, radioactive iodine ablation of the thyroid remnant and metastases was almost universally recommended. Radioactive iodine ablation is generally well tolerated, but bone marrow suppression and gonadal toxicity may occur with higher ^{131}I doses, particularly with repeated administrations. Pediatric patients with pulmonary metastases can develop pulmonary fibrosis. Pawelczak et al[91] reviewed the outcomes of children and adolescents with well-differentiated thyroid carcinoma and pulmonary metastases and showed that although many do not achieve complete response to therapy, most still have very low disease-related morbidity and mortality. Because well-differentiated pediatric thyroid cancers have an excellent prognosis and there has been no evidence that radioactive iodine ablation has decreased the long-term risk for death, recent recommendations have called for a shift toward more conservative use of radioactive iodine.[79,81]

MEDULLARY THYROID CANCER AND FAMILIAL MEDULLARY THYROID CANCER SYNDROMES

Medullary thyroid carcinoma is a well-differentiated thyroid tumor that maintains the biochemical and pathologic features of the parafollicular, calcitonin-producing C cells of the thyroid.[92] It is rarely seen in adolescents. Its presentation is similar to that of other well-differentiated thyroid cancers with a neck mass with or without lymphadenopathy, but because of the location, patients with these tumors have a higher likelihood of experiencing hoarseness as well as symptoms as a result of hypocalcemia from the release of calcitonin.[93]

In children and adolescents, medullary thyroid cancer almost always is part of an inherited syndrome.[94,95] These consist of multiple endocrine neoplasia type 2A (MEN2A, Sipple syndrome), multiple endocrine neoplasia type 2B (MEN2B), and familial medullary thyroid carcinoma (FMTC). The cause of these inherited medullary thyroid cancer syndromes has been demonstrated to be mutations in the RET (REarranged during Transfection) proto-oncogene. The most common of these syndromes is MEN2A, which is characterized by medullary thyroid carcinoma, pheochromocytoma, and primary hyperthyroidism. Familial medullary thyroid carcinoma is a variant of MEN2A, with multigenerational MTC without pheochromocytoma or primary hyperparathyroidism. Nearly 90% of carriers will develop medullary thyroid cancer, and, depending on the mutation, the risk can be earlier or later. Multiple endocrine neoplasia type 2B is rare but aggressive, and it presents the earliest. Patients with MEN2B have a marfanoid habitus and present with medullary thyroid cancer, ganglioneuromas of the gut and oral mucosa, pheochromocytomas, and medullated corneal nerve fibers.[95]

Management of suspected medullary thyroid cancer because of suspicious findings on FNA or significant elevation of calcitonin level with the presence of a thyroid nodule first involves ultrasound to evaluate for signs of metastasis. Calcitonin, carcinoembryonic antigen (CEA), and calcium levels should be obtained. All patients, particularly pediatric patients, should be offered RET mutation analysis. This is particularly relevant for planning prophylactic thyroidectomy in family members. Thyroidectomy is recommended as early as 1 year of age for those with the extremely high-risk mutation. Pheochromocytoma should be ruled out by appropriate testing.

Medullary thyroid carcinoma has a much poorer prognosis compared to the other well-differentiated types of thyroid cancer, with a 10-year survival rate of 50% to 75% reported in adult patients.[94,95] Adolescent survival rates are not expected to be much higher. Total thyroidectomy and compartmental dissection are recommended. A palliative neck operation and experimental clinical trials should be considered in patients with extensive metastases.[95]

CONCLUSION

The prognosis of most adolescent thyroid disorders is excellent and has improved in recent years. These improvements are the result of research evaluating the effects of a variety of medications on the adolescent thyroid gland, breakthroughs in genetic testing, and longer-term follow-up data. As evidenced by this article, however, additional studies are required for us to continue optimizing the management and treatment of adolescent thyroid disorders.

References

1. Cunningham SA, Kramer MR, Narayan KMV. Incidence of childhood obesity in the United States. *N Engl J Med*. 2014;370:403-411
2. Gogakos AI, Bassett JHD, Williams GR. Thyroid and bone. *Arch Biochem Biophys*. 2010;503:129-136
3. American Diabetes Association. Standards of medical care in diabetes 2013. *Diabetes Care*. 2013;36:S11-S66
4. Ivan DL, Cromwell P. Clinical practice guidelines for management of children with Down syndrome: part I. *J Pediatr Health Care*. 2014;28:105-110
5. Bondy CA; Turner Syndrome Study Group. Care of girls and women with Turner syndrome: a guideline of the Turner Syndrome Study Group. *J Clin Endocrinol Metab*. 2007;92:10-25
6. Gies I, Unuane D, Velkeniers B, et al. Management of Klinefelter syndrome during transition. *Eur J Endocrinol*. 2014;171:R67-R77
7. Kibririge D, Luzinda K, Ssekitoleko R. Spectrum of lithium induced thyroid abnormalities: a current perspective. *Thyroid Res*. 2013;6:3
8. Lazarus JH. Lithium and thyroid. *Best Pract Res Clin Endocrinol Metab*. 2009;23:723-733
9. Brownlie BD, Turner JG. Lithium associated thyrotoxicosis. *Clin Endocrinol (Oxf)*. 2011;75:402-403
10. Bogazzi F, Bartalena L, Martino E. Approach to the patient with amiodarone induced thyrotoxicosis. *J Clin Endocrinol Metab*. 2010;95:2529-2535
11. Guccione P, Paul T, Garson A. Long-term follow-up of amiodarone therapy in the young: continued efficacy, unimpaired growth, moderate side effects. *J Am Coll Cardiol*. 1990;15:1118-1124
12. Costigan DC, Holland FJ, Daneman D, et al. Amiodarone therapy effects on childhood thyroid function. *Pediatrics*. 1986;77:703-708
13. Bogazzi F, Tomisti L, Bartalena L, et al. Amiodarone and the thyroid: a 2012 update. *J Endocrinol Invest*. 2012;35:340-348
14. Kundra P, Burman K. The effects of medication on thyroid function. *Med Clin North Am*. 2012;96:283-295

15. Robison LM, Sylvester PW, Birkenfeld P, et al. Comparison of the effects of iodine and iodide on thyroid function in humans. *J Toxicol Environ Health*. 1998;55:93-106
16. Uyttersprot N, Pelgrims N, Carrasco N, et al. Moderate doses of iodide in vivo inhibit cell proliferation and the expression of thyroperoxidase and the Na+/I- symporter mRNAs in dog thyroid. *Mol Cell Endocrinol*. 1997;131:195-203
17. Leung AM, Braverman LE. Iodine induced thyroid dysfunction. *Curr Opin Endocrinol Diabetes Obes*. 2012;19:414-419
18. Vobecky M, Babicky A, Lerner J, et al. Interaction of bromine with iodine in the rat thyroid gland at enhanced bromide intake. *Biol Trace Elem Res*. 1996;54:207-212
19. Barceloux DG. Cobalt. *J Toxicol Clin Toxicol*. 1999;37;201-206
20. Gupta P, Kar A. Role of ascorbic acid in cadmium-induced thyroid dysfunction and lipid peroxidation. *J Appl Toxicol*. 1998;18:317-320
21. Blount BC, Pirkle JL, Osterloh JD, et al. Urinary perchlorate and thyroid hormone levels in adolescent and adult men and women living in the United States. *Environ Health Perspect*. 2006;114:1865-1871
22. Environmental Protection Agency. Drinking water: regulatory determination on perchlorate. *Fed Regist*. 2011;76:7762-7767
23. Council on Environmental Health, Rogan WJ, Paulson JA, Baum C, et al. Iodine deficiency, pollutant chemicals, and the thyroid: new information on an old problem. *Pediatrics*. 2014;133:1163-1166
24. Zamfirescu I, Carlson HE. Absorption of levothyroxine when coadministered with various calcium formulations. *Thyroid*. 2011;21:483-486
25. Walker HK, Hall WD, Hurst JW, eds. *Clinical Methods: The History, Physical, and Laboratory Examinations*. 3rd ed. Boston: Butterworths; 1990
26. Jatana KR, Zimmerman D. Pediatric thyroid nodules and malignancy. *Otolaryngol Clin North Am*. 2015;48:47-58
27. Pearce EN, Leung AM. The state of US iodine nutrition: how can we ensure adequate iodine for all? *Thyroid*. 2013;23;924-925
28. Brown RS. Autoimmune thyroiditis in children. *J Clin Res Pediatr Endocrinol*. 2013;5(Suppl 1):45-49
29. Rizos CV, Elisaf MS, Liberopoulos EN. Effects of thyroid dysfunction on lipid profile. *Open Cardiol Med J*. 2011;5:76-84
30. Churilov LP, Stroev YI, Serdyuk IY, et al. Autoimmune thyroiditis: centennial jubilee of a social disease and its comorbidity. *Pathophysiology*. 2014;12:135-145
31. Rho MH, Kim DW, Hong HP, et al. Diagnostic value of antithyroid peroxidase antibody for incidental autoimmune thyroiditis based on histopathologic results. *Endocrine*. 2012;42:647-652
32. McLeod DSA, Cooper DS. The incidence and prevalence of thyroid autoimmunity. *Endocrine*. 2012;42:252-265
33. Lee HS, Hwang JS. The natural course of Hashimoto's thyroiditis in children and adolescents. *J Pediatr Endocrinol Metab*. 2014;17:807-812
34. Brown RS. Autoimmune thyroiditis in children. *J Clin Res Pediatr Endocrinol*. 2013;5(Suppl 1):45-49
35. Williams JL, Paul DL, Bisset G III. Thyroid disease in children: part 1. State-of-the-art imaging in pediatric hypothyroidism. *Pediatr Radiol*. 2013;43:1244-1253
36. Kambalapalli M, Gupta A, Prasad UR, et al. Ultrasound characteristics of the thyroid in children and adolescents with goiter: a single center experience. *Thyroid*. 2015;25:176-182
37. Antonelli A, Ferrari SM, Corrado A, et al. Autoimmune thyroid disorders. *Autoimmun Rev*. 2015;14:174-180
38. Davies TF, Latif R, Yin X. New genetic insights from autoimmune thyroid disease. *J Thyroid Res*. 2012:623852
39. Minamitani K, Murata A, Ohnishi H, et al. Attainment of normal height in severe juvenile hypothyroidism. *Arch Dis Child*. 1994;70:429-431

40. Watanabe T, Minamitani K, Minagawa M, et al. Severe juvenile hypothyroidism: treatment with growth hormone and GnRH agonist in addition to thyroxine. *Endocr J.* 1998;45(Suppl):S159-S162
41. Nebesio TD, Wis MD, Perkins SM, et al. Does clinical management impact height potential in children with severe acquired hypothyroidism? *J Pediatr Endocrinol Metab.* 2011;24:893-896
42. Gillett M. Subclinical thyroid disease: scientific review and guidelines for diagnosis and management. *JAMA.* 2004;291:228-238
43. Garin MC, Arnold AM, Lee JS, et al. Subclinical thyroid dysfunction and hip fracture and bone mineral density in older adults: the cardiovascular health study. *J Clin Endocrinol Metab.* 2014;99:2657-2664
44. Santos OC, Silva NA, Vaisman M, et al. Evaluation of epicardial fat tissue thickness as a marker of cardiovascular risk in patients with subclinical hypothyroidism. *J Endocrinol Invest.* 2015; 38:421-427
45. DiMase R, Cerbone M, Improda N, et al. Bone health in children with long-term idiopathic subclinical hypothyroidism. *Ital J Pediatr.* 2012;38:56
46. O'Grady MJ, Cody D. Subclinical hypothyroidism in childhood. *Arch Dis Child.* 2011;96:280-284
47. Catli G, Abaci A, Buyukgebiz A, et al. Subclinical hypothyroidism in childhood and adolescence. *J Pediatr Endocrinol Metab.* 2014;27:1049-1057
48. Langham S, Hindmarsh P, Krywawych S, et al. Screening for congenital hypothyroidism: comparison of borderline screening cut-off points and the effect on the number of children treated with levothyroxine. *Eur Thyroid J.* 2013;2:180-186
49. Ford G, LaFranchi SH. Screening for congenital hypothyroidism: a worldwide view of strategies. *Best Pract Res Clin Endocrinol Metab.* 2014;28:175-187
50. Donaldson M, Jones J. Optimising outcome in congenital hypothyroidism: current opinions on best practice in initial assessment and subsequent management. *J Clin Res Pediatr Endocrinol.* 2013;5(Suppl 1):13-22
51. Leger J. Congenital hypothyroidism: a clinical update of long-term outcome in young adults. *Eur J Endocrinol.* 2015;172:R67-R77
52. Bagattini B, Cosmo CD, Montanelli L, et al. The different requirement of L-T4 therapy in congenital athyreosis compared with adult-acquired hypothyroidism suggests a persisting thyroid hormone resistance at the hypothalamic-pituitary level. *Eur J Endocrinol.* 2014;171:615-621
53. de Tristan J, Zenk J, Künzel J, et al. Thyroglossal duct cysts: 20 years' experience (1992-2011). *Eur Arch Otorhinolaryngol.* 2014 Aug 19;[Epub ahead of print]
54. Pietruszewska W. Wagrowska-Danielewicz M, Jozefowicz-Korczynska M. Papillary carcinoma in the thyroglossal duct cyst with uninvolved thyroid. Case report and review of the literature. *Arch Med Sci.* 2014;10:1061-1065
55. Sperling MA, ed. *Pediatric Endocrinology.* Pittsburgh, PA: Saunders Elsevier; 2008
56. Leger J, Kaguelidou F, Alberti C, et al. Graves' disease in childhood. *Best Pract Res Clin Endocrinol Metab.* 2014;28:233-243
57. Kazanavicius G, Lasaite L, Graziene A. Syndrome of isolated FT3 toxicosis. *J Diabetes Endocrinol.* 2012;3:1-5
58. Lazar L, Kalter-Leibovici O, Pertzelan A, et al. Thyrotoxicosis in prepubertal children compared with pubertal and postpubertal patients. *J Clin Endocrinol Metab.* 2000;85:3678-3682
59. Goldstein S, Katowitz WR, Moshan T, et al. Pediatric thyroid-associated orbitopathy: The Children's Hospital of Philadelphia experience and literature review. *Thyroid.* 2008;18:997-999
60. Eha J, Pitz S, Pohlenz J. Clinical features of pediatric Graves' orbitopathy. *Int Ophthalmol.* 2010;30:717-721
61. Kaguelidou F, Carel JC, Leger J. Graves' disease in childhood: advances in management with antithyroid drug therapy. *Horm Res.* 2009;71:310-317
62. Yasude T, Kishida D, Tazawa K, et al. ANCA associated vasculitis with central retinal artery occlusion developing during treatment with methimazole. *Intern Med.* 2012;51:3177-3180
63. Climenti M, Di Gianantonio E, Cassina M, et al. Treatment of hyperthyroidism in pregnancy and birth defects. *J Clin Endocrinol Metab.* 2010;95: E337-E341

64. Douchement D, Rakza T, Holder M, et al. Choanal atresia associated with tracheoesophageal fistula: the spectrum of carbimazole embryopathy. *Pediatrics.* 2011;128:e703-e706
65. Stagnaro-Green S, Abalovich M, Alexander E, et al. Guidelines of the American Thyroid Association for the diagnosis and management of thyroid disease during pregnancy and postpartum. *Thyroid.* 2011;21:1081-1125
66. Bauer AJ. Approach to the pediatric patient with Graves' disease: when is definitive therapy warranted? *J Clin Endocrinol Metab.* 2011;96:580-588
67. Vaidya B, Wright A, Shuttleworth J, et al. Block & replace regime versus titration regime of antithyroid drugs for the treatment of Graves' disease: a retrospective observational study. *Clin Endocrinol (Oxf).* 2014;81:610-613
68. Sato H, Minamitani K, Minagawa M, et al. Clinical features at diagnosis and responses to antithyroid drugs in younger children with Graves' disease compared with adolescent patients. *J Pediatr Endocrinol Metab.* 2014;27:677-683
69. Chao M, Jiawei X, Guoming W, et al. Radioiodine treatment for pediatric hyperthyroid Graves' disease. *Eur J Pediatr.* 2009;168:1165-1169
70. Breur C, Tuggle C, Solomon D, et al. Pediatric thyroid disease: when is surgery necessary, and who should be operating on our children? *J Clin Res Pediatr Endocrinol.* 2013;5:79-85
71. Ronga G, Filesi M, D'Apollo, et al. Autonomous functioning thyroid nodules and ^{131}I in diagnosis and therapy: after 50 years of experience what is still open to debate? *Clin Nucl Med.* 2013;38:349-353
72. Nabhan ZM, Kreher NC, Eugster EA. Hashitoxicosis in children: clinical features and natural history. *J Pediatr.* 2005;146:533-536
73. Wasniewska M, Corrias A, Salerno M. Outcomes of children with hashitoxicosis. *Horm Res Paediatr.* 2012;77:36-40
74. Gupta A, Castroneves LA, Frates MC, et al. How are childhood thyroid nodules discovered: opportunities for improving early detection. *J Pediatr.* 2014;164:658-660
75. Hayles AB, Kennedy RL, Woolner LB, et al. Nodular lesions of the thyroid gland in children. *J Clin Endocrinol Metab.* 1956;16:1580-1594
76. Hegedus L. Clinical practice: the thyroid nodule. *N Engl J Med.* 2004;351:1764-1881
77. Niedziela M. Pathogenesis, diagnosis and management of thyroid nodules in children. *Endocr Rel Cancer.* 2006;13:427-453
78. Gupta A, Ly S, Castroneves LA, et al. A standardized assessment of thyroid nodules in children confirms higher cancer prevalence than in adults. *J Clin Endocrinol Metab.* 2013;98:3238-3245
79. Cooper D, Doherty GM, Haugen BR, et al. Revised American Thyroid Association management guidelines for patients with thyroid nodule and differentiated thyroid cancer. *Thyroid.* 2009;19:1167-1214
80. Gharib H, Papini E, Paschke R, et al. American Association of Clinical Endocrinologists, Associazione Medici Endocrinology, and European Thyroid Association medical guidelines for clinical practice for the diagnosis and management of thyroid nodules. *Endocr Pract.* 2010;16(Suppl 1):1-43
81. Francis GL, Waguespack MD, Bauer AJ, et al. The American Thyroid Association guidelines Task Force on Pediatric Thyroid Cancer. Management guidelines for children with thyroid nodules and differentiated thyroid cancer. *Thyroid.* 2015 Apr 21 [Accepted for Publication]
82. Baloch ZW, LiVolsi VA, Asa SL, et al. Diagnostic terminology and morphologic criteria for cytologic diagnosis of thyroid lesions: a synopsis of the National Cancer Institute Thyroid Fine-Needle Aspiration State of the Science Conference. *Diagn Cytopathol.* 2008;36:425-437
83. Bernet V, Hupart KH, Parangi S, et al. AACE/ACE disease state commentary: molecular diagnostic testing of thyroid nodules with indeterminate cytopathology. *Endocr Pract.* 2014;20:360-363
84. Bauer AJ. Thyroid nodules and differentiated thyroid cancer. *Endocr Dev.* 2014;26:183-201
85. Siegel DA, King J, Tai E, et al. Cancer incidence rates and trends among children and adolescents in the United States, 2001-2009. *Pediatrics.* 2014;134:e945-e955

86. Vergamini LB, Frazier AL, Abrantes FL, et al. Increase in the incidence of differentiated thyroid carcinoma in children, adolescents, and young adults: a population based study. *J Pediatr.* 2014;164:1481-1485
87. Fridman M, Savva N, Krasko O, et al. Initial presentation and late results of treatment of post-Chernobyl papillary thyroid carcinoma in children and adolescents of Belarus. *J Clin Endocrinol Metab.* 2014;99:2932-2941
88. Journy N, Ancelet S, Rehel JL. Predicted cancer risks induced by computer tomography examinations during childhood, by a quantitative risk assessment approach. *Radiat Environ Biophys.* 2014;43:39-54
89. Fallah M, Pukkala E, Tryggvadottir L, et al. Risk of thyroid cancer in first-degree relatives of patients with non-medullary thyroid cancer by histology type and age at diagnosis: a joint study from five Nordic countries. *J Med Genet.* 2013;50:373-382
90. Markovina S, Grigsby PW, Schwarz JK, et al. Treatment approach, surveillance, and outcome of well-differentiated thyroid cancer in childhood and adolescence. *Thyroid.* 2014;24:1121-1126
91. Pawelczak M, David R, F Bonita, et al. Outcomes of children and adolescents with well-differentiated thyroid carcinoma and pulmonary metastases following ^{131}I treatment: a systematic review. *Thyroid.* 2010;20:1095-1101
92. Hazard JB, Hawk WA, Grile G Jr. Medullary (solid) carcinoma of the thyroid: a clinicopathologic entity. *J Clin Endocrinol Metab.* 1959;19:152-161
93. Roy M, Chen H, Sippel R. Current understanding and management of thyroid cancer. *Oncologist.* 2013;18:1093-1100
94. Elisei R, Alvezaki M, Conte-Devolx B, et al. European Thyroid Association guidelines for genetic testing and its clinical consequences in medullary thyroid cancer. *Eur Thyroid J.* 2012;1:216-231
95. Kloos RT, Eng C, Evans D, et al. Medullary thyroid cancer: management guidelines of the American Thyroid Association. *Thyroid.* 2009;19:565-612

Update on Diabetes in Children and Adolescents

Clifford A. Bloch, MD[a]*; Sunil Nayak, MD[b]

[a]*Clinical Professor of Pediatrics, University of Colorado School of Medicine, Pediatric Endocrine Associates, P.C., Greenwood Village, Colorado;* [b]*Assistant Clinical Professor of Pediatrics, University of Colorado School of Medicine, Pediatric Endocrine Associates, P.C., Greenwood Village, Colorado*

INTRODUCTION

According to the Centers for Disease Control and Prevention (CDC), diabetes mellitus is one of the most common chronic diseases in children in the United States. The prevalence of this disease varies by the type of diabetes, age, race, and ethnicity. According to the American Diabetes Association (ADA),[1] there are 4 main categories of diabetes:

1. Type 1 diabetes (T1DM; associated with β-cell destruction and insulin deficiency); subclassified into T1 A (immune destruction) and T1 B (non-immune destruction; rare)[2]
2. Type 2 diabetes (T2DM; associated with insulin resistance, insulin hypersecretion, and subsequent β-cell failure)
3. Other specific types of diabetes associated with genetic defects in glucose transport, β-cell function, insulin action, diseases of the exocrine pancreas (eg, cystic fibrosis), and drug- or chemical-induced β-cell failure
4. Gestational diabetes mellitus (GDM)

Additionally, there is a subtype having elements of both T1DM and T2DM, the maturity-onset diabetes of youth (MODY) syndrome, in which genetic abnormalities result in insulin resistance and β-cell failure.[1,3]

T1DM accounts for only 10% of diabetes in adults, with T2DM accounting for most of the rest of the cases. Much of the information about the prevalence of

---

*Corresponding author
E-mail address: Cbloch7435@msn.com

T1DM in childhood and adolescence comes from National Institutes of Health (NIH)-sponsored T1DM diabetes registries in Colorado and Pennsylvania. These registries are limited by a lack of accurate information on diagnoses and a limited geographic scope (and therefore limited racial/ethnic mix) of the study population. These registry studies were followed by a long-term, proactive NIH-sponsored study, entitled SEARCH for Diabetes in Youth, in which the diagnoses were verified by immunologic testing and, in some cases, by dynamic tests of islet-cell insulin reserves.[4,5] The SEARCH study included an estimated 3.5 million children and adolescents younger than 20 years. They were drawn from 5 carefully chosen areas of relatively stable populations from which records could be accessed with the help of participating medical professionals. Thus, the group was drawn from certain counties in Colorado, Ohio, South Carolina, and Washington; from Health plan members of Kaiser Permanente in Southern California; and from Native Americans living on reservations in Arizona and New Mexico. The prevalence rates in 1999 are summarized in Table 1.[6]

In a subset of children from the SEARCH cohort from Colorado, we determined that there had been a 1.6-fold increase in the incidence of T1DM in children younger than 18 years from 1978-1988 to 2002-2004.[5] The reasons for this increased incidence remain unclear. With the exception of a few isolated communities, more than 95% of all children younger than 10 years with diabetes mellitus have T1DM.[6] Because of the increased prevalence of obesity in children and adolescents, there has been an increased incidence of T2DM in these age groups. According to the medical literature and popular media, we are supposedly facing an "epidemic" of T2DM in the pediatric and adolescent age groups.[7,8] Is this really true? We certainly see more children and adolescents with insulin resistance and metabolic syndrome as a complication of sedentary lifestyle and overeating. However, with the exception of a few communities, only a small percentage of children with metabolic syndrome actually progress to T2DM by the

Table 1

Prevalence of diabetes mellitus in children and adolescents under 20 years of age

Race/ethnicity	Type 1 diabetes mellitus Prevalence (per 1000)	Type 2 diabetes mellitus Prevalence (per 1000)
Non-Hispanic White	2.55	0.09
Black	1.63	0.56
Hispanic	1.29	0.40
Asian/Pacific Islander	0.60	0.19
American Indian/Alaskan native	0.35	0.63
Total	1.93	0.24

Adapted from Pettitt DJ, Talton J, Dabelea D, et al; for the SEARCH for Diabetes in Youth Study Group. Prevalence of diabetes in U.S. youth in 2009: The SEARCH for Diabetes in Youth Study. *Diabetes Care*. 2014;37:402-408.

end of adolescence.[9] Thus, although the incidence of T2DM has increased in children and adolescents, the numbers have yet to translate into a nationwide epidemic.

ETIOLOGY OF T1DM

There has been much research into genetic factors that may play a role in the genesis of T1DM. From the Boston and London twin/triplet studies, we know that there is a strong genetic component to the etiology of diabetes, with a concordance rate of approximately 40% to 50% for T1DM in monozygotic twins/triplets after the index case has developed T1DM.[10,11] Because the concordance rate is not 100%, as one would expect if T1DM were purely a genetic disease, the conclusion was drawn that there must be an environmental component as well that influences disease expression in genetically susceptible individuals.[12] There is epidemiologic evidence supporting a role of environment, with disease prevalence varying geographically within racial and ethnic groups living in one country versus another. Because of these observations, there has been an impetus to understand the relative roles of genetics and environment in the etiology/pathogenesis of T1DM in children. Epidemiologic studies have linked certain high-risk tissue haplotypes to an increased risk for developing T1DM. In particular, human leukocyte antigen (HLA) class II genes, located on chromosome 6p, are thought to confer approximately 50% of the genetic risk. Thus, in a newborn study in Colorado (the DAISY study), HLA DR3/4-DQ2/8 was present in 2.3% of neonates but in more than 30% of children who develop T1DM.[13] Thus, although the prevalence of T1DM is approximately 1 in 300 in childhood/adolescence, the prevalence is estimated to be approximately 1 in 20 if this haplotype combination is present. The haplotypes with the strongest association seem to be HLA DQA1*0301, DQB1*0302, DQA1*0501, and DQB1*0201. More recently, genomewide association studies (GWAS) have found novel candidate genes, numbering more than 60 as of 2012.[14] These include 11p15.5 (VNTR [variable number of tandem repeats on the insulin gene]), 1p13 (PTPN22), and many others. The exact etiologic role of these genes remains to be determined. A variety of islet cell and insulin autoantibodies have been found to be associated with T1DM, including GAD-65, IA-2 (ICA512), IAA, and ZnT8.[14] Whether these antibodies are etiologic or simply epigenetic phenomena that are found after the immune process has commenced remains to be determined.

Years of painstakingly thorough diabetes registry studies in Colorado and Pennsylvania have failed to shed much light on any compelling major environmental factors. Casein milk proteins were suspected at one time because the incidence of T1DM is lower in children who were breastfed as infants. Certain viruses were once implicated, and many other factors, including vaccines, food dyes, pesticides, food preservatives, and hydrocarbons in drinking water, have been considered. One by one, however, they have all been excluded, leaving us with many unanswered questions. For the sake of brevity, however, we will not detail the many studies that have examined excess or deficiency of various trace elements, minerals, vitamins, nitrosamines, and free oxygen radicals.

Because it is abundantly clear that there is a huge chasm in our understanding of the etiology and pathophysiology of T1DM, it is our opinion that it is premature to perform any clinical intervention studies/diabetes prevention trials until we fully understand the etiology and pathophysiology of the disease. We fully endorse the allocation of research funds to determine the etiology and pathophysiology of T1DM but decry the allocation of funding to conduct intervention studies at this time, none of which have yet proven to be successful. We realize that this statement goes against the tide of current diabetes research. However, we believe that the same funds would be better spent studying the genetics, immunology, islet cell biology, and physiology of islet cell function and islet cell disease.

SCREENING FOR T1DM

Our statements regarding funding for intervention studies apply equally to screening studies at this time. Unless we have an intervention strategy to offer patients who are immunologically at high risk for progressing to T1DM, any reasonable hope of averting the disease by use of screening studies seems to us to be a waste of scarce funding resources. In our opinion, these studies raise false hope for patients and their families and generate unnecessary anxiety if the immunologic studies are positive. When the etiology of the disease is better understood, it would then be reasonable to undertake large-scale screening studies as well as case-finding studies for enrollment of high-risk patients or patients with preclinical disease into randomized controlled clinical trials. It will be essential that such trials be conducted with rigorous scientific principles, which include adoption of the null hypothesis and inclusion of a double-blind control group. Anything less will prolong our current lack of knowledge regarding the ability to either prevent the onset of disease or limit progression to overt clinical disease.

DIAGNOSIS OF T1DM

Before discussing the role of tests, which may provide laboratory support for the diagnosis, we would like to state quite unequivocally that the diagnosis of T1DM is a clinical diagnosis. Thus, most children and adolescents present with symptoms that include nocturia, polyuria, polydipsia, polyphagia, and unexplained weight loss. In some instances, the symptoms progress to emesis, dehydration, Kussmaul respiration, and shock. The duration of symptoms typically is short, varying from a few days to a couple of months. Most cases are diagnosed by the primary care physician, with a confirmatory capillary plasma glucose (PG) greater than 200 mg/dL. Although this may appear quite simple, the diagnosis presents a unique challenge to the primary care physician because some of the symptoms of T1DM are common to other diseases. Thus, during a community outbreak of enteroviral (EV) illness, many children may present with emesis, weight loss, and dehydration, and some may progress to Kussmaul respiration and shock. In most of these cases, the glucose concentration will be normal or only modestly increased. A clinical clue to EV illness is oliguria, not polyuria. Most children and adolescents with T1DM are ketotic (positive urine or serum ketones) and have not decompensated to ketoacidosis at diagnosis.

Because most children and adolescents are not ketoacidotic at diagnosis, they may be managed as outpatients in clinics or offices that are set up with a specially trained team to initiate treatment and life skills training (see section on Management of T1DM). Those who have signs of ketoacidosis need to be referred to an emergency room or urgent care center for immediate management. These settings must include facilities for stat laboratory testing, administration of intravenous (IV) fluids and insulin, and equipment and staff for intensive monitoring and intervention.

A small cohort of children or adolescents presents atypically, providing a unique diagnostic challenge. In some cases of acute illness, including EV illness, patients present with "stress hyperglycemia." In these cases, simple administration of rehydrating IV fluids will resolve the hyperglycemia. Urine ketones are usually low or absent, the hemoglobin A_{1c} (HbA_{1c}) concentration is normal, and these patients lack the antecedent history of nocturia, polyuria, and polydipsia. In these cases, measurement of islet cell antibodies will usually be negative, thereby obviating the need for continued endocrine evaluation. However, it may take up to a week or more to obtain a result. If antibodies are positive, there is a 90% likelihood that the child or adolescent has diabetes or is likely to progress to diabetes. The child will require glycemic monitoring and intervention with insulin if necessary. Occasionally, some children or adolescents present with symptoms of urinary frequency, which may be confused with polyuria, unless a meticulous history is obtained.

With regard to diagnostic testing, islet cell antibody testing is usually not clinically useful and is seldom required, except in unusual cases, such as the atypical examples cited earlier. Although HLA haplotyping has been performed in epidemiologic population studies, it has no utility in the diagnosis of T1DM. An HbA_{1c} test is helpful at diagnosis when symptoms are present, and the test can be performed routinely. However, it has not been useful as a stand-alone screening test for diabetes in asymptomatic children and adolescents because of possible false-positives and false-negatives. There is very little role for oral glucose tolerance testing for diagnosis of T1DM in children and adolescents. Although the World Health Organization and the American Diabetes Association have adopted criteria for diagnosis (including symptoms and a casual PG >200 mg/dL, a fasting PG ≥126, or a PG >200 2 hours after an OGTT),[3] these criteria are seldom required to establish a diagnosis because most children and adolescents present with symptoms and PG greater than 200. An OGTT may be useful in diagnosing T2DM in high-risk individuals.

MANAGEMENT OF T1DM

Despite considerable progress in the management of children and adolescents with T1DM over the past 20 years, the core objectives remain unchanged, namely, to provide adequate nutrition for growth, administration of exogenous insulin, and participation in physical activity in a manner that avoids hyperglycemia, hypoglycemia, and other acute complications, including ketoacidosis, while permitting a normal lifestyle and physical and emotional growth and development. Additionally, the intent is to prevent long-term microvascular, macrovascular, and neurologic complications. All of these goals were found to be feasible upon publication of the compelling results of the Diabetes Control and Complications Trial (DCCT), in which the outcomes of "conventional insulin therapy" were compared with those of "intensive insulin therapy."[15,16]

The DCCT results taught us that the core goals of diabetes management were attainable in adults and adolescents. Since then, there have been several advances in accomplishing these goals more effectively and safely (ie, decreasing the risks of severe hypoglycemia).[17-19] These advances include the use of customized human insulin, providing modified insulin pharmacokinetics and pharmacodynamics, improved insulin delivery systems (eg, insulin pens and programmable insulin pumps), and enhanced glucose monitoring capabilities. The latter include improved accuracy of standard glucose meters, glucose meters coupled to insulin pumps, continuous glucose monitoring systems (CGMS), and CGMS sensor-augmented insulin pump therapy with automated insulin suspension.

With all of these new management tools available, it is important to recognize that they have to be used judiciously, customizing therapy for each patient. Such customization requires knowledge and experience of the physician and an education team, which typically includes a certified diabetes educator and registered dietitian, and support of others, including knowledgeable parents/guardians, nurses, nurse practitioners, physician assistants, medical assistants, counselors, a school nurse or nurse surrogate, teachers, babysitters, and coaches. Other contributors include ophthalmologists, podiatrists, and other specialists as needed. The team is usually spearheaded by a diabetes specialist, such as a pediatric endocrinologist, in partnership with a PCP.[3]

Examples of customized insulin therapy are given for consideration. For therapy to be successful, glycemic targets need to be set with 2 major considerations in mind. First, tight metabolic control is associated with a lower risk of long-term microvascular and macrovascular complications. Second, lower glycemic targets are associated with a greater potential for acute hypoglycemia. Therefore, the enthusiasm in advocating for lower glycemic targets needs to be tempered by caution that hypoglycemia may ensue. For tight metabolic control to be successful and safe, one needs to take into consideration the age and cognitive and emotional maturity of the patient and the support of family before planning a strategy for the best modality of outpatient therapy.

In a younger child or adolescent or one who lacks the required adult support or has emotional or cognitive impairments, the recommendation should be a simplified twice-daily regimen of "conventional insulin therapy" with insulin lispro or aspart insulin mixed with NPH insulin at breakfast and dinnertime. Glycemic target ranges are raised and HbA_{1c} expectations are set to higher target numbers, and the diet is relatively fixed with regard to carbohydrate content and timing of meals and snacks.

In adolescents who have all the required elements to be successful, one may consider starting with a basal-bolus regimen with 24-hour acting insulin (eg, glargine) administered once per day or long-acting insulin (eg, detemir) administered once or twice per day, with insulin lispro or aspart administered before meals and snacks. This regimen requires accurate carbohydrate counting, more frequent injections, and the ability to calculate and adjust doses using a simple formula. This typically involves use of an "insulin-to-carb ratio" to bolus for carbohydrates that are about to be eaten and the addition of a "correction factor" to account for higher or lower PG concentrations. This regimen ought to be more liberating because carbohydrate counts and meal timing can be varied.

Any child or adolescent who is managed as an outpatient at diagnosis requires a physician who is skilled in the management of diabetes and is available via phone at all times. In our experience, outpatient management on the day of diagnosis only permits the teaching of essential survival skills ("life skills management"), which include instruction on glycemic monitoring using a glucose meter, insulin administration, and rudimentary aspects of diet, before returning over the next few days for systematic teaching with the rest of the diabetes team. Because the patient will need some time to learn the concepts of carbohydrate counting, the physician will need to be able to provide assistance with carb counting at mealtimes. Insulin pump therapy requires careful planning because a process is typically required to obtain insurance authorization for coverage before initiation of training and therapy. For pump therapy, the adolescent needs to be able to count carbs accurately, insert subcutaneous insulin infusion catheters independently if there is a site occlusion, and calculate insulin doses using similar formulae. Adjustments may need to be made to accommodate exercise. If these criteria are not met, there needs to be a plan for adult supervision to be available at all times to assist with these tasks. In addition to parental supervision at home, the child will need assistance from a school nurse and his or her surrogate.

Basal-bolus therapy or insulin pump therapy is typically the standard of care for most adolescents with established T1DM because they can usually perform the necessary tasks independently. Of note is the emotional toll that typically accompanies the diagnosis of chronic illness in adolescents. It may influence the choice of therapy because some teenagers indicate that they are not ready for insulin pump therapy. Some adolescents express displeasure with "having something attached to me" and want no involvement with pump therapy. Such patients are best managed with basal-bolus therapy or conventional insulin therapy, as necessary.

As indicated by these examples, insulin therapy needs to be customized to each child's circumstances.[3] Unfortunately, these considerations sometimes are derailed by patient self-advocacy. Some patients will choose to embark on insulin pump therapy before they are ready for it, resulting in failure to master the skills, attain the glycemic goals, and meet the safety requirements. Of course, regardless of the prescribed insulin dose regimen, glycemic monitoring is required. The usual standard of care is to use a glucose meter, which typically measures plasma capillary glucose on a small drop of blood. Meters have improved over the years, requiring smaller drops of blood, and are more accurate and faster at producing results. Most diabetes specialists require use of uploadable glucose meters, from which the glycemic data can be entered into a computer linked to an electronic medical record and analyzed. As pediatric endocrinologists we decry the use of non-uploadable, store-brand glucose meters because they represent a downgrade in the quality of diabetes care. Unfortunately, use of these less expensive glucose meters has become more prevalent of late in an attempt to decrease the costs of health care. With the addition of CGMS, children and adolescents now have the capability of supplementing standard glycemic monitoring with a continuous glucose sensor. Initially approved by the United States Federal Drug Administration (FDA) for use in adolescents older than 16 years, it has also been used effectively in younger children, as documented in the STAR 3 study, which included 78 children, ages 11.7 ± 3 years.[18] Based upon this study, many pediatric endocrinologists have prescribed CGMS in younger and younger children, using it "off label." However, although CGMS may be helpful by triggering an alarm when glucose concentrations fall outside of preset limits, the full benefit of real-time glycemic monitoring and insulin dose adjustment is only realized by older children and adolescents who are capable of checking their CGMS meter and making the requisite changes. Per FDA labeling, insulin dose changes are to be made only after the low or high glucose concentration on a capillary PG is confirmed by a glucose meter.

More recently, the FDA-approved CGMS sensor-augmented insulin pump therapy with automated insulin suspension.[19] This represents state-of-the-art diabetes management, in which the child wears a glucose sensor/transmitter and an insulin pump, linked together via Bluetooth technology. CGMS glucose measurements are recorded in the insulin pump. An insulin infusion may be suspended automatically if the glucose concentration declines too rapidly such that it is likely to progress to hypoglycemia, or automatic insulin suspension may occur if a preset, low glycemic threshold is reached. Use of this system was reported in 46 and 49 study and control children, adolescents, and adults, aged 4 years and older.[19] In this study, the adjusted incidence rate of moderate or severe hypoglycemia was reduced from 34.2 to 9.5 per 100 patient months in the pump-only group versus the low-glucose suspension group after 6 months of therapy. The HbA_{1c} concentrations were identical for both groups, which means that glycemic goals could be met with a lower risk of serious hypoglycemia. We see this as the most exciting and potentially life-changing new therapy over the past 5 years, with the potential to prevent serious hypoglycemia and neuroglycopenia, which are the feared, short-term risks of diabetes insulin management. At the time of writing, this system has only been FDA-approved for adults and adolescents older than 16 years. Although this system is not an FDA-approved form of therapy at this time, a recently published report from Israel of 56 pre-teens and teens aged 10 to 18 years using their MD-Logic, closed-loop insulin pump (the "artificial pancreas") demonstrated improved nocturnal glycemic control compared to that with the open-loop, sensor-augmented insulin pump.[20]

DIABETES EDUCATION

Because diabetes care has become more complex with the advent of new technology, the role of professional diabetes education has become greater than ever before. Typically, every child and adolescent undergoes comprehensive one-on-one teaching with a team of diabetes educators at diagnosis and initiation of therapy. Together with the family, the child or adolescent is taught the skills necessary for diabetes self-management, including basic information about the disease, glycemic goals, the relationship between glycemic control and acute and long-term complications, hypoglycemia and its management, the principles of insulin dose adjustment for high and low glucose concentrations, ketone testing, exercise, and management of diabetes at school. Additionally, the child or adolescent is taught about diet, including carbohydrate counting. Current consensus recommends a healthy, balanced diet that is high in carbohydrates (preferably unrefined), high in fiber, and low in saturated fat. The child or adolescent will need to have a line of communication with his/her caregivers 24 hours a day, 7 days a week, because he/she will require backup support. Typically, communication is frequent shortly after diagnosis and is infrequent thereafter if the teaching is successful. The goal of teaching is to render the child or adolescent and his/her family self-sufficient and proficient in self-management, such that they can manage the disease independently. When pump therapy and CGMS are introduced, he/she will need to meet with a pump trainer to explain the use and application of the technology. Once again, backup phone support needs to be available at all times.

GLYCEMIC GOALS

The ADA recommends considering patient age in the establishment of glycemic goals, with different targets for pre-meal and bedtime/overnight glucose concentrations in patients aged 0 to 6, 6 to 12, and 13 to 19 years of age.[3] Glycemic targets for HbA_{1c} have been adjusted to a single target of less than 7.5%, regardless of age.[3] However, it issues a disclaimer that "individualization is still encouraged".

EXERCISE

No activity restrictions are imposed on children and adolescents with T1DM.[3] Patients are advised to make physical activity a consistent part of their day. Insulin dosing can be adjusted to accommodate activity of any intensity and duration. Patients, their families, and their coaches must be able to recognize and treat symptoms of hypoglycemia. Hypoglycemia may occur during exercise or several hours later, after stress hormone concentrations have decreased. This can be anticipated and prevented by adjusting insulin or having the adolescent eat a "booster snack" before exercise, such as a protein bar or crackers and cheese or peanut butter or a piece of fruit.

MANAGEMENT OF DIABETES IN SCHOOLS

As diabetes management has become more complex, the burden on school staff has become greater to ensure that the child or adolescent is safe at school. Various states have developed their own school programs, some limited and others quite sophisticated. First, it is important to note that it is not the job of the school to manage a child's or adolescent's diabetes at school. The school staff may assist the child or adolescent in executing a written plan, which may include assistance with glycemic testing, carbohydrate counting, calculation of insulin dose, assistance with insulin administration, and documentation of these tasks. It is the school's job to ensure that the child is safe and to intervene if any complications arise. Thus, the school needs to ensure that a child or adolescent with diabetes has a written plan detailing when and where he/she is able to perform glycemic monitoring. If hypoglycemia should arise, the plan ought to detail how it should be managed. Younger children may require assistance from the school staff to count carbohydrates, communicate with a parent, and administer insulin via syringe, injection pen, or pump. Adolescents, in particular, should be taught the skills to manage their diabetes independently. Thus, they should acquire the skills to administer and adjust their doses of insulin, use their CGMS to monitor their interstitial glucose, confirm CGMS readings with a capillary PG check, and make pump adjustments in basal or bolus insulin infusion on the fly. This means having a liberal school plan that allows the pump-savvy adolescent to make changes independently if state law permits. For those who are less sophisticated, the assistance of school personnel may be required. In Colorado, we believe that we have one of the most comprehensive school plans in the country. It involves school nurse education, proficiency training of nurse surrogates, and state and board of nursing legislation to permit nurses and surrogates to perform functions for which they are trained, including administration of insulin boluses via an insulin syringe, insulin injection pen or insulin pump, and injection of glucagon for serious hypoglycemia. These guidelines follow those published by the National Diabetes Education Program (NDEP) in 2012,[21] which were modified and customized for use in schools in Colorado.[22]

T2DM

The focus of this diabetes update has been predominantly on T1DM. With the increasing prevalence of childhood obesity, insulin resistance, and metabolic syndrome, many had predicted that there would be a marked increased incidence of T2DM in children and adolescents. As noted previously, although T2DM in children and adolescents has increased in incidence, it has yet to reach epidemic proportions.[9,23,24] The Pediatric Endocrine Society recently published guidelines for management of children and adolescents with T2DM.[25] A large intervention study of lifestyle modification and use of insulin-sensitizing drugs (the TODAY study) was published recently, with disappointing results.[26] Unlike in adult studies, children and adolescents in the TODAY study failed to attain the treatment glycemic goals, which has set us back in determining how to optimally manage those in these age groups with T2DM.

FUTURE DIRECTIONS

Although progress has been slow, there is hope that future studies will uncover the etiology of diabetes. That holds the promise of ushering in a host of intervention studies using novel approaches to prevent diabetes or halt its progression to clinical disease when it is diagnosed in its preclinical phase. Although CGMS sensor-augmented insulin pump therapy with automated insulin suspension is the current state of the art for management of T1DM, we can look forward to enhanced technology, using closed-loop insulin pumps (the "artificial pancreas") in the future. However, we urge the reader to temper his/her enthusiasm for this new technology at this time given that the closed-loop study focused only on nocturnal control. This is because it has proved difficult to regulate diabetes postprandially using closed-loop pumps during the day.

CONCLUSION

Although we have learned much about the pathophysiology of autoimmune T-cell–mediated islet cell destruction, the etiology of T1DM remains elusive. Until we learn more about the etiology, we believe that any intervention studies are premature because they are unlikely to be successful. We discussed the new developments in diabetes care, particularly in the area of continuous glucose monitoring and CGMS sensor-augmented insulin pump therapy with automated insulin suspension. This latest technology has opened a new avenue for improved diabetes management. Although at this point we have minimal published information on closed-loop pump automation at night, we are hopeful that the next 5 years will usher in an era of continuous, closed-loop pump automation, day and night, and that this will significantly improve care for children and adolescents in the upcoming years.

References

1. American Diabetes Association. Diagnosis and classification of diabetes mellitus. *Diabetes Care.* 2014;37(Suppl 1):S81-S90
2. Concannon P, Rich SS, Nepom GT. Genetics of type 1A diabetes. *N Engl J Med.* 2009;360:1646-1654
3. American Diabetes Association. Standards of medical care in diabetes—2015: summary of revisions. *Diabetes Care.* 2015;38 Suppl:S4
4. Writing Group for the SEARCH for Diabetes in Youth Study Group; Dabelea D, Bell RA, et al. Incidence of diabetes in youth in the United States. *JAMA.* 2007;297:2716-2724
5. Vehik K, Hamman RF, Lezotte D, et al. Increasing incidence of type 1 diabetes in 0- to 17-year-old Colorado youth. *Diabetes Care.* 2007;30:503-509
6. Pettitt DJ, Talton J, Dabelea D, et al; for the SEARCH for Diabetes in Youth Study Group. Prevalence of diabetes in U.S. youth in 2009: The SEARCH for Diabetes in Youth Study. *Diabetes Care.* 2014;37:402-408
7. Kaufman FR. Type 2 diabetes in children and young adults: a "new epidemic." *Clin Diabetes.* 2002;20:217-218
8. Alberti G, Zimmet P, Shaw J, et al; for the International Diabetes Federation Consensus Workshop. Type 2 diabetes in the young: the evolving epidemic. *Diabetes Care.* 2004;27:1798-1811
9. Goran MI, Davis J, Kelly L, et al. Low prevalence of pediatric type 2 diabetes: where's the epidemic? [NHANES III]. *J Pediatr.* 2008;152:753-755
10. Srikanta S, Ganda OP, Jackson RA, et al. Type 1 diabetes mellitus in monozygotic twins: chronic progressive beta cell dysfunction. *Ann Intern Med.* 1983;99:320-326
11. Metcalfe KA, Hitman GA, Rowe RE. Concordance for type 1 diabetes in identical twins is affected by insulin genotype. *Diabetes Care.* 2001;24:838-842
12. The TEDDY Study Group. The environmental determinants of diabetes in the young (TEDDY) study. *Ann N Y Acad Sci.* 2008;1150:1-13
13. Rewers M, Bugawan TL, Norris JM, et al. Newborn screening for HLA markers associated with IDDM. Diabetes Autoimmunity Study in the Young (DAISY). *Diabetologia.* 1996;39:807-812
14. Bakay M, Pandey R, Hakonarson H. Genes involved in type 1 diabetes: an update. *Genes.* 2013;4:499-521
15. The DCCT Research Group. The effect of intensive treatment of diabetes on the development and progression to long-term complications in insulin-dependent diabetes mellitus. *N Engl J Med.* 1993;329:977-986
16. White NH, Cleary PA, Dahms W, et al; the Diabetes Control and Complications Trial (DCCT)/Epidemiology of Diabetes Interventions and Complications (EDIC) Research Group. Beneficial effects of intensive therapy of diabetes during adolescence: outcomes after the conclusion of the diabetes and complications control trial (DCCT). *J Pediatr.* 2001;139:804-812
17. Seaquist ER, Anderson J, Childs B, et al. Hypoglycemia and diabetes: a report of a Workgroup of the American Diabetes Association and The Endocrine Society. *Diabetes Care.* 2013;36:1384-1395
18. Bergenstal RM, Tamborlane, WV, Ahmann A, et al; for the STAR 3 Study group. Effectiveness of sensor-augmented insulin-pump therapy in type 1 diabetes. *N Engl J Med.* 2010;363:311-320
19. Ly TT, Nicholas JA, Retterath A, et al. Effect of sensor-augmented insulin pump therapy and automated insulin suspension v standard insulin pump therapy on hypoglycemia in patients with type 1 diabetes. A randomized clinical trial. *JAMA.* 2013;310:1240-1247
20. Phillip M, Battelino T, Atlas E, et al. Nocturnal glucose control with an artificial pancreas at a diabetes camp. *N Engl J Med.* 2013;368:824-833

21. National Diabetes Education Program. Helping the Student with Diabetes Succeed: A Guide for School Personnel. Available at: ndep.nih.gov/publications/PublicationDetail.aspx?PubId=97#main. Accessed May 13, 2015
22. Bobo N, Wyckoff L, Patrick K, et al. A collaborative approach to diabetes management: the choice made for Colorado schools. *J School Nursing*. 2011;27:269-281
23. Dabelea D, Mayer-Davis EJ, Saydah S, et al; for the SEARCH for Diabetes in Youth Study. Prevalence of type 1 and type 2 diabetes among children and adolescents from 2001 to 2009. *JAMA*. 2014;311:1778-1786
24. D'Aadamo E, Caprio S. Type 2 diabetes in youth: epidemiology and pathophysiology. *Diabetes Care*. 2011;34(Suppl 2):161-165
25. Copeland KC, Silverstein J, Moore KR, et al. Management of newly diagnosed type 2 diabetes mellitus (T2DM) in children and adolescents. *Pediatrics*. 2013;131:364-382
26. Zeitler P, Hirst K, Pyle L, et al; TODAY Study Group. A clinical trial to maintain glycemic control in youth with type 2 diabetes. *N Engl J Med*. 2012;366:2247-2256

Update on Puberty and Its Disorders in Adolescents

Amit Lahoti, MD[a]*; Irene Sills, MD[b]

[a]Division of Pediatric Endocrinology, Le Bonheur Children's Hospital, University of Tennessee Health Science Center, Memphis, Tennessee; [b]Professor of Pediatrics, Pediatric Endocrinologist, SUNY Upstate Medical University, Syracuse, New York

INTRODUCTION

Puberty, the process of transformation of a child into a young adult, involves both physical and psychosocial maturation. It is characterized by secretion of gonadal hormones, development of secondary sexual characteristics, and maturation of gametogenesis and reproductive functions. This developmental stage is also characterized by a period of rapid growth, the pubertal growth spurt. Pubertal onset and progression are important because they are closely linked to optimum and timely growth during this phase and an adolescent's ability to fit in among his peers. It is also associated with long-term health outcomes not immediately apparent to the adolescent and the physician. This review focuses on newer developments over the past few years, which have allowed us to better understand the genetic and epigenetic determinants of pubertal development and its underlying processes, the pathophysiology of deviations from normal, and the management of patients with these deviations. Epidemiologic studies evaluating a change in the timing of puberty are also reviewed. An update on our current knowledge of determinants of puberty, and its secular trends and variations (especially delayed puberty), will help those who provide care to adolescents to distinguish the normal from the abnormal. Appropriate and timely evaluation and referral to a pediatric endocrinologist for management of identified or suspected disorders of puberty in this patient population are vital for a good outcome.

*Corresponding author
E-mail address: alahoti@uthsc.edu

PHYSIOLOGY OF PUBERTY AND PUBERTAL GROWTH

Linear growth in humans is the outcome of a complex interplay of a variety of factors, including genetics, nutrition, hormones, and the environment. The relative importance of these individual factors varies during different phases of life, beginning in utero and extending through infancy, childhood, and puberty. Growth and puberty are closely linked. Sex hormones, which bring about the secondary sexual characteristics that mark puberty, are the most important determinants of growth during this phase of life.[1]

In an average child, pubertal growth accounts for 15% of total final adult height in a relatively short span and is the fastest period of growth after the first 1 to 2 years of life. Most pubertal growth occurs as part of the pubertal growth spurt. Endochondral bone formation at the growth plate responsible for longitudinal bone growth is tightly regulated by a multitude of endocrine signals. Estrogen (produced by the ovaries in females and by aromatization of androgens in males) is a crucial factor for the accelerated growth during puberty and growth plate fusion, for males as well as for females. Indirect effects of sex hormones on growth are mediated by their effects on the growth hormone (GH) axis: increased secretion of GH, increased end-organ sensitivity to GH, and increased serum insulin like growth factor-1 (IGF-1) levels.[1] The growth spurt is an early pubertal event in the development of girls that coincides clinically with the onset of breast development and reaches a peak growth velocity of 8 cm/year. Peak growth velocity (ie, the growth spurt) in boys occurs at a testicular volume of 10 to 12 mL, reaches 10 cm/year, and is a late pubertal event, occurring an average of 2 years later than in girls. The exact reason for this difference in timing of the growth spurt in boys and girls is not well known; however, the additional years of prepubertal growth and the larger magnitude of the growth spurt in boys are the physiologic bases for boys being taller than girls on average.[1]

The hormonal changes that form the basis of puberty begin before the physical signs. A vital event in this process is the release of gonadotropin-releasing hormone (GnRH) from the hypothalamus. Pulsatile GnRH secretion from hypothalamic neurons stimulates the gonadotropes in the pituitary, leading to release of luteinizing hormone (LH) and follicle-stimulating hormone (FSH), which in turn stimulate growth and maturation of the gonads and release of testosterone in males and estrogens in females. Animal studies and studies in patients and their families with single gene deletions causing gonadotropin deficiency or extreme variations in pubertal onset have improved our understanding of the factors regulating gonadotropic axis activation. Previously considered the first step in the start of the pubertal process, GnRH release now seems to be the final common pathway of several factors upstream of the GnRH neurons that have recently been discovered. It is now known that activation of the gonadotropic axis at puberty involves increased excitatory and decreased inhibitory inputs, as well as secretory factors (eg, transforming growth factor-α [TGF-α] and prostaglandins), from the glial cells, which are important for pubertal onset. This was a particularly important discovery because glial cells were previously believed to not play any role in neuronal regulation. Leptin and ghrelin, hormones secreted by adipose tissue and the gastrointestinal tract, respectively, have been known to be involved in energy homeostasis and have recently been found to play an important role in the regulation of both puberty and reproduction. Stimulatory neuronal factors upstream to the GnRH neurons include kisspeptins, neurokinin B, and glutamate. Inhibitory factors include gamma-amino butyric acid (GABA) and opioid peptides. Kisspeptins are a family of neuropeptides encoded by the *Kiss1* gene in neurons located in the arcuate nucleus of the hypothalamus that are now known to stimulate GnRH neurons through their actions on their G-protein–coupled receptor GPR54.[2,3]

TIMING OF PUBERTY

Implications for Health

Puberty is a crucial physiologic process in the life of an individual, and the timing of puberty has lately been identified to play an important role in psychological development and in the pathophysiology of several conditions that extend beyond the adolescent age. Boys and girls undergoing early pubertal maturation have lower social competence in 6th grade and are more likely to smoke cigarettes in 9th grade compared to their later maturing peers.[4] These findings highlight the psychological effect of earlier pubertal timing in both boys and girls.

Menarche is a significant pubertal event in the reproductive life of women. Epidemiologic studies from as early as the 1960s and 1970s had shown a link between early age at menarche (AAM) and the risk of developing breast and endometrial cancer later in life.[5,6] Age at menarche also has a curvilinear relationship (U-shaped) with the metabolic syndrome and oligomenorrhea in adulthood. Whereas early AAM (10 years) is associated with high childhood body mass index (BMI) and the metabolic syndrome, late AAM (16 years) is associated with low childhood BMI and the metabolic syndrome. However, both early and late AAM are associated with the metabolic syndrome and cardiometabolic abnormalities in adults.[7] Data linking timing of puberty and long-term health outcomes in boys are sparse and not as definite.

Determining Factors and Change in Normal Standards

The timing of menarche is influenced by a combination of genetic and environmental factors. Although 70% to 80% of variability in the timing of menarche can be explained by heritable factors, specific common genetic variants that influence the timing of puberty were not known until recently and hence have been the basis of several studies in the past few years.[8,9] Newer technologies, including genome wide association studies (GWAS) and copy number variations (CNVs), have been used to conduct epidemiologic studies on large samples of populations to answer these questions.[10] Among the new genetic targets identified by investigators is the common C allele of rs314276 in the *LIN28B* gene on the 6q21 region, which is associated with earlier breast development and menarche in girls, earlier voice breaking and more advanced pubic hair development in boys, a faster tempo of height growth in girls and boys, and shorter adult height in men and women because of earlier cessation of growth.[9] A subsequent meta-analysis has identified the association of 30 novel loci with AAM. Several of these factors have previously been associated with BMI, energy homeostasis, and hormonal regulation, further reinforcing the linkage between genetic and environmental factors and their influence on AAM.[11] More recently, a CNV-based GWAS study identified a novel locus in the 2q14.2 region, upstream of the diazepam binding inhibitor (*DBI*) gene. This gene is known to regulate estrogen levels, a key factor in menarche. Subjects with a 1-copy variant of this CNV have a mean AAM of 14 years, whereas those with 2 copies have a mean AAM of 12.9 years.[10]

Environmental factors affecting puberty and AAM include nutrition and environmental exposures. Heavy (>20 cigarettes per day) prenatal tobacco smoke exposure via maternal smoking and childhood environmental tobacco smoke exposure are associated with a later age of menarche (>12 years) compared to no exposure (age of menarche <12 years).[12] In recent years, body fat and a group of chemicals that interfere with steroid hormone activity known as endocrine disrupting chemicals have attracted attention as factors influencing pubertal development and menarche. Several recent studies have found a positive association between higher body fat and earlier timing of puberty in girls; however, more studies are needed to evaluate whether earlier puberty is the cause or effect of the higher body fat.[13] Findings of studies evaluating endocrine disrupting chemicals such as phthalates and bisphenol-A (BPA) for an association with pubertal timing have been somewhat variable, although it seems that age at exposure (including in utero exposure) may be an important determinant. Higher levels of in utero phthalate exposure seems to influence prepubescent hormonal concentrations and the timing of sexual maturation.[14] Data from 12- to 16-year-old female participants in the National Health and Nutrition Examination Survey (NHANES) for the years 2003 to 2008 showed an association between exposure to 2,5-dichlorophenol (2,5-DCP) and earlier age of menarche in the general US population.[15] More longitudinal studies with samples collected at different stages of development are needed to strengthen these associations and establish causality.

Secular trends on pubertal timing over the past century have been evaluated by large epidemiologic studies from both the developed and the developing world. Most of these studies were performed in females. Although menarche is a rather late event in the pubertal development of a girl, AAM is more often used when studying pubertal onset than other events, such as age at thelarche, because the former tends to be better remembered and well defined for the general population. Although studies on this subject have been published since the 1980s, the number of reports has increased significantly in the past 2 decades and more so in the past few years. Almost all studies noted a downward trend in AAM over the past century, although the degree of change and the periods of maximum change have been variable. Several European studies and some US studies showed a steady decline in AAM until the mid-20th century birth cohorts, after which the decline stopped in some countries and even increased slightly in other countries.[16,17] Most of the recent studies evaluating AAM in birth cohorts from the latter half of the 20th century and early 21st century again noted a decline in AAM, even in countries that seemed to have shown a stabilization earlier.[18,19] The studies found a variable rate of decline in AAM ranging from 0.12 to 0.65 years per decade.[20,21] The mean AAM in the most recent reports from Europe and the United States in the 21st century ranges from 12.2 to 13.05 years,[22] with a greater proportion of girls reaching menarche at an age younger than 12 years. Within the United States, the few studies that looked at this issue found a trend of declining AAM, and significant racial differences were noted (with black girls reaching menarche 0.25–1 year earlier than their white counterparts).[23,24] However, the last US birth-cohort year for which AAM data were published to date was 1994.[24] Because of the scarcity of data analyzed for subsequent birth-year cohorts, the most recent AAM trends in the United States are not yet known.

Data on changes in puberty are much more sparse for boys than for girls.[13] Even when available, the data between different studies and between different time periods are not comparable because of differences between the criteria used to define the onset of puberty in boys as testicular enlargement (>3 mL), pubic hair (Tanner 2), or age at voice breaking, along with differences in training of the investigators.[24] However, 1 recent large study on this topic, performed in pediatric offices across the United States and using testicular enlargement (>3 mL) as the marker of pubertal onset in boys, concluded that the mean age of genital and pubic hair growth was 6 months to 2 years earlier than in past studies, with black boys maturing sooner than their white and Hispanic counterparts.[25] However, the age cutoff for precocious puberty in boys (testicular enlargement earlier than 9 years) is not yet changed and remains a topic of further discussion. Causes and future implications of this apparent shift in age of puberty among US boys requires further investigation.

VARIANTS OF GROWTH: DELAYED PUBERTY

Puberty is considered delayed if there are no physical signs of pubertal maturation (testicular enlargement in boys, breast development in girls) by an age that is 2 to 2.5 standard deviations (SDs) above the mean for the population. These cutoff ages traditionally have been 14 years for boys and 13 years for girls. However, some experts have called for updating these ages toward younger cutoffs in view of the downward trend in pubertal timing discussed earlier and differences between different racial and ethnic groups.[26]

Constitutional Delay of Growth and Puberty

Constitutional delay of growth and puberty (CDGP) is considered an extreme end of the normal spectrum of pubertal timing and is the most common cause of delayed puberty (Figure 1). However, CDGP should be a diagnosis of exclusion after other more serious causes of delayed puberty have been ruled out by

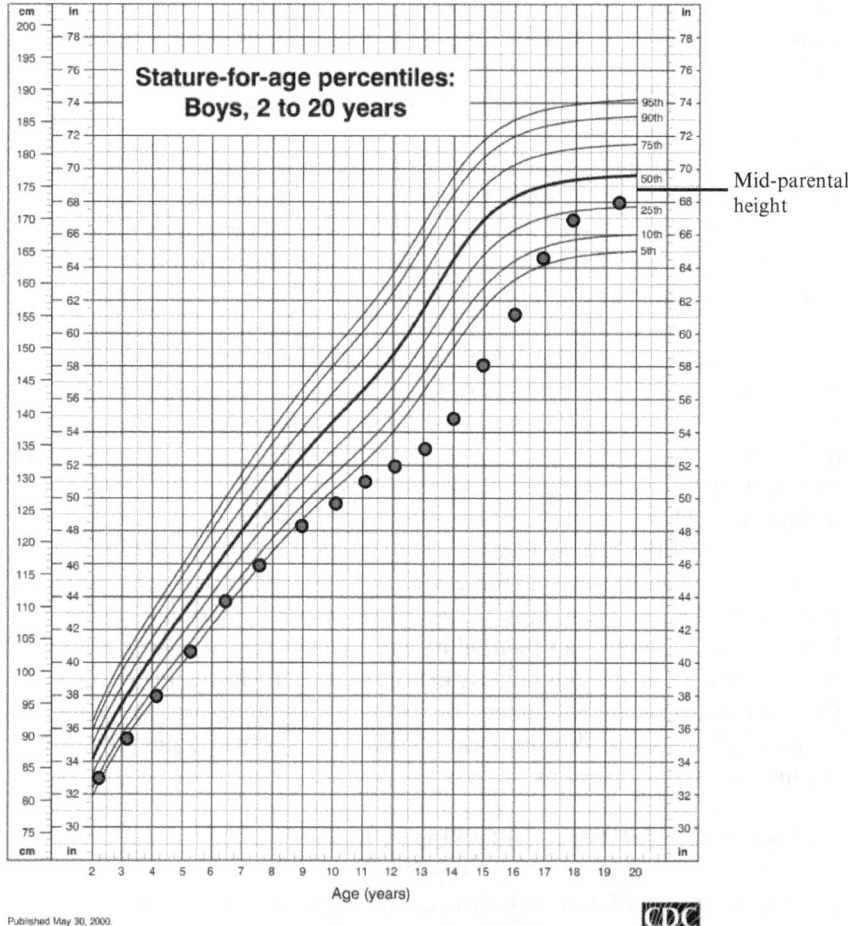

Fig 1. Growth chart representing growth pattern of boys with constitutional delay of growth and puberty compared to males with average timed puberty. Note the growth deceleration apparent at 10-14 years followed by a delayed growth spurt between 14-17 years and a final height usually in range for target height.

careful evaluation and close follow-up of the patient. Approximately 65% of males and 30% of females with delayed puberty in a large case series had CDGP, although this may be an underestimate because the study was done in a tertiary-care hospital and a higher number of CDGP patients may be seen by primary care physicians and not always referred to subspecialists.[27] Although some studies have shown an almost equal prevalence of CDGP in males and females, boys present with delayed puberty more often than girls, perhaps because the social pressures of delayed maturation and short stature are more problematic for boys than for girls.[28] Most of the studies, and hence the following discussion, pertains to boys with CDGP.

Studies have shown that 50% to 80% of variability in pubertal timing is genetically determined, and 50% to 75% of patients with CDGP have a family history of pubertal delay with a trend toward autosomal dominant inheritance.[28,29] Despite recent discoveries of genes that influence the timing of puberty, the search for the genetic basis of CDGP has been difficult so far. Variations or mutations in the coding regions of *LIN28B, FGFR1, GNRHR, TAC3, TACR3,* and leptin or leptin receptor polymorphisms have not been found to underlie CDGP.[30-32] On the other hand, pleomorphisms in estrogen receptor alpha (ESR1) and mutations in the growth hormone secretagogue receptor (GHSR) have been found in CDGP, highlighting the need for a continued search for the genetic basis of this condition.[33,34] Over the past decade, leptin (secreted by adipocytes) and ghrelin (primarily secreted by distinctive endocrine cells called *P/D1* cells lining the fundus of the stomach) have been identified as playing an important role in the initiation and progress of puberty. Ghrelin has been found to inhibit GnRH secretion, whereas leptin facilitates it. A recent study found that in adolescent boys with CDGP, ghrelin levels were significantly higher and leptin levels significantly lower than in pubertal boys of the same age, supporting our current knowledge of the actions of these hormones on puberty.[35]

The major differential diagnoses for CDGP are hypergonadotropic hypogonadism (characterized by elevated FSH and LH because of the absence of negative feedback from the gonads) and hypogonadotropic hypogonadism (characterized by low FSH and LH). Laboratory findings of hypogonadotropic hypogonadism (low FSH and LH, low testosterone in males, low estradiol in females) usually are indistinguishable from those seen in CDGP and hence pose a diagnostic challenge. A delay in bone age can also be seen in both conditions. Because the treatment of the 2 varies significantly, alternative markers to differentiate them have been studied and recently reviewed.[36] Inhibin B (INHB) is a hormone produced by Sertoli cells upon FSH stimulation. A baseline INHB concentration of 35 pg/mL or less had sensitivity and specificity of 100% in a study on identifying Tanner stage I boys with hypogonadotropic hypogonadism (either isolated or as part of combined pituitary hormone deficiency). Although another study did not find such high sensitivity or specificity for INHB, that study evaluated subjects at variable Tanner stages, so its results may not be as reliable. In a different study, a combination of the GnRH stimulation test and 3-day and 19-day human chorionic gonadotropin (HCG) stimulation tests gave 100% sensitivity and specificity in differentiating CDGP and hypogonadotropic hypogonadism in adolescent boys.[36]

The most commonly accepted approach for management of a child with CDGP is to "wait and watch" because these patients are considered to have variants of normal growth. However, different growth-promoting agents have been tried in these patients to improve their final height and in the short term to improve their growth and relieve the psychological stress sometimes associated with being significantly shorter and more immature appearing than their peers. The question has arisen whether it is possible to predict which boys with CDGP will attain adult heights less than -2.25 SD (or <160 cm) without intervention and hence may be considered for recombinant human growth hormone (rhGH) therapy under the indication of idiopathic short stature. A study evaluated the final adult height of 69 young men, aged 22.6 ± 3.5 years, who were diagnosed with CDGP at a mean age of 14.9 ± 1.2 years. Final height was less than 160 cm in 6 subjects (8.7%). When the height predictions made by various height prediction rules and target heights with actual adult heights were compared, none of the methods identified the 6 subjects with sufficient sensitivity. Hence, rhGH candidates among 14- to 16-year old boys with CDGP cannot be accurately identified by the currently available height prediction methods.[37]

Oxandrolone (a nonaromatizing androgen) and aromatase inhibitors (agents that block conversion of androgens to estrogens, eg, letrozole) have also been investigated as growth-promoting agents in this population. Several trials, including randomized placebo controlled trials performed as early as the 1980s using oxandrolone in patients with CDGP, have shown improvement in the growth velocity (an increase of 3.5-4.5 cm/year from baseline) and height of treated patients.[38-40] The improved effects have lasted in most studies, even up to 1 year after treatment with oxandrolone.[39] However, several of these studies had relatively small sample sizes, and almost all had short treatment and follow-up durations. Studies comparing oxandrolone to rhGH treatment have found that the increase in growth velocity and IGF-1 levels were comparable. In some studies, growth velocity was even better in the oxandrolone group.[38,41] More recently, oxandrolone was compared to letrozole for treatment of CDGP in a double-blind placebo controlled trial. Both treatments improved height to a similar degree (mean increase ~ 0.6 ± 0.3 SD) after a 2-year treatment, but letrozole caused less bone age advancement. The letrozole group also had a higher increase in predicted adult height (PAH) but less pubertal advancement and bone mineral loss.[42] However, the use of aromatase inhibitors in CDGP is still off-label, and long-term studies are needed to assess their safety.[43]

A short course (3-6 months) of testosterone therapy, usually in boys older than 13 years, has been used to induce puberty, although the mechanism remains unclear. It is proposed that testosterone treatment primes the hypothalamic-pituitary-gonadal axis for a brisk increase in FSH secretion or a faster testicular response to FSH than would occur in the natural course in patients with CDGP. A single (and sometimes a second) treatment course can serve as a diagnostic test as well as therapy for CDGP and can rule out hypogonadism and true GH deficiency. Patients with CDGP show an increase in growth velocity during the treatment, as well as an increase in testicular size (often soon after the testosterone course), whereas patients with hypogonadism do not show testicular growth, and true GH-deficient patients do not have the brisk growth response.[44] Different testosterone dosing regimens have been proposed, with some studies, especially the older ones, using doses upward of 200 mg every 3 weeks. However, more recently, lower doses have been proposed: monthly intramuscular doses of 50 to 100 mg of testosterone enanthate, cypionate, or propionate.[29,45,46] Using higher testosterone doses for a long duration raises concerns of promoting growth in the short term but earlier skeletal maturation and eventual closure of epiphyses with consequent short stature. However, the newer regimens have been shown to be effective (increasing growth velocity) and safe (no significant bone age advancement or other side effects) when used in selected male adolescents with CDGP.

Hypergonadotropic Hypogonadism and Hypogonadotropic Hypogonadism

The term hypergonadotropic hypogonadism implies (1) the hypothalamic-pituitary component of puberty has been activated, and (2) the negative feedback of sex steroids to the hypothalamus is not present. Hence, this biochemical state of elevated FSH and LH with low estradiol (in girls) and low testosterone (in boys) reflects gonadal dysfunction of various etiologies. Hypergonadotropic hypogonadism is always pathologic. Essential parts of assessment include a history of gonadal trauma, infection, surgery, or exposure to chemotherapeutic drugs or irradiation, along with an examination for clinical features suggestive of Turner syndrome (TS), Klinefelter syndrome (KS), Noonan syndrome, and consideration of performing a karyotype.

Hypogonadotropic hypogonadism, on the other hand, implies a failure of activation of the hypothalamus or pituitary. In the absence of stimulation by gonadotropins, the gonads, which are otherwise usually normal in this condition, do not produce sex steroids.

A detailed discussion of individual causes of hypogonadism can be found elsewhere[2] and is beyond the scope of this discussion. We will focus our discussion on recent updates in the pathophysiology, diagnosis, and treatment of these conditions in boys and girls separately, with a few notable examples.

Males

HYPERGONADOTROPIC HYPOGONADISM

Causes of hypergonadotropic hypogonadism in males include several congenital/genetic causes, as well as acquired causes, which have been discussed in detail elsewhere.[2] Notable among the genetic causes is KS, which has an estimated prevalence of more than 150 per 100,000 live-born males and is the most common chromosomal anomaly in males. Most patients have a 47,XXY karyotype, but other variations include 48,XXXY, 48,XXYY, and 49,XXXYY.[2,47] However, epidemiologic studies from different parts of the world report that only 20% to 25% of these patients are diagnosed during their lifetime. Diagnostic activity seems to be higher in Australia, where up to 50% of expected cases are diagnosed. However, only 10% of these patients are diagnosed before puberty, highlighting a significant delay in diagnosis, underdiagnosis, and nondiagnosis.[47] The relatively mild phenotype is proposed as one of the reasons why so many KS patients go through their lives without being diagnosed. There are no firm guidelines for diagnosis; however, the cardinal features include small testes in almost all patients, hypergonadotropic hypogonadism, gynecomastia, learning difficulties, and infertility. Other typical features include tall stature, disproportionate long limbs, poor muscle development, and a variable degree of masculinization, leading to decreased sexual hair and a feminine fat distribution. The clinical features in KS are presumed to be a consequence of extra genes from the X chromosome (despite inactivation of 1 of the X chromosomes, as in women, some genes remain non inactivated). More than 10% of genes on the X chromosome are expressed in testes and hence probably play a role in KS. Patients with 3 or 4 X chromosomes have a more severe phenotype. In addition to the features mentioned, these patients have an increased risk of developing abdominal adiposity, the metabolic syndrome, autoimmune disease, osteopenia, and cancers (breast cancer in adults and mediastinal cancer in children) and hence require regular monitoring and periodic screenings.

Most patients with KS begin puberty spontaneously and at a normal time. Bilateral testes grow to approximately 6 mL and shrink thereafter to a pathologic size less than 6 mL by the time patients reach adulthood. The underlying mechanism of this shrinkage is thought to be hyalinization of the seminiferous tubules, which likely starts at midpuberty. Although germ cell loss, Leydig cell hyperplasia, and seminiferous tubule hyalinization occur in the testes, focal spermatogenesis may be found, with the possibility of surgically extracting viable sperm. Levels of LH, FSH, and testosterone are normal at the beginning of puberty. Subsequently, FSH and LH begin to increase and testosterone levels decline compared to normal boys. The hypogonadism that these patients develop is relative rather than absolute. Testosterone levels typically are in the lower normal range or subnormal.[47]

Hypogonadotropic Hypogonadism

Hypogonadotropic hypogonadism can be congenital or acquired; the latter can be secondary to trauma, malignancies, surgery, systemic illness, or other insults to the hypothalamic-pituitary axis. Either congenital or acquired hypogonadotropic hypogonadism can be isolated or may be associated with other pituitary hormone deficiencies. Congenital hypogonadotropic hypogonadism (either isolated or with other pituitary hormone deficiencies) can present in the neonatal period in boys with micropenis, with or without cryptorchidism, or later on with pubertal delay.

With the newer insights on the genes regulating puberty, there has been a great deal of interest in congenital isolated hypogonadotropic hypogonadism (from here on referred to as HH) and we will review its etiopathogenesis in detail. A genetic mutation has been reported in 25% to 30% cases of HH. However, with our increasing knowledge of genes regulating puberty, this percentage is expected to increase in the coming years. HH can be subdivided into normosmic HH or hypoanosmic HH, depending on normal or low/absent sense of smell, respectively. Normosmic HH is caused by a congenital dysfunction in the synthesis, release, or ability of GnRH to induce pulsatile release of gonadotropins. Knowledge from studies of affected families have shown normosmic HH to be caused by mutations causing decreased/absent activity of 6 genes so far: *GnRH1, GnRH receptor (GnRHR), KiSS1, KiSS1 receptor (KiSS1R), TAC3* encoding neurokinin B, and its receptor *TACR3*. All of these are autosomal recessive conditions.[48]

HH with hypoanosmia is Kallmann syndrome, and it has a variable inheritance. It affects 1 in 8000 men. Although it can affect women as well, the prevalence is approximately 5 times lower. Clinical features are variable and may include midline facial defects and renal anomalies. Magnetic resonance imaging of the brain usually shows aplasia or hypoplasia of the olfactory bulbs and defective GnRH neuron migration through the cribriform plate. Inactivating mutations of the *KAL1* gene (which encodes for protein anosmin-1) located on the X chromosome was the first identified gene for Kallmann syndrome. Since then, several autosomal genes have also been identified: *FGFR1/Kal2* (fibroblast growth factor-1 receptor), *PROK2/Kal4* (prokineticin 2), *PROKR2/Kal3* (prokineticin 2 receptor), *FGF8* (fibroblast growth factor-8), *NELF* (nasal embryonic LHRH factor), *WDR11* (WD repeat-containing protein 11), and *SEMA3A* (semaphorin 3A).[48]

Mutations in the *CHD7* gene are found in 60% to 70% of patients with the CHARGE (Coloboma, Heart defects, choanal Atresia, Retardation of growth and/or development including intellectual disability, Genital hypoplasia, and external Ear anomalies) syndrome. Over the past few years, *CHD7* mutations have also been reported in 5% to 11% of patients with Kallmann syndrome, and there is increasing interest in further characterizing these patients for clinical and genetic counseling purposes.[49]

Treatment of Males with Hypogonadism

Treatment of hypogonadism involves hormone replacement therapy with testosterone, beginning at puberty and after reaching a skeletal age of more than 12 years. However, depending on the underlying etiology, additional interventions may be needed. For example, in patients with KS, delays in speech development and learning problems may begin in early childhood, so timely referral to speech therapists or appropriate adjustments in school for an optimum learning experience are needed much earlier before puberty.

Because most adolescents with KS enter puberty spontaneously, a universal consensus on when to start testosterone replacement therapy (TRT) is lacking. Some experts recommend beginning testosterone supplementation as soon as LH and FSH levels begin to rise,[47] but others believe that the benefits are unclear for patients with normal or slightly low testosterone levels. Benefits of testosterone therapy include advancement and maintenance of pubertal changes and preserved bone mineral density (BMD). Advantages can also include improving the metabolic profile, increasing muscle mass, and improving neurocognitive function, which have been shown in small observational studies, although definite evidence is lacking. Irrespective of when treatment is started, future fertility should be discussed, preferably before treatment is started. The effect of TRT on future fertility of KS individuals is largely unknown, although there is a theoretical concern that exogenous testosterone may further suppress testicular function in preexisting primary testicular failure. Referral to a fertility specialist or urologist would be appropriate, and treatment can be postponed until after viable sperm is retrieved.

The most accepted and widely used mode of beginning TRT is with monthly injections of testosterone esters (undecanoate, cypionate, or enanthate) in gradually increasing doses. Although testosterone injections usually are well tolerated, they may cause local pain at the injection site, require visits to the physician's office, and cause fluctuating levels of testosterone and its metabolites. Smaller doses at shorter intervals help level out fluctuations. A transdermal gel (testosterone gel 1%) preparation is being evaluated as a treatment modality for beginning TRT in adolescents with KS or other causes of hypergonadotropic hypogonadism. In a relatively short (6-month) observational study, 1% testosterone gel was shown to be effective in raising and maintaining testosterone levels in those in the pubertal range and in causing only mild treatment-emergent adverse effects, including cough, acne, and headaches.[50] A reversible, nonsteroidal aromatase inhibitor (letrozole) has also been used in KS patients to normalize the testosterone-to-estradiol ratio and offset the hyperestrogenic state; a higher response rate to aromatase inhibitors has been linked to higher rates of surgical sperm retrieval.[51] However, this is not a standard practice, and uniform guidelines on dose and duration of treatment are lacking.

In boys who present with delayed puberty and nonelevated gonadotropins, broad differential diagnoses are CDGP and hypogonadotropic hypogonadism. Although newer studies on tests such as Inhibin B and HCG stimulation, as discussed in the section on CDGP, show some promise, none are widely accepted to differentiate between the 2 conditions at this point. A short course of low-dose testosterone (4-6 months of depot testosterone, 50-100 mg per dose intramuscularly per week) can be both diagnostic and therapeutic for CDGP. This therapy has been shown not to reduce final height in boys with a skeletal age more than 12 years. Testosterone levels should be measured several weeks after the last dose and, if clearly within the pubertal range (>50 ng/dL), confirm CDGP. These patients should be serially followed to ensure adequate progression of puberty by endogenous testosterone production. Testosterone levels that remain low are indicative of hypogonadotropic hypogonadism. After the diagnosis of hypogonadotropic hypogonadism has been made, TRT should be continued. Appropriate genetic studies may be obtained based on clinical presentation for prognostic and genetic counseling purposes. Gradually increasing doses of testosterone are used to induce pubertal changes.

Once the patient is at full replacement doses of androgens, continuation of therapy is needed to maintain physical and sexual maturity. This can be accomplished by continuing with intramuscular testosterone ester injections, which may be needed at 2- to 3-week intervals, or by changing over to transdermal preparations with a gel or patch. In some patients, biosynthetic LH and FSH, GnRH, or HCG administration can stimulate spermatogenesis, endogenous testosterone production, and fertility. However, the expense and frequency of administration of these treatments usually limit their use to adult men desiring fertility. Until then, testosterone replacement is the most accepted treatment of choice.[2]

Females

Hypergonadotropic Hypogonadism

Hypergonadotropic hypogonadism in females can be caused by chromosomal/syndromic/genetic or congenital causes such as TS (45,X and its variants), galactosemia, and complete gonadal dysgenesis, or acquired causes such as autoimmune ovarian failure, the effects of irradiation or chemotherapy, and iron overload in transfusion-dependent patients. A detailed discussion of these several causes can be found elsewhere[2]; here we will focus our discussion on TS. TS affects approximately 1 in 3000 live-born female infants and is the result of a sex chromosome aneuploidy in which some critical segments of the X chromosome are missing. About half of TS patients have a karyotype of 45,X; the other half show mosaicism of 45,X cells with normal cells or cells with a structurally abnormal second X chromosome.[2,52] Patients with this syndrome can have several abnormalities, including dysmorphic features (short webbed neck, midface hypoplasia, high arched palate), cardiac abnormalities (bicuspid aortic valve, coarctation of aorta), structural renal anomalies, and hypertension (either essential or related to renal anomalies). Beyond the immediate period after birth, the most common reasons for TS patients to seek medical attention are progressive short stature and absent or arrest of puberty (because of gonadal failure), which is discussed in detail in the next paragraph. The mechanism of growth failure in TS is not well understood, although contributing factors likely include sex chromosome aneuploidy, leading to loss of a copy of the short stature homeobox-containing gene on the X chromosome (the *SHOX* gene), a primary skeletal dysplasia, mild dysfunction in GH secretion, and estrogen deficiency. In TS patients with genetic tall stature, growth may track along the fifth percentile of normal female height curves, and growth failure may not be evident until 9 years of age. In general, without treatment, TS adults will be approximately 20 cm shorter than expected from their midparental target height (Figure 2). Growth hormone therapy has been shown to increase growth velocity in these patients and improve the final height outcome. Although the benefit in height outcome is variable across studies, it is greatest when GH therapy is started early, continued for a substantial duration, and given at a reasonably aggressive dose.[52]

More than 90% of 45,X TS patients have gonadal dysgenesis and gonadal failure, which is a cardinal feature of TS. However, approximately 20% to 30% of patients may start puberty spontaneously (more common among girls with mosaic karyotype), although only 2% to 5% have spontaneous menarche.[53] Hence, almost all TS patients require hormone replacement therapy for either failure to start puberty or arrest of progression. Low levels of estrogen are secreted by the ovaries even before puberty in normal women but are theoretically absent in patients with TS. While the utility of low dose estrogen replacement beginning in early life is being actively studied in research setting, based on current evidence, estrogen therapy in preadolescent patients plays no role in growth therapy and hence should not be started. Estrogen therapy should typically be delayed in patients with TS until 3 or more years of GH therapy and a skeletal age of 12 to 14 years to gain maximum growth benefit.[52]

Hypogonadotropic Hypogonadism

Hypogonadotropic hypogonadism is caused by a defect at the hypothalamus-pituitary level. These defects can be permanent because of a genetic condition (eg, Kallmann syndrome, mutations in GnRH receptor), or to structural lesions or tumors of the pituitary/hypothalamic region (eg, craniopharyngioma, hyperprolactinoma, after head trauma, surgery, central nervous system infections).[2]

On the other hand, hypogonadotropic hypogonadism can be temporary, with potential for normal function, in patients who have chronic illnesses, are in an

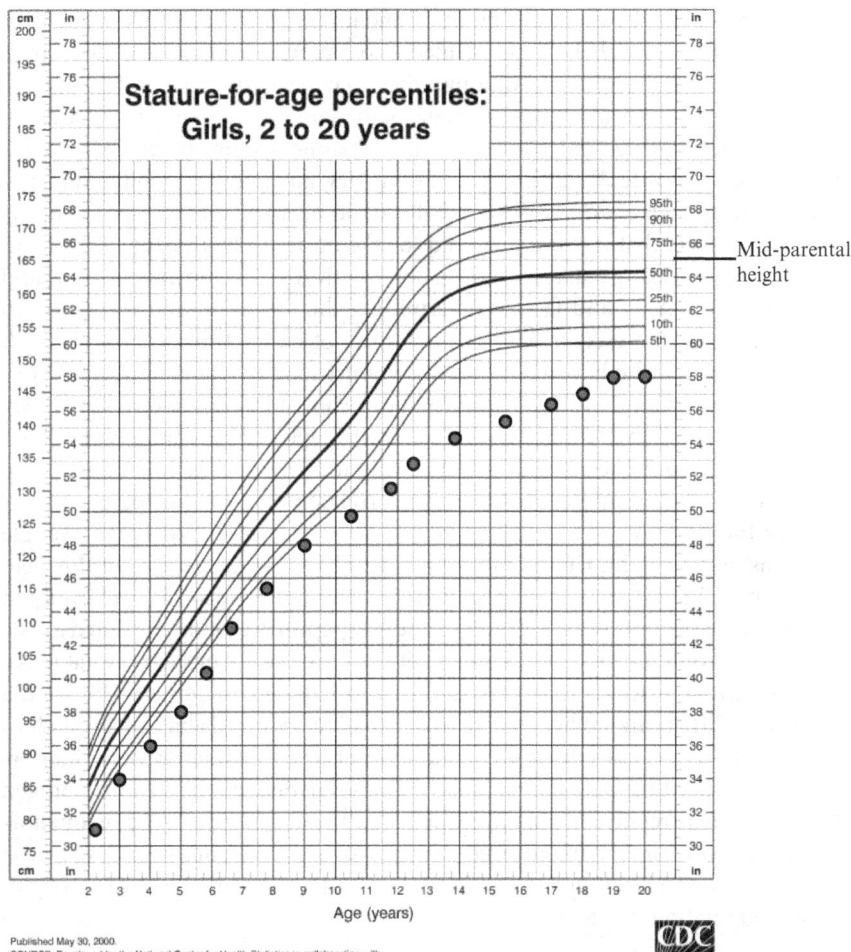

Fig 2. Growth chart representing growth pattern of untreated Turner Syndrome girls compared to normal females. Note a steady growth decline beginning in early childhood, absence of a pubertal growth spurt and a mean final height of approximately 147 cm.

undernourished state, are experiencing excess emotional stress, have an imbalance of other hormones, or are undergoing unusual intense physical activity. Most of these states are reversible with correction of the underlying condition. Among the reversible causes of hypogonadotropic hypogonadism in females, anorexia nervosa (AN) and other anorexia syndromes are a major cause. With a prevalence of 0.2% to 4% in adolescent girls and young women, AN is estimated to be the third most common chronic illness among adolescent girls in western societies.[54,55] Another term frequently used in this context is functional hypothalamic amenorrhea (FHA), defined as hypogonadotropic hypogonadism related to dysfunction of the pulsatile GnRH release from the hypothalamus. This leads to disturbed LH pulses from the pituitary and low estrogen levels. Depending on the underlying cause, FHA is subdivided into 3 types: weight loss related, stress related, and exercise related. Although they may have different underlying etiologies, FHA and AN are considered part of the same clinical spectrum based on psychological testing, and patients with AN show a more profound psychopathological disorder.[56,57] Primary or secondary amenorrhea is often an early and enduring sign of AN.[54,55] This is believed to be an adaptive response of the body to indicate that it is not prepared to take on reproductive functions in an overall negative energy state. Not all patients with AN develop amenorrhea, and the pathophysiology and factors determining the causation and resolution of amenorrhea in adolescents with AN are still not clear. Adolescents and adult women with AN who have amenorrhea demonstrate a hypogonadotropic hypogonadism-like picture. It has previously been shown in adult women with AN that the normal pubertal pulsatile LH pattern is replaced by a prepubertal (low-amplitude LH pulses) or early pubertal (nighttime LH pulses) pattern.[55] The degree of LH pulse suppression does not correlate well with the degree of thinness or the duration of illness, and return of menses does not show a simple relationship to weight. Hence, in recent years the focus of research in this field has been on identifying factors regulating GnRH (and hence LH) pulsatility in amenorrheic patients with AN. Leptin and kisspeptin are being evaluated as key factors. As would be expected, women with AN, as a result of their low fat mass, have, on average, lower leptin levels than normal-weight women. However, a leptin cutoff that can predict amenorrhea in patients with AN has not been identified, and there is considerable overlap in levels seen in amenorrheic and normally menstruating patients with AN.[54] Amenorrhea results in low estrogen levels as well as relative hypoandrogenemia. The effects of the latter in amenorrheic women with AN are not well known; however, low androgen levels have been associated with symptoms of depression and anxiety, irrespective of weight, in this population.[54]

Treatment of Females with Hypogonadism

In patients with pubertal delay resulting from systemic disease or chronic illness or in those with certain tumors such as prolactinoma, treatment of the primary illness can restore normal hypothalamic-pituitary-ovarian axis function and spontaneous puberty. For most other causes of hypogonadism, puberty can be induced using low doses of estrogen therapy beginning at age 10 to 12 years, with the rationale of inducing breast development without causing undue bone age advancement and not having any significant negative effect on final height. Puberty induction in patients with TS, however, usually is delayed to 12 to 14 years in order to allow for optimum benefit from GH therapy. Treatment of patients with hypogonadotropic hypogonadism (as a result of genetic causes described in the section on hypogonadotropic hypogonadism) may often be delayed until closer to 12 to 13 years of age because of difficulty in distinguishing these conditions from CDGP and because the latter usually is managed by a wait and watch approach in girls.

The goal of estrogen replacement therapy is to induce a pubertal increase in the size of the breasts and uterus, and to replicate a tempo of puberty and timing of menarche comparable to those of peers. However, as in patients with TS, sometimes, in order to strike a balance between growth and puberty, hormone replacement may have to be delayed. Estrogen replacement can be provided by an oral or transdermal route. Oral estrogen preparations include ethinyl estradiol, conjugated equine estrogens, and 17-beta estradiol. Because oral ethinyl estradiol is no longer available as a single agent in the United States and formulations of conjugated equine estrogens contain a mixture of multiple estrogenic substances with varying biologic potencies that are not optimal for puberty induction, in recent years the preference has been for the use of micronized 17-beta estradiol (E_2), which can be given via an oral or transdermal route, because estradiol is identical to the ovarian product and the most physiologic form of estrogen currently available. Oral estrogen undergoes first-pass metabolism in the liver, leading to a higher serum estrone concentration, whereas transdermal preparations do not have this effect.[53,58] Transdermal preparations also can be cut in halves and quarters, allowing for beginning estradiol concentrations as low as 6 to 7 μg/d, with an increase in dose every 6 to 12 months based on clinical response and a goal of achieving adult replacement doses over 2 to 3 years of therapy.

Once full estrogen replacement doses (100-200 μg/d of transdermal estradiol) are reached, cyclical progesterone as medroxyprogesterone acetate (5-10 mg) or micronized progesterone (200-400 mg) daily can be added for 10 to 12 days per month to induce menstrual bleeding. Cyclic therapy with estrogen-progesterone may be given as the combined oral contraceptive pill with low-dose estrogen, or as oral or transdermal estrogen therapy for 21 days with the addition of progesterone for 12 days (days 10-21, followed by a week without hormones or on days 20-30 of the monthly cycle). When at full adult replacement doses, the oral preparations offer the advantage of being a simpler regimen. However, recent studies are evaluating whether continuing transdermal preparations may offer other advantages. In a randomized controlled trial, oral and transdermal 17-beta-estradiol were studied for a year to evaluate the metabolic effects and changes in body composition with both preparations. Serum E_2 doses were periodically monitored and doses adjusted to maintain levels similar to those of normally menstruating adolescents. Both treatments had comparable effects on bone mineral content accrual, lipoprotein profiles, inflammatory markers, and glucose and insulin concentrations. However, the oral formulation was associated with lower IGF-1 levels and significantly higher estrone levels, resulting in a less physiologic state.[58] At this time, none of the hormone replacement regimens can be considered as "one size fits all," so there remains a need to individualize the regimens, especially the progestational agents that are used and the mode of delivering the estrogen component.

Adolescents with AN who have amenorrhea often have resumption of menses (ROM) within 3 to 6 months of achieving a BMI between the 14th and 39th percentiles. Resumption of menses is often used as a marker of recovery from AN. However, the clinical predictors of ROM during weight gain in AN remain poorly understood. A recent study found that along with an increase in BMI, a higher percentage of body fat, as measured by dual-energy X-ray absorptiometry scan, was associated with ROM. However, there is no universal "ideal" percentage body fat for ROM. It likely varies based on factors such as levels of physical activity/exercise, with patients who are more active requiring greater body fat for ROM.[59] Another study on factors determining ROM in patients with AN requiring a first hospital admission found that the diagnosis of AN before menarche and a longer duration of hospital treatment predicted a more prolonged time of amenorrhea. Also, a higher premorbid BMI correlated with protracted amenorrhea, probably because the BMI at which menstruation was suspended was higher than the BMI often used as a treatment target (15th-20th age-adjusted BMI percentile).[60]

Another major concern in those with AN, especially amenorrheic patients, is low bone mass because of a lack of estrogen during adolescence, which is a period of peak bone accrual. Although restoration of weight and ROM is the currently accepted strategy to improve bone accrual in AN, the recovery may not be complete. Also, despite maximal efforts by the treating team, weight gain and ROM may not occur. Hence, hormone replacement therapy with oral contraceptive pills has been studied and is often used (especially in young adults) with the hope of improving bone mineral content or preventing further loss. However, giving relatively high estrogen doses has not been shown to improve BMD. It also may give a false sense of normalcy to patients with AN while the underlying pathology remains untreated and masks the true recovery of the hypothalamic-pituitary-ovarian axis. Hence, the evidence and experts advise against the use of oral contraceptive pills in patients with AN. A recent randomized, placebo controlled study, however, used physiologic oral/transdermal estrogen replacement in amenorrheic adolescent girls with AN (girls with skeletal age >15 years were also given cyclic progesterone, whereas those with skeletal age <15 years were only given estrogen at progressively increasing doses). This study showed that physiologic estrogen replacement significantly increased spine and hip BMD in girls with AN over an 18-month period compared to those who received placebo, highlighting a potential treatment modality and the need for further research.[61]

Leptin replacement was tried in 1 study as a treatment of amenorrhea in non-AN patients with hypothalamic amenorrhea. Three of 8 women studied had ovulatory cycles with treatment, raising the possibility of a pathophysiologic role of leptin in hypothalamic amenorrhea. However, a reduction in weight (attributed to reduction in fat mass) was observed in the women treated with leptin, consistent with the anorexigenic effects of leptin.[54] Although this theoretically limits utility of leptin as a treatment modality in AN, therapeutic trials with leptin have not been conducted in AN patients. Low leptin levels in AN are considered to be an adaptive response. Some experts, however, believe that leptin could ameliorate hyperactivity and depression in acutely ill patients and possibly have beneficial effects on the psychopathologic features of starvation in acutely ill patients with AN, including the obsession with food, weight, and body shape. Hence, although there are both potential side effects and benefits of leptin therapy in patients with AN, the overall picture will not be clear until more carefully designed clinical trials are performed.[62]

Kisspeptin, an endogenous ligand for the kisspeptin receptor on GnRH neurons, has been proposed to regulate reproductive function in women with FHA. In 1 study, kisspeptin therapy led to gonadotropin release acutely; however, the effect did not last with chronic therapy. There are no published studies using kisspeptin therapy in patients with AN.[54] Hence, there continues to be a need for further research on the pathophysiology of amenorrhea in AN, and newer therapeutic trials are required.

CONCLUSION

A carefully elicited history and skillfully performed physical examination can help target the assessment of youth who have slower pubertal onset and progression. Increased understanding of genetic etiologies and acquired disorders aids in choosing appropriate therapies. However, much more knowledge is needed to further define optimal ways to help these patients.

References

1. Murray PG, Clayton PE. Endocrine control of growth. *Am J Med Genet C Semin Med Genet.* 2013;163C:76-85
2. Lee PA, Houk CP. Puberty and its disorders. In: Lifshitz F, ed. *Pediatric Endocrinology.* Volume 2. 5th ed. New York: Informa Healthcare; 2009:273-303
3. Pinilla L, Aguilar E, Dieguez C, et al. Kisspeptins and reproduction: physiological roles and regulatory mechanisms. *Physiol Rev.* 2012;92:1235-1316
4. Westling E, Andrews JA, Peterson M. Gender differences in pubertal timing, social competence, and cigarette use: a test of the early maturation hypothesis. *J Adolesc Health* 2012;51:150-155
5. Shapiro S, Strax P, Venet L, et al. The search for risk factors in breast cancer. *Am J Public Health Nations Health.* 1968;58:820-835
6. Elwood JM, Cole P, Rothman KJ, et al. Epidemiology of endometrial cancer. *J Natl Cancer Inst.* 1977;59:1055-1060
7. Glueck CJ, Morrison JA, Wang P, et al. Early and late menarche are associated with oligomenorrhea and predict metabolic syndrome 26 years later. *Metabolism* 2013;62:1597-1606
8. Parent AS, Teilmann G, Juul A, et al. The timing of normal puberty and the age limits of sexual precocity: variations around the world, secular trends, and changes after migration. *Endocr Rev.* 2003;24:668-693
9. Ong KK, Elks CE, Li S, et al. Genetic variation in LIN28B is associated with the timing of puberty. *Nat Genet.* 2009;41:729-733

10. Liu YZ, Li J, Pan R, et al. Genome-wide copy number variation association analyses for age at menarche. *J Clin Endocrinol Metab.* 2012;97:E2133-E2139
11. Elks CE, Perry JR, Sulem P, et al. Thirty new loci for age at menarche identified by a meta-analysis of genome-wide association studies. *Nat Genet.* 2010;42:1077-1085
12. Ferris JS, Flom JD, Tehranifar P, et al. Prenatal and childhood environmental tobacco smoke exposure and age at menarche. *Paediatr Perinat Epidemiol.* 2010;24:515-523
13. Euling SY, Selevan SG, Pescovitz OH, et al. Role of environmental factors in the timing of puberty. *Pediatrics.* 2008;121(Suppl 3):S167-S171
14. Watkins DJ, Tellez-Rojo MM, Ferguson KK, et al. In utero and peripubertal exposure to phthalates and BPA in relation to female sexual maturation. *Environ Res.* 2014;134C:233-241
15. Buttke DE, Sircar K, Martin C. Exposures to endocrine-disrupting chemicals and age of menarche in adolescent girls in NHANES (2003-2008). *Environ Health Perspect.* 2012;120:1613-1618
16. Morris DH, Jones ME, Schoemaker MJ, et al. Secular trends in age at menarche in women in the UK born 1908-93: results from the Breakthrough Generations Study. *Paediatr Perinat Epidemiol.* 2011;25:394-400
17. Nichols HB, Trentham-Dietz A, Hampton JM, et al. From menarche to menopause: trends among US Women born from 1912 to 1969. *Am J Epidemiol.* 2006;164:1003-1011
18. Flash-Luzzatti S, Weil C, Shalev V, et al. Long-term secular trends in the age at menarche in Israel: a systematic literature review and pooled analysis. *Horm Res Paediatr.* 2014;81:266-271
19. Ahn JH, Lim SW, Song BS, et al. Age at menarche in the Korean female: secular trends and relationship to adulthood body mass index. *Ann Pediatr Endocrinol Metab.* 2013;18:60-64
20. Prentice S, Fulford AJ, Jarjou LM, et al. Evidence for a downward secular trend in age of menarche in a rural Gambian population. *Ann Hum Biol.* 2010;37:717-721
21. Jaruratanasirikul S, Sriplung H. Secular trends of growth and pubertal maturation of school children in Southern Thailand. *Ann Hum Biol.* 2014:1-8
22. Talma H, Schonbeck Y, van Dommelen P, et al. Trends in menarcheal age between 1955 and 2009 in the Netherlands. *PloS One.* 2013;8:e60056
23. Freedman DS, Khan LK, Serdula MK, et al. Relation of age at menarche to race, time period, and anthropometric dimensions: the Bogalusa Heart Study. *Pediatrics.* 2002;110:e43
24. Euling SY, Herman-Giddens ME, Lee PA, et al. Examination of US puberty-timing data from 1940 to 1994 for secular trends: panel findings. *Pediatrics.* 2008;121(Suppl 3):S172-S191
25. Herman-Giddens ME, Steffes J, Harris D, et al. Secondary sexual characteristics in boys: data from the Pediatric Research in Office Settings Network. *Pediatrics.* 2012;130:e1058-e1068
26. Susman EJ, Houts RM, Steinberg L, et al. Longitudinal development of secondary sexual characteristics in girls and boys between ages $9^{1}/_{2}$ and $15^{1}/_{2}$ years. *Arch Pediatr Adolesc Med.* 2010;164: 166-173
27. Sedlmeyer IL, Palmert MR. Delayed puberty: analysis of a large case series from an academic center. *J Clin Endocrinol Metab.* 2002;87:1613-1620
28. Wehkalampi K, Widen E, Laine T, et al. Patterns of inheritance of constitutional delay of growth and puberty in families of adolescent girls and boys referred to specialist pediatric care. *J Clin Endocrinol Metab.* 2008;93:723-728
29. Palmert MR, Dunkel L. Clinical practice. Delayed puberty. *N Engl J Med.* 2012;366:443-453
30. Tommiska J, Wehkalampi K, Vaaralahti K, et al. LIN28B in constitutional delay of growth and puberty. *J Clin Endocrinol Metab.* 2010;95:3063-3066
31. Banerjee I, Trueman JA, Hall CM, et al. Phenotypic variation in constitutional delay of growth and puberty: relationship to specific leptin and leptin receptor gene polymorphisms. *Eur J Endocrinol.* 2006;155:121-126
32. Vaaralahti K, Wehkalampi K, Tommiska J, et al. The role of gene defects underlying isolated hypogonadotropic hypogonadism in patients with constitutional delay of growth and puberty. *Fertil Steril.* 2011;95:2756-2758
33. Kang BH, Kim SY, Park MS, et al. Estrogen receptor alpha polymorphism in boys with constitutional delay of growth and puberty. *Ann Pediatr Endocrinol Metab.* 2013;18:71-75

34. Pugliese-Pires PN, Fortin JP, Arthur T, et al. Novel inactivating mutations in the GH secretagogue receptor gene in patients with constitutional delay of growth and puberty. *Eur J Endocrinol.* 2011;165:233-241
35. El-Eshmawy MM, Abdel Aal IA, El Hawary AK. Association of ghrelin and leptin with reproductive hormones in constitutional delay of growth and puberty. *Reprod Biol Endocrinol.* 2010;8:153
36. Harrington J, Palmert MR. Clinical review: distinguishing constitutional delay of growth and puberty from isolated hypogonadotropic hypogonadism: critical appraisal of available diagnostic tests. *J Clin Endocrinol Metab.* 2012;97:3056-3067
37. Krajewska-Siuda E, Malecka-Tendera E, Krajewski-Siuda K. Are short boys with constitutional delay of growth and puberty candidates for rGH therapy according to FDA recommendations? *Horm Res.* 2006;65:192-196
38. Loche S, Pintor C, Cambiaso P, et al. The effect of short-term growth hormone or low-dose oxandrolone treatment in boys with constitutional growth delay. *J Endocrinol Invest.* 1991;14:747-750
39. Papadimitriou A, Wacharasindhu S, Pearl K, et al. Treatment of constitutional growth delay in prepubertal boys with a prolonged course of low dose oxandrolone. *Arch Dis Child.* 1991;66:841-843
40. Stanhope R, Buchanan CR, Fenn GC, et al. Double blind placebo controlled trial of low dose oxandrolone in the treatment of boys with constitutional delay of growth and puberty. *Arch Dis Child.* 1988;63:501-505
41. Buyukgebiz A, Hindmarsh PC, Brook CG. Treatment of constitutional delay of growth and puberty with oxandrolone compared with growth hormone. *Arch Dis Child.* 1990;65:448-449
42. Salehpour S, Alipour P, Razzaghy-Azar M, et al. A double-blind, placebo-controlled comparison of letrozole to oxandrolone effects upon growth and puberty of children with constitutional delay of puberty and idiopathic short stature. *Horm Res Paediatr.* 2010;74:428-435
43. Dunkel L. Off-label use of aromatase inhibitors to promote taller stature: is it safe. *Horm Res Paediatr.* 2010;74:436-437
44. Kaplowitz PB. Diagnostic value of testosterone therapy in boys with delayed puberty. *Am J Dis Child.* 1989;143:116-120
45. Kelly BP, Paterson WF, Donaldson MD. Final height outcome and value of height prediction in boys with constitutional delay in growth and adolescence treated with intramuscular testosterone 125 mg per month for 3 months. *Clin Endocrinol.* 2003;58:267-272
46. Lampit M, Hochberg Z. Androgen therapy in constitutional delay of growth. *Horm Res.* 2003;59:270-275
47. Groth KA, Skakkebaek A, Host C, et al. Clinical review: Klinefelter syndrome—a clinical update. *J Clin Endocrinol Metab.* 2013;98:20-30
48. Villanueva C, Argente J. Pathology or normal variant: what constitutes a delay in puberty? *Horm Res Paediatr.* 2014;82:213-221
49. Marcos S, Sarfati J, Leroy C, et al. The prevalence of CHD7 missense versus truncating mutations is higher in patients with Kallmann syndrome than in typical CHARGE patients. *J Clin Endocrinol Metab.* 2014;99:E2138-E2143
50. Rogol AD, Swerdloff RS, Reiter EO, et al. A multicenter, open-label, observational study of testosterone gel (1%) in the treatment of adolescent boys with Klinefelter syndrome or anorchia. *J Adolesc Health.* 2014;54:20-25
51. Mehta A, Clearman T, Paduch DA. Safety and efficacy of testosterone replacement therapy in adolescents with Klinefelter syndrome. *J Urol.* 2014;191(5 Suppl):1527-1531
52. Neely EK, Fechner PY, Rosenfeld RG. Turner syndrome. In: Lifshitz F, ed. *Pediatric Endocrinology.* Volume 2. 5th ed. New York: Informa Healthcare; 2009:305-324
53. Gonzalez L, Witchel SF. The patient with Turner syndrome: puberty and medical management concerns. *Fertil Steril.* 2012;98:780-786
54. Miller KK. Endocrine dysregulation in anorexia nervosa update. *J Clin Endocrinol Metab.* 2011;96:2939-2949

55. Misra M, Klibanski A. Neuroendocrine consequences of anorexia nervosa in adolescents. *Endocr Dev.* 2010;17:197-214
56. Bomba M, Corbetta F, Bonini L, et al. Psychopathological traits of adolescents with functional hypothalamic amenorrhea: a comparison with anorexia nervosa. *Eat Weight Disord.* 2014;19:41-48
57. Meczekalski B, Katulski K, Czyzyk A, et al. Functional hypothalamic amenorrhea and its influence on women's health. *J Endocrinol Invest.* 2014 [Epub ahead of publication]
58. Torres-Santiago L, Mericq V, Taboada M, et al. Metabolic effects of oral versus transdermal 17beta-estradiol (E(2)): a randomized clinical trial in girls with Turner syndrome. *J Clin Endocrinol Metab.* 2013;98:2716-2724
59. Pitts S, Blood E, Divasta A, et al. Percentage body fat by dual-energy X-ray absorptiometry is associated with menstrual recovery in adolescents with anorexia nervosa. *J Adolesc Health.* 2014;54:739-741
60. Dempfle A, Herpertz-Dahlmann B, Timmesfeld N, et al. Predictors of the resumption of menses in adolescent anorexia nervosa. *BMC Psychiatry.* 2013;13:308
61. Misra M, Katzman D, Miller KK, et al. Physiologic estrogen replacement increases bone density in adolescent girls with anorexia nervosa. *J Bone Miner Res.* 2011;26:2430-2438
62. Hebebrand J, Albayrak O. Leptin treatment of patients with anorexia nervosa? The urgent need for initiation of clinical studies. *Eur Child Adolesc Psychiatry.* 2012;21:63-66

Bone Health in Adolescence

Dennis E. Carey, MD[a]; Neville H. Golden, MD[b]

[a]*Division of Pediatric Endocrinology, Cohen Children's Medical Center of New York, Associate Professor of Pediatrics, Hofstra–North Shore LIJ School of Medicine, New Hyde Park, New York;* [b]*Chief, Division of Adolescent Medicine, The Marion and Mary Elizabeth Kendrick Professor of Pediatrics, Stanford University School of Medicine, Palo Alto, California*

As the understanding of osteoporosis in adults expands, there is an increasing awareness that the antecedents of adult osteoporosis exist in children and adolescents, as do various forms of childhood bone disease and osteoporosis. Osteoporosis in children and adolescents can be associated with fractures and significant morbidity. In childhood, the rate of fractures increases with increasing age, with a peak incidence during the pubertal growth spurt. It has been suggested that the increase in fractures is the result of rapid growth outpacing the increase in bone strength. Children and adolescents who sustain fractures, especially those who sustain fractures repeatedly, may have an underlying bone disorder. It is not unexpected for children and adolescents to sustain fractures from trauma as a result of sports injuries or accidents. It is the nontraumatic or so-called *fragility fractures* in childhood and adolescence that are pathologic and suggestive of an underlying disorder that may be associated with osteoporosis in later life. Fractures of the forearm are common in children.[1] Fractures at other sites, especially the femur and vertebrae, are rare.[2] Occurrence at the latter sites are of particular concern, especially if trauma is relatively minor. There is an increasing awareness of vertebral fractures being part of underlying bone pathology in children and adolescents with chronic diseases.[3] It is well within the purview of those caring for adolescents not only to diagnose and treat osteoporosis but also to work toward prevention of osteoporosis in later life by addressing issues related to bone development in the early stages of life.

BONE DEVELOPMENT

Strategies for prevention and treatment of osteoporosis are based on an understanding of normal bone physiology and development. The skeleton both provides a source of calcium for bodily functions and acts as a supportive superstructure. The skeleton is a dynamic organ that grows rapidly in early life and continues to remodel itself after full linear growth has been achieved. The accumulation of calcium, as well as phosphorus, into the fetal skeleton begins during the third trimester, and the mineral content of bone increases more than 40-fold from birth until adulthood.

There are 2 main types of bones: flat bones, such as the skull, mandible and scapula; and long bones, such as the femur, tibia, and humerus. Flat bones develop by membranous bone formation; long bones develop by a combination of endochondral bone formation and membranous bone formation. Long bones consist of a central tube, termed the diaphysis, which widens at both ends to form the metaphyses, the regions below the growth plate, and the epiphyses, the regions above the growth plate. The diaphysis is composed primarily of cortical bone, whereas the metaphyses and epiphyses contain trabecular (cancellous) bone surrounded by a shell of cortical bone. Approximately 80% of the skeleton is cortical bone and 20% is trabecular bone.

Pluripotential precursor cells can differentiate into either bone-forming cells (osteoblasts) or cartilage-forming cells (chondrocytes). Differentiation into osteoblasts occurs in areas of membranous ossification, including the subperiosteal bone-forming layer of the long bones. Differentiation into chondrocytes occurs in the remaining skeleton at sites in which the cartilage will develop into future bone by the process of endochondral ossification. The formed skeleton undergoes a continuous process of renewal that is lifelong. Bone remodeling has 4 phases: activation, resorption, reversal, and formation (Figure 1). Activation involves transformation of a previously quiescent bone surface into a remodeling surface. Preosteoclasts create bone-resorbing compartments next to the organic matrix. Enzymes activated in the acidic microenvironment dissolve and digest the mineral and organic phases of the matrix, producing resorption cavi-

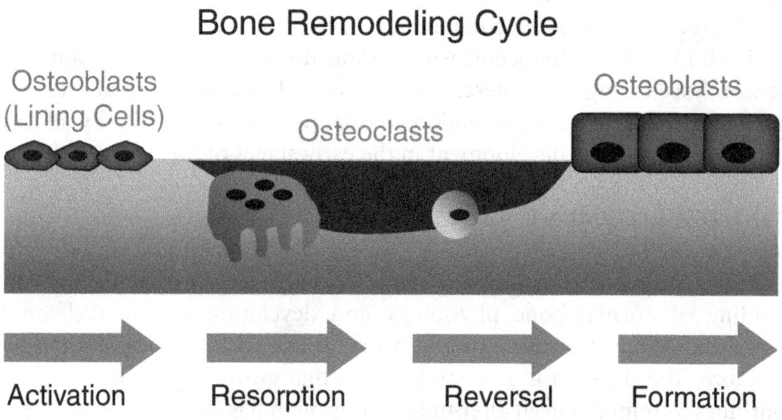

Fig 1. Bone remodeling cycle. (From Carey DE, Golden NH. Bone health and disorders. In: Fisher MM, Alderman EM, Kreipe RE, Rosenfeld WD, eds. *Textbook of Adolescent Health Care*. Elk Grove Village, IL: American Academy of Pediatrics; 2011: 728-742.)

ties, or lacunae, on the surface of cancellous bone and cylindrical tunnels within the cortex. The resorption phase ends with osteoclast apoptosis and is followed by reversal. During reversal, local signaling leads to recruitment of bone-forming cells. The coupled process is completed when osteoblasts lead to synthesis of a new matrix and regulate its mineralization. A third cell type, the osteocyte, has been underappreciated for its role in bone metabolism. In the adult skeleton, osteocytes make up 90% to 95% of all bone cells, compared to 4% to 5% osteoblasts and 1% to 2% osteoclasts.[4] Osteocytes are regularly dispersed throughout the mineralized matrix, connected to each other, the bone marrow, and cells on the bone surface through dendritic processes. Osteocytes function as a network of sensory cells, mediating the effects of mechanical loading and thus regulating bone resorption and formation. Osteocytes have been demonstrated to secrete the receptor activator of nuclear-factor-κB ligand (Rank-L), sclerostin, and macrophage–colony-stimulating factor (M-CSF), in addition to other cytokines.[5]

Osteoblast and osteoclast formation, activation, and activity all are regulated by local cytokines and systemic hormones, such as parathyroid hormone (PTH), 1,25-dihydroxyvitamin D [1,25(OH)$_2$D], and calcitonin. Calcitonin primarily inhibits the osteoclastic pathway. PTH and 1,25(OH)$_2$D influence both the osteoblastic and osteoclastic pathways. Fundamental to an understanding of postmenopausal osteoporosis is an understanding of how loss of estrogen leads to increased osteoclastic activity. Decreased serum estrogen levels lead to increased production of osteoclastic cytokines, such as interleukin-1, interleukin-6, and tumor necrosis factor (TNF) by circulating macrophages. These molecules enhance bone resorption via a circulating protein, RANK-L, which activates its receptor RANK and promotes osteoclast formation, activation, and activity. A circulating antiosteoclastogenic factor, osteoprotegerin (OPG), competes with RANK-L for the RANK receptor, thus modulating the RANK-L effect. The WNT signaling pathway stimulates differentiation toward the osteoblast lineage and plays an essential role in bone formation. Sclerostin is an osteocyte-derived WNT pathway antagonist.[4]

Bone Mass Acquisition

Peak bone mass is a concept that promotes the idea that bone mass reaches a maximum, after which it decreases. Achievement of an adequate peak bone mass during adolescence is a prerequisite for bone health in adulthood. Osteoporosis in adulthood is the result of either failure to achieve an adequate peak bone mass, rapid loss of bone, or both (Figure 2). Before peak bone mass is achieved, bone formation exceeds bone resorption, resulting in net acquisition. Once peak bone mass is accomplished, bone resorption outpaces bone formation and bone mass declines. If a low bone mass threshold is reached, osteoporosis is considered to be present. Implicit in the concept of peak bone mass is

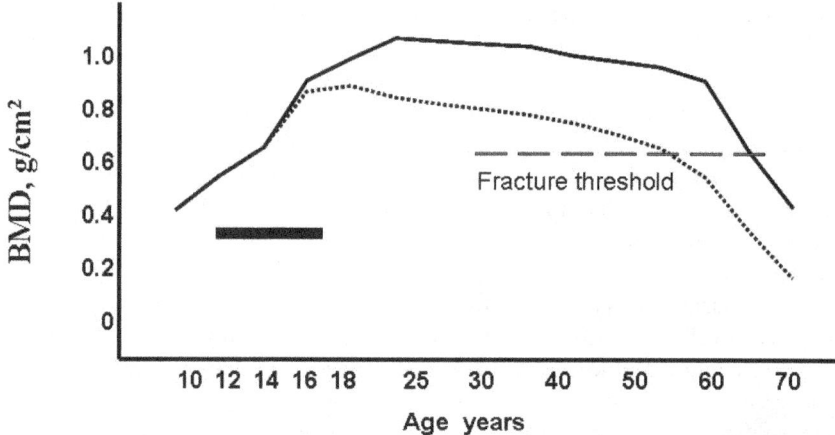

Fig 2. Impact of a disease such as anorexia nervosa *(solid bar)* on achievement of peak bone mass. Rather than following the normal expected pattern *(solid line)*, the patient *(short dashed line)* does not achieve peak bone mass and reaches the fracture threshold *(long dashed line)* much earlier. (From Golden NH. Osteopenia and osteoporosis in anorexia nervosa. *Adolesc Med State Art Rev.* 2003;14(1):98-108.)

that osteoporosis, a disease of adulthood, has its antecedents in childhood and adolescence, and therefore an understanding of the determinants of bone accumulation is an important facet in the prevention of osteoporosis.

The increase in bone mass that occurs during childhood and puberty results from a combination of growth of bone at the endplates (endochondral bone formation) and of change in bone shape (modeling and remodeling). These processes occur at primary and secondary sites of bone formation. Between 40% and 60% of peak bone mass is acquired during adolescence, and 25% of peak bone mass may be acquired during the 2-year period around peak height velocity.[6] Up to 90% of net peak bone mass is acquired by age 18, and net gain in bone mass during young adulthood may not be significant.[7] The density of trabecular bone is more strongly influenced than cortical bone by the hormonal factors associated with sexual development. It is likely that the increase in pubertal bone mass accumulation is related to sex steroids and sex steroid–induced increases in growth hormone and insulinlike growth factor (IGF)-1.

ASSESSMENT OF BONE HEALTH IN ADOLESCENTS

Dual-Energy X-Ray Absorptiometry

The preferred method of assessing bone mass in clinical practice is dual-energy X-ray absorptiometry (DXA) because of its availability, speed, precision, low cost, and low dose of radiation (5-6 microSievert [μSv] for the lumbar spine, hip, and total body, less than the radiation exposure of a transcontinental flight and one-tenth that of a standard chest radiograph).[8] The usual sites measured are the posteroanterior lumbar spine (L1-L4), hip (femoral neck and total hip), and total body. In younger children, the hip is not a reliable site for measurement of bone mineral density (BMD) because of variability in skeletal development in this age group, which can lead to difficulties in positioning that result in reduced precision of measurements at this site. Measurements of the hip can be reliably assessed starting in mid to late adolescence. For total body measurements in children, the head represents a sizeable portion of the skeleton but does not respond to physical activity or other interventions that increase BMD. Therefore, the total body, not including the head, is the preferred site to scan.[9] Scanning time of the spine is less than 1 minute and of the total body is approximately 5 minutes. In addition to measurement of BMD, the total body scan can also assess body composition (fat mass, lean body mass, and percent body fat).

Bone mass measured by DXA is reported as bone mineral content (BMC) or BMD. Dual-energy X-ray absorptiometry measures the difference in absorption of high-energy and low-energy X-rays as they pass through the body. High-density X-rays penetrate both soft tissue and bone, whereas low-energy X-rays can only penetrate soft tissue. The difference in absorption of high-energy and low-energy X-rays gives a measure of BMC. The BMD is then calculated from BMC by dividing BMC by the projected area in the coronal plane of the region scanned. This value gives a measure of 2-dimensional areal BMD (aBMD, expressed as g/cm^2). Robust pediatric reference databases are now available for children older than 5 years and are included with the software of the major DXA manufacturers.[9-13]

However, measurement of aBMD does have some limitations, especially in children and adolescents. In contrast to measurement of true volumetric density (vBMD, expressed as g/cm^3), measurement of aBMD can underestimate true volumetric density in small children and adolescents and overestimate it in larger children and adolescents. Therefore, a correction should be made that adjusts for size, either by estimating bone mineral apparent density (BMAD) or by adjusting for the height Z-score, particularly in those with short stature or growth delay.[9] Based on data in postmenopausal women, a 1 standard deviation (SD) reduction in aBMD compared to young adult norms (T-score $<$ -1.0) is associated with a 2-fold increase in fracture risk. In children and adolescents, Z-scores (number of SD below the age-matched mean) should be used instead of T-scores. A low BMD T-score in a 14-year-old adolescent who has not yet achieved peak bone mass may be perfectly normal compared with age-matched controls.

Unlike studies in adults in whom a T-score in the osteoporotic range is associated with an increased fracture rate, in children and adolescents there is no specific Z-score below which fractures are more likely to occur. However, there is a growing body of evidence demonstrating an association between low aBMD and increased fracture risk.[14-16] The International Society for Clinical Densitometry (ISCD) recommends that in patients younger than 20 years, the term *osteopenia* should no longer be used and the term *osteoporosis* should not be based on bone densitometry results alone. The ISCD defines low BMD for chronologic age as an age, sex, and body size-adjusted BMD Z-score of -2 or less.[9,17] The ISCD further recommends that in those younger than 20 years, the diagnosis of "osteoporosis" requires *both* a low BMD or BMC for age (Z-score ≤ -2) *plus* a clinically significant fracture history, defined as 2 or more long bone fractures by age 10 years, or 3 or more fractures at any age up to age 19 years, or a vertebral compression fracture.[17] Osteoporosis can also be considered to be present if there is a vertebral fracture even if BMD is normal. Fractures of digits or toes are not included in the definition of clinically significant fractures.[18] Similarly, a child or adolescent with low BMD for chronologic age but without a clinically significant fracture history does not meet criteria for osteoporosis.

Who should undergo DXA? Per the 2013 ISCD statement, the main purpose of performing a bone density study is to "identify children and adolescents who may benefit from intervention to decrease elevated risk of a clinically significant fracture." In addition, DXA studies may be performed during follow-up of an intervention but not more frequently than every 6 to 12 months. The decision to perform a DXA study should be based on clinical judgment and could be considered for adolescents with a single long bone fracture after minimal trauma, recurrent fractures, bone pain, or osteopenia on radiograph, especially if there is a family history of osteoporosis. Some authorities recommend performing DXA as a baseline in adolescents with conditions associated with reduced bone mass (see section on Conditions Associated with Low Bone Mass).

Quantitative Computed Tomography

Quantitative computed tomography (QCT) uses a clinical whole-body CT scanner equipped with special software to measure true volumetric BMD. Bone size and geometry also can be assessed. However, QCT machines are costly, are not readily available, and use high doses of radiation (30-7000 μSv).[19]

Newer modalities such as peripheral QCT (pQCT) can measure volumetric BMD of the appendicular skeleton with much lower doses of radiation (<3 μSv). The pQCT machines are smaller, more mobile than clinical whole-body scanners, and can also measure cortical thickness, cortical density, and trabecular density from cross-sectional images generated. Usual sites measured are the nondominant distal tibia and distal radius. High-resolution pQCT (HR-pQCT) measures small regions of the distal tibia and radius and can evaluate bone microstructure as well as bone strength. Use of HR-pQCT, although still limited to research, shows great promise for clinical use and has the potential to better predict fracture risk than DXA. Unfortunately, HR-pQCT machines are found in only a few select bone research centers.

Radiography

Standard skeletal radiographs generally are unreliable for assessment of bone density because significantly reduced BMD may be present in bones that appear normal by radiography. On the other hand, radiographs of the spine may have significant utility to determine the extent of osteoporosis leading to frank vertebral fractures (as assessed by Genant score).[20]

Biochemical Markers of Bone Metabolism

Measurement of proteins involved in bone turnover has been used to assess levels of bone formation and bone resorption. Table 1 lists biochemical markers of bone metabolism.

Osteoblasts synthesize a number of proteins, including type I collagen, alkaline phosphatase, and osteocalcin. Alkaline phosphatase is essential for mineralization, but its precise role in this process has still not been elucidated. Alkaline phosphatase levels are much higher in normal children than in adults and are particularly high during the adolescent growth spurt. They are also elevated in rachitic disorders. This enzyme is also found in liver, intestine, spleen, placenta, and bone. Bone-specific alkaline phosphatase can be measured for research, although it is not widely used in clinical practice.

Table 1

Biochemical markers of bone metabolism

Marker	Abbreviation	Sample source
Bone Formation		
Osteocalcin	OC	Serum
Bone-specific alkaline phosphatase	BSAP	Serum
Procollagen type I C-terminal peptide	PICP	Serum
Procollagen type I N-terminal peptide	PINP	Serum
Bone Resorption		
Deoxypyridinoline	DPD	Urine/serum
Pyridinoline	PYD	Urine
Cross-linked N-telopeptide	NTX	Urine/serum
Cross-linked C-telopeptide	CTX	Urine/serum
Type I collagen C-terminal telopeptide	ICTP	Serum

Osteocalcin is considered a marker of bone formation but, because it is incorporated into bone matrix and later released into the circulation during bone resorption, it more properly should be considered a marker of bone turnover. Like alkaline phosphatase, circulating levels of osteocalcin are higher in children than in adults.

Type I collagen is the major collagen of bone and the most abundant product of the osteoblast. Type I collagen is produced as a precursor molecule with carboxy-terminal and amino-terminal propeptides, which are cleaved before release into the circulation. Assays have been developed to measure both the C-terminal propeptide of collagen (PICT) and the N-terminal propeptide of collagen (PINP). As with alkaline phosphatase and osteocalcin, levels of type I collagen in serum are much greater in growing children than in adults. However, because type I collagen is not exclusive to bone, circulating levels represent total type I collagen synthesis from all tissues, including skin.

Collagen degradation products can be measured as biochemical markers of bone resorption. Collagen molecules form fibrils that are joined by covalent cross-links. These consist of hydroxylsyl-pyridinolines (PYDs) and lysyl-pyridinolines (DPDs). Upon bone breakdown by osteoclasts, by-products are released into the circulation and both free and peptide-bound PYD and DPD can be measured in urine. The amino-terminal (NTX) and the carboxy-terminal (CTX) telopeptides of collagen cross-links can be measured in urine as well as in blood.

The clinical use of biochemical markers has expanded from the research field, mainly in the care of adults with osteoporosis. Measurement of bone markers before and during treatment is being increasingly used to monitor effectiveness of antiresorptive therapy. Failure to exhibit the expected reduction in bone resorptive markers can be taken to indicate therapeutic failure, improper administration, or poor adherence. Use of biochemical markers in children has been primarily in follow-up care of children treated for osteogenesis imperfecta (OI).

FACTORS THAT AFFECT BONE MASS

Factors affecting bone mass are listed in Table 2. Genetic factors play an important role, with 70% to 80% of the variability in peak bone mass accounted for by heredity.[21-23] A fundamental need is the ability to identify those at risk for osteoporosis and fragility fractures so that preventive measures can be initiated. Attainment of peak bone mass and early treatment of developing bone loss both are critical. Osteoporosis runs in families. Daughters of women with osteoporosis have reduced bone mass, and women whose mothers have experienced a hip fracture exhibit a 2-fold increase in risk of hip fracture compared to controls.[24] However, the genotype-phenotype relationship is complex. There likely are many "osteoporosis genes," with an ever-expanding candidate list, such as vita-

Table 2
Factors influencing bone mass

Nonmodifiable
  Gender
  Ethnicity
  Heredity
Modifiable
  Diet: calcium, vitamin D
  Body type: body weight, body mass index
  Hormonal status: estrogen, testosterone, growth hormone, cortisol
  Exercise
  Lifestyle choices: smoking, alcohol

min D receptor gene, calcium-sensing receptor gene, TNF ligand superfamily members, *WNT10B*, collagen 1α1 gene, transforming growth factor (TGF)-β genes, and others, being investigated.

Osteoporosis and fragility fractures occur much more frequently in women than in men. For example, there is a 4- to 8-fold higher incidence of vertebral fractures in women. The cross-sectional area of a vertebral body is 11% smaller in prepubertal girls compared to boys, and this gender discrepancy widens to 25% by the time of skeletal maturity. Therefore, the higher fracture rate in women may be more dependent on vertebral area than actual BMD.[25] Race is a factor determining bone mass. Blacks suffer fewer fractures than whites and other racial groups. Larger bone size and greater volumetric bone density in blacks likely accounts for this difference.[26] Differences in bone density between whites, Hispanics, and Asian children are eliminated when corrected for height and weight.[7]

Calcium is the principal cation of bone mineral, and the skeleton constitutes a reserve of calcium for bodily functions. Sustained withdrawal from this reserve can lead to decreases in bone mass and poses a threat to skeletal health. Low calcium intake early in life can predispose to fragile bones in childhood and adolescence and lead to osteoporosis later in life. Calcium intake is positively correlated with bone mass at all ages, and calcium supplementation has been shown to increase BMD in healthy adolescents.[27] Adequate vitamin D intake is essential for utilization of calcium. Excessive intake of carbonated beverages has been shown to be associated with fractures in athletic adolescent girls.[28]

Hormonal status plays an important role in maintaining bone mass. Testosterone, IGF-1, and growth hormone all promote bone formation, whereas hypoestrogenemia and cortisol excess increase bone resorption, leading to a reduction in net bone mass. Body weight is a major determinant of BMD, both in healthy adolescents and in those with anorexia nervosa (AN). Weight restoration in girls with AN is associated with improvement in BMD.[29]

Weight-bearing exercise is protective of BMD. Immobilization is associated with reduced BMD. Smoking and alcohol are associated with reduced BMD.

CONDITIONS ASSOCIATED WITH LOW BONE MASS

Conditions associated with low bone mass are either primary or secondary. A list of those conditions is given in Table 3.

Osteogenesis Imperfecta

Osteogenesis imperfecta is a somewhat rare (incidence 1:10,000) osteoporotic disorder of childhood. In the past it had been referred to as "brittle bone disease." OI is most often an autosomal dominant genetic disorder of type I collagen in connective tissue, with a wide range of clinical severity dependent on the specific type. Types I to IV represent disorders characterized in the original clinical classification of Sillence.[30] Type II OI, the most severe form, usually is lethal in the perinatal period, and fractures occur in utero. Types III and IV OI are intermediate in severity. Patients with type III OI exhibit a very high number of fractures over their lifetime and suffer with severe disability and extreme short stature. Patients with type IV tend to have less disability, a lesser degree of short stature, and a decreasing rate of fractures after puberty. Type I is the mildest form of OI, and the diagnosis is often missed in childhood. It presents as early-onset adult osteoporosis with normal stature and little or no deformity. It should be suspected in patients with a history of fractures and low bone density who also have blue sclerae, easy bruising, or hearing loss. Types V to XI OI are very rare, and all but type V are autosomal recessive. Approximately 95% of the mutations in individuals with OI are found in the 2 type I collagen genes: *COL1A1* and *COL1A2*; hence, genomic sequencing of *COL1A1* and *COL1A2*

Table 3
Low bone mass in adolescents

Primary
  Osteogenesis imperfecta
  Idiopathic juvenile osteoporosis
Secondary
  Anorexia nervosa
  Female athlete triad
  Contraceptive use
  Glucocorticoid excess
  Inflammatory bowel disease
  Celiac disease
  Cystic fibrosis
  Rheumatologic conditions
  Malignancy
  Endocrine disorders
  Cerebral palsy/immobilization

is the screening test of choice. If a mutation is not found, gene sequencing for type V or autosomal recessive forms may be pursued. Using cultured dermal fibroblasts for OI screening has been replaced, for the most part, by gene sequencing.[31]

Idiopathic Juvenile Osteoporosis

Idiopathic juvenile osteoporosis (IJO) is another primary form of osteoporosis of childhood. It usually presents in prepubertal boys and girls, typically between 8 and 12 years of age, and it resolves spontaneously postpubertally. The classic form of IJO was described by Dent and Friedman in 1965.[32] In a recent review of the topic, Rauch and Bishop[33] suggested that children with unexplained low bone mass and fractures who do not fit the classic description should still be considered to have "IJO in the wider sense" or what one might call nonclassic IJO. In their experience, IJO is approximately 10-fold less common than OI. They further distinguished IJO from children in late prepuberty and early puberty who exhibited low bone mass and fractures, mainly of the forearm, whom they considered healthy but undergoing "an adaptational bone problem." They proposed that "IJO should only be diagnosed when vertebral compression fractures are present (with or without extremity fractures)."

Classic IJO is characterized by metaphyseal and vertebral compression fractures with collapsed or biconcave vertebrae on lateral spine films and radiolucent areas in the metaphyses of long bones, termed *neo-osseous osteoporosis*. The latter represents new osteoporotic bone with callus formation. Unlike the thin long bones of OI, the long bones of patients with IJO have a normal diameter and cortical width. Bone histomorphometric studies show that in IJO there is a disturbance of bone formation mainly in trabecular bone and possibly in the cortical surface adjacent to the marrow cavity. There is no biochemical marker specific for IJO.

Anorexia Nervosa and Eating Disorders

Eating disorders constitute the third most common chronic disease of adolescence after obesity and asthma. Both girls and boys with AN have reduced BMD for age at multiple sites.[29,34-39] The lumbar spine is affected more than the appendicular skeleton because of the greater proportion of metabolically active trabecular bone in the spinal vertebrae. Studies using biochemical markers of bone metabolism have demonstrated reduced bone formation as well as increased bone resorption, and an episode of AN during adolescence can interfere with peak bone mass acquisition. Cross-sectional studies from the United States and Europe have demonstrated a 2- to 3-fold increased incidence of fractures in those who previously had AN.[40,41] In adult patients with AN, the annual rate of bone loss is approximately 2.5%.[42] Contributing factors to low BMD in AN include low body weight, dietary deficiencies of protein, calcium, and vitamin D, hypogonadism, hypercortisolemia, and low IGF-1 levels. Adolescents with bulimia nervosa may also have low BMD if they were previously of low weight or amenorrheic.[43] The effect of AN on achievement of peak bone mass and its implications in later life are illustrated in Figure 2.

Weight restoration with spontaneous resumption of menses in girls is associated with some increases in BMD, but levels may not return to normal.[20,36,40,44] Weight gain without resumption of menses is not associated with significant increases in BMD.[45] Although calcium and vitamin D supplementation increase BMD in healthy adolescents, no randomized controlled trials have been conducted in adolescents with AN. Oral contraceptives do not increase BMD in this condition.[30,46,47] One study found that transdermal physiologic doses of estrogen increased BMD compared to controls.[48] Current recommendations for low BMD in AN include weight restoration with resumption of spontaneous menses in girls, optimal calcium and vitamin D intake, and treatment of vitamin D deficiency.

Female Athlete Triad

Female athletes who are amenorrheic may have reduced BMD and can be at increased risk for development of stress fractures. The female athlete triad refers to 3 interrelated conditions found in female athletes: reduced energy availability (previously called *disordered eating*), menstrual dysfunction (previously called *amenorrhea*), and low BMD for age (previously called *osteoporosis*). The revised terminology reflects the fact that each of the components of the triad exists as a spectrum ranging from optimal health to disease.[49] The cause of the triad is an imbalance of energy intake and energy output, resulting in an energy deficit. This imbalance may be intentional or unintentional. In some instances the athlete may have an underlying eating disorder or disordered eating, but in other cases the energy deficit may result from a lack of knowledge about the increased energy requirements for the sport. The female athlete triad is more prevalent in elite athletes and in those who participate in individual sports that emphasize a lean appearance or low body weight, but it can occur in recreational athletes and in participants of all sports.[50] Although the prevalence of all 3 components of the triad in high school athletes is only about 1%, the prevalence of individual components of the triad is approximately 20%.[51] As the number of triad-related risk factors increases so does the risk of bone stress injuries in adolescent and young adult female athletes.[52]

Contraceptive Use

Depo-Provera
Depot medroxyprogesterone acetate (Depo-Provera [DMPA]) is a very effective long-acting injectable contraceptive that has been associated with reduced BMD in adolescent girls.[53] Reduced bone mass is thought to occur as result of hypo-

thalamic suppression after prolonged use. However, the reduction in BMD is rapidly reversible after discontinuation of the medication.[54] The Society for Adolescent Health and Medicine (SAHM) recommends continuing to prescribe DMPA to adolescent girls needing contraception, but it also recommends providing an explanation of the risks and benefits.[55] The American College of Obstetricians and Gynecologists further states that concerns about the effects of DMPA on BMD should neither prevent practitioners from prescribing it nor limit its use to 2 consecutive years.[56]

Oral Contraceptives
Low-dose oral contraceptives containing less than 30 μg of ethinyl estradiol may interfere with peak bone mass acquisition in adolescent girls compared with oral contraceptives containing 30 μg or more of ethinyl estradiol.[57,58] Despite a possible reduction in BMD, a recent Cochrane review found no association between oral contraceptive use and increased fracture risk.[59]

Glucocorticoid-Induced Osteoporosis

Pharmacologic doses of glucocorticoids are widely used in pediatric patients, especially for the treatment of inflammatory disorders. Chronic glucocorticoid therapy probably is the most common cause of osteoporosis in children.[60] At high doses, glucocorticoids stimulate osteoclastic activity, which is followed by a decrease in bone formation by suppression of osteoblastic activity and promotion of apoptosis in osteoblasts and osteocytes.[61-63] The negative effect of glucocorticoids on bone is mainly through inhibition of bone formation, with the increase in bone resorption being a transient phenomenon. Indirect negative effects occur through inhibition of growth factors, sex steroids, calcium absorption, and decreased "mechanical strain" on bone from weakened muscle.[64] Glucocorticoids increase the risk of bone fractures throughout the skeleton, but especially in the spine and ribs. A meta-analysis in adults treated with the equivalent of 5 mg or more per day of prednisolone was associated with significant decreases in BMD and an increased fracture risk within 3 to 6 months of starting therapy.[65] The increased risk for fractures was independent of age and underlying disorder. There seems to be an "at-risk population," as BMD is not lowered as much in some chronically treated patients as it is in others, and it has been postulated that genetic variations in the glucocorticoid receptor account for this difference.[66] Whether or not an individual will have fractures as a result of glucocorticoid therapy depends on several factors, in addition to possible variations in the glucocorticoid receptor. These include the pretherapy BMD, the disease for which the glucocorticoid is being used, glucocorticoid dose, and length of treatment. A lower starting BMD, higher dose, longer administration, and more severe underlying disorder would be expected to be accompanied by a higher fracture risk. A relatively short course of glucocorticoid therapy leading to bone loss is likely to be readily reversible upon discontinuation, whereas a longer course may reduce bone mass to a point at which recovery is not likely even after cessation of therapy. Children and adolescents are more likely than adults to recover from glucocorticoid-induced osteoporosis, but glucocorticoid therapy possibly could prevent achievement of peak bone mass. Obtaining vertebral radiographs should be considered in any chronically ill child on glucocorticoid therapy for 6 months or longer.

Osteonecrosis (avascular necrosis), especially in the knee or hip, is being increasingly reported in children treated for acute lymphocytic leukemia (ALL) and non-Hodgkin lymphoma with glucocorticoids. The risk is greater with higher dosing or longer treatment, but the condition can occur with a low dose or after short-term exposure. Routine imaging studies should be considered.[60]

Chronic Childhood Illness

A number of chronic illnesses of childhood and adolescence, such as juvenile idiopathic arthritis (JIA), inflammatory bowel disease (IBD), celiac disease, cystic fibrosis (CF), and childhood cancer may predispose to low BMD, either because of the underlying disorder or because of treatment. Whether disease-induced low BMD in such circumstance leads to osteoporosis in adulthood remains unclear. Rationales for intervention with bone-specific therapy have become clearer in recent years, as discussed here.

Inflammatory Bowel Disease
Low BMD is reported to be common in IBD.[67] Decreased BMD may occur in IBD secondary to malnutrition, nutrient malabsorption, decreased activity, delayed puberty, inflammation, and glucocorticoid therapy. Population studies in adults with either Crohn disease or ulcerative colitis suggest that the risk of fractures is not elevated relative to age- and sex-matched controls in the absence of glucocorticoid therapy.[68,69] There are no studies on the relationship between fractures and BMD in children with IBD, but one might expect a lack of an association, paralleling the adult data. On the other hand, there are reports of silent vertebral fractures in adults with IBD possibly not related to glucocorticoids.[70]

Celiac Disease
Celiac disease is an autoimmune malabsorptive disorder of the gastrointestinal tract. The prevalence of celiac disease in populations of European ancestry in North America is reported to be approximately 1%.[71] Bone disease in celiac disease patients has been reported for more than 70 years.[72-74] The mechanisms underlying low bone density in adult celiac disease are secondary hyperparathyroidism and osteomalacia as a result of calcium and vitamin D malabsorption. This does not seem to be the case in children. Other mechanisms, primarily immunologic and inflammatory changes, may also contribute to bone mass reduction. At the time of presentation, approximately one-third of adults with celiac disease have osteoporosis, one-third have osteopenia, and one-third have normal BMD.[75,76] In children, low bone density has been reported at the time of

presentation; Turner et al[77] reported that 16% of children with newly diagnosed celiac disease have a lumbar spine BMD Z-score of -2 SD or less. A Position Statement of the Canadian Gastroenterological Association concluded that adults with celiac disease have a significant risk of fractures.[78] Although data regarding fractures in the pediatric and adolescent population are limited, a Swedish national registry found 6 hip fractures per 100,000 patient-years for children with celiac disease compared to 2 per 100,000 patient-years among the reference population.[79] It is important to note that children with celiac disease who have an abnormal BMD at the time of diagnosis normalize their BMD status after initiation of a gluten-free diet.[78] Hence, therapy is directed primarily at the underlying disease, with the Canadian Gastroenterological Association stating that there is no indication for performing a BMD test in pediatric patients with celiac disease if they adhere to the dietary therapy.[78] The International Society for Clinical Densitometry does not include celiac disease as an indication to perform a DXA scan in children and adolescents.[80]

Cystic Fibrosis

Low BMD and fractures occur in both pediatric/adolescent and adult patients with CF,[81] and the term CF-related bone disease (CF-RBD) has been coined to describe this condition.[82,83] Although traditional factors such as nutritional deficiencies, lack of exercise, hypogonadism, and various treatments have been considered contributory to CF-RBD, recent evidence supports a hypothesis that the inflammatory response to chronic pulmonary infection plays a significant role in the pathophysiology.[84,85] The degree of osteoporosis correlates with the degree of disease severity. Papaioannou et al[86] found approximately 20% of an adult cohort with CF to have 1 or more vertebral fractures. Vertebral fractures not only accelerate the decline in lung function but also are a contraindication to lung transplant.[84,85] In 1 study, treatment with human growth hormone for 1 year was shown to increase total-body BMC in poorly growing children with CF.[87] It remains to be determined whether similar changes in site-specific BMD occur and whether increases are sustained and are not simply a result of increased bone growth.

Rheumatologic Conditions

Both low BMD and localized bone loss are seen in rheumatologic conditions. Poor functional state, leading to decreased activity, and therapeutic interventions, especially with glucocorticoids, contribute to the decrease in BMD. Low BMD is influenced by local and systemic cytokines that stimulate and support osteoclastic activity.[88,89] In children with JIA, bone formation is also likely affected.[65] Patients with JIA often have low BMD before initiation of glucocorticoid therapy. One study found that 30% of mildly to moderately ill prepubertal patients had low BMD.[90] Although fractures of the long bones occur in children with rheumatic diseases, asymptomatic vertebral compression fractures have also been increasingly recognized as a cause of morbidity, at times being present before glucocorticoid use.[91,92] As part of the Canadian STOPP consortium,

LeBlanc et al[93] studied 136 children with rheumatic diseases and found 13% had sustained an incident vertebral fracture within 3 years after the start of glucocorticoid therapy. Cumulative dose, average daily dose, and recent average daily dose all were significant risk factors.

Childhood Malignancy

Osteoporosis and fragility fractures are part of the sequelae of childhood cancer and survival. Fractures have been reported in 18% to 25% of children with acute lymphoblastic leukemia (ALL)[94] and occur in other forms of childhood cancer, including lymphoma and solid tumors. Fractures can occur at any time during and after treatment. Decreased BMD occurs as a result of multiple factors, including radiotherapy, cytotoxic agents, glucocorticoids, decreased activity, impaired nutrition, and hormone deficiencies, especially deficiency of sex steroids. Male sex and white race are factors associated with a higher risk for osteoporosis in survivors of ALL.[95] Mostoufi-Moab et al[96] described a prospective longitudinal pQCT study of children and young adults with ALL followed for 1 year after completion of therapy that did not include cranial radiation. Both trabecular and cortical BMD Z-scores improved significantly, with a suggestion that cortical bone density took longer to increase. Interestingly, total glucocorticoid dose, leukemia risk status, and cytotoxic medication were not associated with outcomes in this study.

Endocrine Disorders

Endocrine disorders may result in low BMD. Excess endogenous glucocorticoid secretion, as in Cushing syndrome, can affect the skeleton similarly to exogenous glucocorticoid excess. Thyrotoxicosis, as well as overtreatment with thyroid hormone, can cause low BMD. Growth hormone deficiency slows not only linear growth but also the accretion of bone mineral. There has been a recent move toward considering growth hormone therapy in growth hormone-deficient patients beyond the closure of growth plates for the anticipated augmentation of peak bone mass. Some have recommended growth hormone therapy up to age 25 years in patients with severe growth hormone deficiency (eg, those with postsurgical growth hormone deficiency). Achievement of optimal peak bone mass may be jeopardized by gonadal failure or even late pubertal development. Girls with AN are particularly at risk. In Turner syndrome (TS), an example of congenital hypogonadism, osteoporosis has been described historically. However, Bakalov et al[97] found that women with TS are often misdiagnosed with osteoporosis because their small size is not taken into account when assessing areal BMD. On the other hand, the same group described the finding of lower forearm cortical BMD but similar trabecular BMD when women with TS were compared to women with primary ovarian failure and suggest that this difference is independent of ovarian hormone exposure and probably is related to X-chromosome gene(s) haploinsufficiency.[98] The effect of therapy with estrogen treatment and growth hormone therapy in girls with TS has been reviewed in depth.[99]

Cerebral Palsy

Osteoporosis and fractures seem to be more common in children with cerebral palsy (CP) than in able-bodied children; however, evidence-based information on BMD, fracture risk and interventions is limited by the great variation in subject disabilities and lack of power of reported studies.[100] Mergler et al[101] reviewed the literature in 2009 and concluded that children with CP who were nonambulatory, had previous fractures, had feeding difficulties, or were taking anticonvulsive medications are at high risk for developing a low BMD and should be monitored for low BMD. Henderson et al[102] evaluated bone density in a population-based cohort of children and adolescents with moderate to severe CP and found a BMD Z-score less than -2.0 in the femur in 77% of subjects. The mean Z-score for the femur (-3.1 ± -0.2) was less than the mean Z-score for the spine (-1.8 ± -0.1). Fractures had occurred in 26% of the children who were older than 10 years. In another study by Henderson, the annual incidence in fractures was 4%, compared to a fracture rate of 2.5% in healthy children, a group in which their high activity level is most likely the greatest contributory factor.[103]

Despite our expanding knowledge of these disorders, more research in the development and natural history of diseases associated with diminished BMD is warranted. From a clinical point of view, due consideration should be given to baseline assessment of site-specific BMD by DXA scanning in children and adolescents who develop a chronic illness. Correct interpretation of BMD in chronically ill adolescents with growth failure or bone age delay requires analysis relative to bone age or height age in addition to chronologic age.

MANAGEMENT

Prevention in Healthy Children

Calcium and Vitamin D

The American Academy of Pediatrics (AAP) report "Optimizing Bone Health in Children and Adolescents" affirms the importance of adequate calcium intake during childhood and adolescence for peak bone mass development, emphasizes the importance of the family in achieving adequate calcium intake in adolescents, and suggests that pediatricians periodically assess calcium intake by questionnaire during the growing years.[104] Survey data have indicated that most American children older than 8 years fail to achieve the recommended daily intake of calcium, with only 10% of adolescent girls doing so.[105,106] Barriers to adequate calcium intake include lactose intolerance, a misconception that dairy products are fattening, and excessive intake of soft drinks, fruit drinks, and fruit juices in lieu of milk. In preadolescents and adolescents aged 9 to 18 years, an intake of elemental calcium of 1300 mg/day is recommended. At intakes above this level some believe there is a plateau effect on calcium retention,[107] whereas others do not.[108] Drinking 4 glasses of milk (8 ounce) will provide the recommended calcium intake for adolescents. As a general rule, flavored milks and reduced fat milks contain similar amounts of calcium as regular milk. Yogurt, cheese, and calcium-fortified juices and cereals are other good dietary sources of calcium but need to be ingested in sufficient quantities to meet recommendations. If the recommended level of calcium cannot be achieved through foodstuffs, calcium supplements should be considered.

Vitamin D is a fat-soluble hormone necessary for the absorption and utilization of calcium. It occurs in 2 forms: vitamin D_2 (ergocalciferol), which is plant derived, and vitamin D_3 (cholecalciferol), which is synthesized by animals. Vitamin D is produced in the skin on exposure to ultraviolet radiation. Synthesis depends on latitude, time of day of exposure, and skin pigmentation. Exposure of the arms and legs to a 0.5 minimal erythemal dose of sunlight for 5 to 15 minutes 2 to 3 times per week produces approximately 3000 IU of vitamin D.[109] Maximal synthesis occurs during the hours of 10:00 a.m. to 3:00 p.m. in the spring, summer, and fall, and synthesis is effectively blocked by sunscreen with a sun protection factor greater than 8. Dietary sources of vitamin D are limited but include cod liver oil, fatty fish such as salmon, sardines, and tuna, and some fortified foods. Milk and orange juice both contain approximately 100 IU per 8-ounce serving.

In the skin, vitamin D_3 is synthesized from 7-dehydrocholesterol, binds to vitamin D-binding protein, and is transported to the liver, where it undergoes hydroxylation to form 25-hydroxyvitamin D (25OHD). The 25OHD is then transported to the kidney, where it undergoes a second round of hydroxylation to form $1,25(OH)_2D$, the most active form of vitamin D. The half-life of $1,25(OH)_2D$ is only 4 hours, whereas the half-life of 25OHD is 2 to 3 weeks. Consequently, measurement of serum 25OHD levels, but not $1,25(OH)_2D$ levels, can be used to assess vitamin D stores.[104]

The recommended daily allowance (RDA) for vitamin D has recently been increased to 600 IU/day for children older than 1 year and for adolescents.[104,110] The upper safety limit for adolescents is 4000 IU/day. The Institute of Medicine determined the RDAs based on the dose of vitamin D required to achieve a serum 25OHD level greater than 20 ng/mL (50 nmol/L) in 98% of the population, assuming minimal exposure to sunlight.[110] The AAP and the Pediatric Endocrine Society both define vitamin D deficiency in healthy children and adolescents as a serum 25OHD level less than 20 ng/mL and sufficiency as a level greater than 20 ng/mL.[104,111] In contrast, in an attempt to address the needs of the adult and geriatric population, the Endocrine Society defines sufficiency as a 25OHD level greater than 30 ng/mL (75 nmol/L), insufficiency as a level between 21 and 29 ng/mL, and deficiency as a level less than 20 ng/mL.[112] Controversy remains as to whether there are specific health benefits to a target of 30 ng/mL in healthy children and adolescents. The recommendation regarding the higher "lower limit of normal" was generated from data in geriatric populations in which high PTH levels were noted, suggesting increased vitamin D requirements in that population.[113] However, with regard to bone health in children no such correlation exists. In a large study of middle school children with a wide range of weights there was no correlation of PTH to decreasing 25OHD levels that remained greater than 20 ng/mL.[114]

The AAP does not recommend universal screening of healthy children for vitamin D deficiency with serum 25OHD levels because the benefits of doing so have not been demonstrated. Universal screening would result in large numbers of dark-skinned or obese children being treated, retested, and possibly retreated without any demonstrable benefit to their bone health. On the other hand, the AAP does recommend screening children and adolescents with conditions associated with reduced bone mass and increased fracture risk and treating them if vitamin D is found to be deficient.[104] One must also take into account the significant variability between various 25OHD assays and the relatively large within-laboratory and between-laboratory variability that hinders conclusive assessments of bias and accuracy. Total 25OHD may be underestimated in some assays and within some ranges but may be overestimated in other assays.[115-118]

Optimal absorption and retention of calcium in preteens and adolescents require a vitamin D intake of 600 IU (15 μg) per day.[104] For those with inadequate dairy intake of vitamin D, supplementation up to 600 IU may be considered.

Although there is some controversy regarding the potency of vitamin D_2 versus vitamin D_3, with the suggestion that D_3 is more potent than D_2,[119] Holick et al[120] reported that D_2 is as effective as D_3 in maintaining circulating concentrations of 25OHD.

Exercise and Lifestyle

Weight-bearing activity should be encouraged for all children and adolescents in order to optimize peak bone mass acquisition. The quantity of soda consumed should be limited, and patients should be counseled about the negative effect of smoking on BMD.

In children, a 10-minute, 3 times per week school-based exercise program conducted in 14 schools in Canada was associated with significant increases in BMD in early pubertal girls compared with a control group that did not participate in the program.[121] This exercise program incorporated high-impact jumping activities during regularly scheduled physical education classes. The same group demonstrated that 10 countermovement jumps 3 times per day (total ~3 min/day) in a program called "Bounce at the Bell" enhanced bone mass at the weight-bearing proximal femur in early pubertal children.[122] In college women randomly assigned to a weight-bearing exercise program, a resistance training program, or no exercise, both weight-bearing and resistance training were associated with increases in BMD of the lumbar spine, whereas in the sedentary controls there was no change in BMD.[123]

Prevention in Children and Adolescents with Chronic Illness

Amounts of vitamin D in excess of the preventive amounts for healthy children and adolescents have been recommended for those with chronic illnesses. For example, for children and adolescents with IBD, up to 1600 mg of elemental calcium and 1000 IU of vitamin D have been recommended to prevent development of vitamin D deficiency.[67]

The Cystic Fibrosis Foundation consensus recommends that all individuals with CF older than 10 years be treated with an initial dose of 800 to 2000 IU vitamin D_3 per day.[124] For children with celiac disease, Fouda et al[78] suggested that with careful adherence to a gluten-free diet, additional vitamin D beyond the IOM recommendation of 600 IU/day was not necessary. For patients taking pharmacologic doses of glucocorticoids, Liu et al[60] recommended vitamin D supplementation to a serum total 25 OH D level of 20 ng/mL (50 nmol/L) or ideally to 30 ng/mL (75 nmol/L).

TREATMENT

Vitamin D

Vitamin D deficiency causes rickets in young children and adolescents. Rickets is defined as poor mineralization of bone in a growing child. Once a child ceases to grow, the mineralization defect is termed osteomalacia. Osteoporosis, on the other hand, is defined as a low bone mass, that is, a decrease in the total amount of mineralized bone and microarchitectural deterioration of bone tissue. Vitamin D deficiency is associated with elevated alkaline phosphatase levels (indicating poor mineralization) and compensatory secondary hyperparathyroidism with hypophosphatemia. Reduced BMD also may present concomitantly with rickets or osteomalacia. One longitudinal prospective study of 6712 physically active girls aged 9 to 15 found that vitamin D status and not dietary calcium intake predicted future fracture risk during 7 years of follow-up.[125]

Deficiency of vitamin D is common in climates north of latitude 33°N or south of latitude 33°S, in dark-skinned individuals, and in those who spend most of their time indoors or cover their skin for religious or other reasons. However, vitamin D deficiency also occurs in sunny climates.[126,127] Cross-sectional studies have identified 25OHD levels to be less than 20 ng/ml (50 nmol/L) in 28% to 54% of American adolescents,[127-129] with higher risks in black and Hispanic teens.[128-130] Powe et al[131] found that black Americans have lower vitamin D-binding protein levels compared to white Americans, potentially explaining why blacks have higher BMD and lower risk for fragility fractures than whites despite lower 25OHD levels. Obese children and adolescents tend to have lower 25OHD levels than lean children, with 25OHD levels being inversely correlated with weight.[129,132,133] As vitamin D is fat soluble, low serum levels are very likely the result of sequestration of vitamin D in adipose tissue. While it could be assumed that the vitamin D in fat tissue is not bio-available, whether it is or not is not really known. Wortsman et al have speculated that vitamin D in adipose tissue is not bio-available;[134] however, there is no evidence that vitamin D deficiency associated with increased body fat has negative consequences on BMD and bone health in the pediatric age group.[135,136]

Adolescents with vitamin D deficiency (ie, 25OHD level <20 ng/mL and elevated plasma PTH) should be provided therapeutic doses of vitamin D. Endocrinologists traditionally use 2000 to 10,000 IU daily of vitamin D_2 or D_3 (alternatively, 50,000 IU of vitamin D_2 or D_3 weekly) for 6 to 8 weeks, followed by a maintenance dose of 600 to 1000 IU/day to achieve a serum 25OHD concentration greater than 20 ng/mL and to normalize PTH levels.[137] The 2014 AAP statement suggests using a daily vitamin D dose of 2000 IU/day for vitamin D deficiency.[104] The higher doses seem to be safe for vitamin D rickets and to normalize laboratory parameters more rapidly.[138]

In children who have limited sunlight exposure, poor nutritional state, a chronic disease, or are undergoing glucocorticoid or anticonvulsant therapy, consideration for provision of additional vitamin D supplementation can be based on abnormal PTH and/or 25OHD concentrations. Several pediatric subspecialties have made suggestions regarding treatment of vitamin D deficiency or insufficiency in children with diseases in their purview. Pappa et al[139] studied the response of 25OHD levels in children and adolescents having IBD with 25OHD vitamin D levels less than 20 ng/mL to 3 different therapeutic regimens of vitamin D. They found 2000 IU/day of oral vitamin D_3 and 50,000 IU/week of oral vitamin D_2 for 6 weeks were superior to 2000 IU/day of vitamin D_2 in raising serum 25OHD levels. Twenty-five percent of subjects treated with the latter regimen failed to achieve a 25OHD level greater than 20 ng/mL compared to only 5% for the 2 other regimens; therefore, they do not recommend using the 2000 IU/day vitamin D_2 therapy.

The CF Foundation recommends that all individuals older than 10 years with CF having a 25OHD level between 20 and 30 ng/mL receive 1600 to 6000 IU/day orally and that those with a level less than 20 ng/mL receive vitamin D_3 increased to a maximum of 10,000 IU/day orally.[121]

Although the AAP does not recommend screening with 25OHD levels in obese adolescents, in practice 25OHD levels are often obtained. It probably is unnecessary to supplement obese adolescents having 25OHD levels less than 20 ng/mL with more than 600 IU of vitamin D if the PTH level is not elevated. Some practitioners may feel more comfortable supplementing with a modestly higher daily intake of vitamin D (eg, 1000 IU); however, use of larger amounts should be guarded because there are no data supporting such a recommendation.

A final note on vitamin D: recent data in the adult literature have indicated that there are side effects of daily calcium supplement intake with and without vitamin D (eg, increased cardiovascular events, increased risk of kidney stones) and have also even called into question the utility of their intake for preventing fragility fractures in postmenopausal women.[140,141] As a result, the report of the United States Preventive Services Task Force, an independent panel of nonfederal experts in preventive and evidence-based medicine, recommended supplementation with 400 IU or less of vitamin D and 1000 mg or less of calcium for primary prevention of fractures in noninstitutionalized, postmenopausal women.[142] Whether and how this applies to bone health and overall health in children and adolescents remains to be determined. Clearly, in an age of low milk intake and high sunscreen protection, adolescents are at risk for vitamin D deficiency, and caregivers should do their best to ensure appropriate intake and supplementation when necessary, according to AAP guidelines.[104] At the same time, we all should be careful not to think "more is better," especially as high vitamin D intake is touted because of "associations" related to non-bone health issues. *Primum non nocere.*

Other Therapies

In most chronic illnesses accompanied by decreased BMD, treatment of the underlying disease process should be the primary intervention along with providing adequate amounts of calcium, vitamin D, and calories. Maintaining activity levels, as tolerated, to prevent the added burden of immobilization-induced bone loss is important in conditions such as juvenile rheumatoid arthritis and CP.

Hormone Therapy
With rare exceptions, hormone therapy is indicated only for children who have permanent hormone deficiencies (eg, hypogonadism, growth hormone deficiency, hypothyroidism). Hormone replacement therapy should not be prescribed routinely to increase BMD in adolescent girls with eating disorders or for the female athlete triad because there is no evidence supporting its efficacy.

In girls with hypergonadotropic hypogonadism (eg, Turner syndrome), the timing of estrogen replacement must be individualized and is sometimes delayed until near final height is achieved because of concern that estrogen will promote premature closure of the growth plate. However, for psychological reasons, estrogen therapy, especially using low-dose transdermal preparations, should not be delayed unduly.

In boys who have idiopathic juvenile osteoporosis and delayed puberty, short-term, low-dose testosterone therapy may be considered. Testosterone therapy should be individualized but can be introduced at a low dose and advanced slowly. Short-term, low-dose testosterone therapy is often recommended for psychological reasons in adolescent boys with constitutional delay of growth and puberty. It was once thought that boys with delayed puberty may have reduced BMD as adults. However, recent studies assessing volumetric BMD indicate that pubertal delay does not adversely affect peak bone mass.[143]

Bisphosphonates

In women with postmenopausal osteoporosis, bisphosphonates have been the mainstay of treatment. However, in recent years other medications have been added to this armamentarium (eg, teriparatide, a PTH analog; and denosumab, a monoclonal antibody). These newer drugs have not been used in children (see sections on Teriparatide and Denosumab). Bisphosphonates have been used sparingly in children and adolescents, but they may be beneficial in some children and adolescents with fragility fractures.

Bisphosphonates are synthetic analogs of naturally occurring pyrophosphates. The osteoblastic enzyme alkaline phosphatase cleaves pyrophosphate, preventing it from interacting with the bone matrix. Bisphosphonates are deposited in bone matrix but are resistant to cleavage by alkaline phosphatase. This results in decreased osteoclast activity, perhaps by inducing programmed osteoclast death and inhibiting the attachment of osteoclasts to bone matrix. At very high dosages, bisphosphonates also inhibit bone mineralization, so doses that favor a predominance of inhibition of bone resorption should be used. Bisphosphonates accumulate in bone and can remain in the bone for decades.

Bisphosphonates of greater potency continue to be developed. Zoledronate, for example, is 10,000 times more potent than the first bisphosphonate, etidronate, and 100 times more potent than the commonly used pamidronate. Bisphosphonates may be administered either parenterally or orally. Alendronate was the first oral bisphosphonate approved for treatment of osteoporosis.

Bisphosphonates have been studied much less extensively in children and adolescents than in adults. A 2005 position paper of the Lawson Wilkins Pediatric Endocrine Society Pharmacy and Therapeutic Committee on Bisphosphonate Treatment of Pediatric Bone Disease stated, "Because of the paucity of long-term studies among children regarding the safety and efficacy of these drugs, it is difficult to formulate strong evidence-based recommendations for their use except perhaps in children with Osteogenesis Imperfecta."[144] However, bisphosphonates are being used in children with severe bone disease (secondary osteoporosis), especially in those with pain and frequent fractures.

The bisphosphonates that have been used most frequently in children with osteoporosis are pamidronate, which is given intravenously, and alendronate, which is an oral preparation. Intravenous zoledronate and oral risedronate have been investigated in recent years. Each of these drugs has been evaluated for the treatment of OI, mainly using the intravenous preparations. A 1998 landmark study using pamidronate, administered in cycles of 1 to 3 months to treat children and adolescents with severe OI, showed rapid relief of bone pain, absence of new vertebral fractures, and reduction in the number of long bone fractures.[145] BMD increased by 50% to 120%. Several other studies support the use of pamidronate in OI.[146,147] Ward et al[148] reported that alendronate administered to subjects with OI for 2 years in a randomized placebo-controlled trial had no significant effect on long bone fracture rates or reshaping of fractured vertebral bodies even though spine BMD increased. A recent randomized placebo-controlled trial using oral risedronate showed increased areal BMD and reduced risk of first and recurrent long bone fractures.[149] An accompanying editorial pointed out that the trial included few subjects with severe OI and low efficacy for prevention of new vertebral fractures.[150]

There are a limited number of clinical trials of bisphosphonates in IJO, and the few existing studies are hampered by the lack of a stringent definition of IJO and the natural history of spontaneous recovery. An increase in BMD and a decrease in fracture rates have been reported.[151]

There have been a number of studies, mainly observational, using intravenous bisphosphonates in children and adolescents with secondary osteoporosis (eg, from glucocorticoids, IBD, or JIA). These reports suggest that therapy can increase BMD, promote vertebral reshaping, and relieve back pain. Current recommendations would limit use of bisphosphonates to children and adolescents with bone fragility or pain in whom spontaneous recovery is unlikely.[152,153] A potential use for preventing glucocorticoid-induced osteoporosis has been suggested, as the most rapid bone loss occurs in the first 6 to 12 months after commencement of high-dose glucocorticoid therapy. Reid et al[154] conducted a multicenter, double-blind, double-dummy, randomized controlled trial comparing zoledronic acid and risedronate in the prevention and treatment of glucocorticoid-induced osteoporosis. They found zoledronic acid was superior to risedronate for increasing lumbar spine BMD in both the treatment and prevention subgroups at 12 months.

Bisphosphonates have been shown to increase BMD in subjects with AN in some studies, but the effect is modest and they are not recommended for general use because of potential side effects.[155,156]

In a systematic review of interventions for low BMD in children with CP, only 3 articles using bisphosphonates were cited.[100] One was a double-blind placebo-controlled trial conducted on 6 pairs of subjects, which demonstrated that BMD increased 89% ± 21% over the 18-month study period in subjects treated with pamidronate compared with 9% ± 6% in the control group.[157] The wide variation in disability in patients with CP and the difficulty in enrolling subjects seem to be major obstacles to performing evidence-based studies of bisphosphonates, as well as various physical interventions, in this population.

At the present time, how long a child or adolescent must stay on bisphosphonate therapy to maintain benefit is unknown. Observations in adults have shown maintenance of benefit following discontinuation of alendronate after 5 years of therapy, suggesting that a "drug holiday" could be given to some patients. This does not seem to be the case in children with OI in whom bisphosphonate therapy must be continued until cessation of growth.[146,158]

Although it might be said that bisphosphonate usage in children and adolescents has been safe overall, much remains to be learned regarding bisphosphonate safety, especially because in theory bisphosphonates remain in bone and continue to be released into the circulation indefinitely. Short-term side effects relate to acute phase reactions to intravenous preparations and gastrointestinal problems with oral preparations. First or second intravenous dosing (but rarely beyond that) is often accompanied by fever and flulike symptoms (so-called *cytokine storm*) within the first 24 hours, and the reaction is generally attenuated by prophylactic antipyretic therapy.

Oral bisphosphonates must be taken in the fasting state in order to ensure absorption. However, because they can cause esophageal irritation, they should be taken with 8 ounces of water, and the patient should remain upright until after eating, which should be delayed at least 30 minutes after ingestion of the medication. Oral bisphosphonates should be used with caution in children and adolescents who cannot remain upright or who have upper gastrointestinal disorders. Similar precautions should be taken with the liquid preparation of alendronate as with the tablet form.

Transient hypocalcemia of a mild degree occurs infrequently with rapid IV administration. Pancreatitis, renal toxicity, and eye disorders (uveitis, conjunctivitis, scleritis) have been reported in adults.[159]

The potential for long-term use of bisphosphonates in children has raised concerns regarding their effects on growth and possible reproductive toxicity. With regard to the former, animal studies using very high doses of pamidronate found poor skeletal development.[160] However, linear growth has not been found to be abnormal in several studies of children receiving bisphosphonates.[161] With regard to the use of bisphosphonates in girls and young women of childbearing age, a recent study reviewed 51 cases of exposure to bisphosphonates before or during pregnancy.[162] No skeletal abnormalities or other congenital malformations were noted in the offspring. Yet, Kauffman et al,[163] reporting in Obstetric Gynecologic Survey stated, "The question remains unanswered as to when bisphosphonate therapy should be terminated before anticipated pregnancy or even if it should be administered at all to the adolescent female considering future pregnancy."

A single case of osteopetrosis (marble bone disease) in a 12-year-old boy treated with 4 times the usual dose of pamidronate has been reported.[164] Poor healing after surgical osteotomy in children previously treated with bisphosphonates for OI has also been reported.[165] The occurrence of osteonecrosis of the jaw (after dental procedures) seen in adults[166] has not been reported in children to date.[167] In general, one needs to remain cautious and judicious in dosing children or adolescents with bisphosphonates.

Calcitonin
Calcitonin, a former mainstay of osteoporosis therapy, has fallen out of favor as newer modalities have proven efficacious and safe. Both injectable and nasal salmon calcitonin have a prominent analgesic effect on the bone pain of acute vertebral fracture.

Future Therapies

Teriparatide
Teriparatide (recombinant human PTH) has emerged as another treatment modality for adult osteoporosis. Teriparatide mainly stimulates bone formation, in contrast to the bisphosphonates, which mainly inhibit bone resorption. Teriparatide has been shown to increase BMD and to decrease fracture rates. Overall it has a therapeutic profile at least comparable to that of alendronate.[168] Teriparatide currently has a black box warning from the United States Federal Drug Administration (FDA) against its use in children and adolescents because of an increased incidence of osteogenic sarcoma in rodents administered high-dose teriparatide. There have been no incidences of osteogenic sarcoma in teriparatide-treated humans to date, and this valuable therapy might be available for children and adolescents in the future, after appropriate investigation.[169]

Denosumab
Denosumab is a fully human monoclonal antibody that inhibits bone resorption by neutralizing RANKL, a key mediator of osteoclast formation, function, and survival. In a multicenter, double-blind study comparing the efficacy and safety of denosumab with alendronate in postmenopausal women with low bone mass, denosumab led to significantly larger gains in BMD and a greater reduction in bone turnover markers compared with alendronate.[170] Overall, the safety profile was similar to that of alendronate.

Sclerostin Antibody
In early phase II trials in postmenopausal women with low bone density, an antibody (AMG 785) against the protein sclerostin, an endogenous inhibitor of bone formation, has been shown to significantly increase BMD.[171] This treatment is novel in that it increases bone density by increasing bone formation rather than decreasing bone resorption.

SUMMARY

Osteoporosis occurs during childhood and adolescence as a heritable condition such as OI, with acquired disease (eg, IBD), or iatrogenically as a result of high-dose glucocorticoid therapy. However, the number of children affected by osteoporosis during youth is small compared to the numbers who will develop osteoporosis in adulthood. Prevention of adult osteoporosis requires that an optimal environment for the achievement of peak bone mass be established during the growing years. Detection of low BMD can be achieved using modalities such as DXA and pQCT. Standard radiologic studies, especially vertebral radiography, may also be helpful in children and adolescents at high risk for osteoporosis. It is critical to the development of healthy bones that adolescents have proper nutrition with adequate calcium and vitamin D intake and that they participate in regular physical activity (especially weight-bearing exercise). In the recent past, the dual goals of proper nutrition and exercise were not being achieved by many, if not most, adolescents. Those caring for adolescents should strive to educate teens and their families on the importance of dietary calcium and vitamin D as well as advocate for supportive environments in schools and communities that foster the development of healthy habits with regard to diet and exercise. In order to help identify the population at risk for osteoporosis, a bone health screen with assessment of calcium intake and determination of family history of adult osteoporosis (hip fracture, kyphosis) should be a routine part of adolescent health care. Universal screening of healthy adolescents with serum 25OHD levels is not recommended. Adolescents with conditions associated with reduced bone mass should undergo bone densitometry or other studies as a baseline, and BMD should be monitored at intervals no more frequently than yearly. Although controversy remains regarding the optimum dose of vitamin D for treatment of osteoporosis, all would agree that vitamin D should be provided, and in doses somewhat higher than previously recommended. Excessive vitamin D should be avoided. The use of bisphosphonates is recommended for the treatment of OI, as well as for treatment of select children with severe osteoporosis associated with chronic conditions that lead to frequent or painful fragility fractures. In such situations, bisphosphonates should be prescribed only in the context of a comprehensive clinical program with specialists knowledgeable in the management of osteoporosis in children.

References

1. Bailey DA, Wedge JH, McCulloch RG, et al. Epidemiology of fractures of the distal end of the radius in children as associated with growth. *J Bone Joint Surg Am.* 1989;71:1225-1231
2. Cooper C, Dennison EM, Leufkens HG, et al. Epidemiology of childhood fractures in Britain: a study using the general practice research database. *J Bone Miner Res.* 2004;19:1976-1981
3. Mäyränpää M, Viljakainen H, Toiviainen-Salo S, et al. Impaired bone health and asymptomatic vertebral compressions in fracture-prone children: a case-control study. *J Bone Miner Res.* 2012; 27:1413-1424

4. Bonewald LF. The amazing osteocyte. *J Bone Miner Res.* 2011;26:229-238
5. Bellido T. Osteocyte-driven bone remodeling. *Calcif Tissue Int.* 2014;94:25-34
6. Bailey DA, Faulkner RA, McKay HA. Growth, physical activity, and bone mineral acquisition. *Exerc Sport Sci Rev.* 1996;24:233-266
7. Bachrach LK. Acquisition of optimal bone mass in childhood and adolescence. *Trends Endocrinol Metab.* 2001;12:22-28
8. Lewis MK, Blake GM, Fogelman I. Patient dose in dual x-ray absorptiometry. *Osteoporos Int.* 1994;4:11-15
9. Crabtree NJ, Arabi A, Bachrach LK, et al. Dual-energy X-ray absorptiometry interpretation and reporting in children and adolescents: the revised 2013 ISCD Pediatric Official Positions. *J Clin Densitom.* 2014;17:225-242
10. Kalkwarf HJ, Zemel BS, Gilsanz V, et al. The bone mineral density in childhood study: bone mineral content and density according to age, sex, and race. *J Clin Endocrinol Metab.* 2007;92:2087-2099
11. Ward KA, Ashby RL, Roberts SA, et al. UK reference data for the Hologic QDR Discovery dual-energy x ray absorptiometry scanner in healthy children and young adults aged 6-17 years. *Arch Dis Child.* 2007;92:53-59
12. Horlick M, Wang J, Pierson RN Jr, et al. Prediction models for evaluation of total-body bone mass with dual-energy X-ray absorptiometry among children and adolescents. *Pediatrics.* 2004;114:e337-e345
13. Zemel BS, Kalkwarf HJ, Gilsanz V, et al. Revised reference curves for bone mineral content and areal bone mineral density according to age and sex for black and non-black children: results of the bone mineral density in childhood study. *J Clin Endocrinol Metab.* 2011;96:3160-3169
14. Goulding A, Grant AM, Williams SM. Bone and body composition of children and adolescents with repeated forearm fractures. *J Bone Miner Res.* 2005;20:2090-2096
15. Clark EM, Ness AR, Bishop NJ, et al. Association between bone mass and fractures in children: a prospective cohort study. *J Bone Miner Res.* 2006;21:1489-1495
16. Kalkwarf HJ, Laor T, Bean JA. Fracture risk in children with a forearm injury is associated with volumetric bone density and cortical area (by peripheral QCT) and areal bone density (by DXA). *Osteoporos Int.* 2011;22:607-616
17. Gordon CM, Leonard MB, Zemel BS; International Society for Clinical Densitometry. 2013 Pediatric Position Development Conference: executive summary and reflections. *J Clin Densitom.* 2014;17:219-224
18. Bachrach LK, Sills IN; American Academy of Pediatrics Section on Endocrinology. Clinical report-bone densitometry in children and adolescents. *Pediatrics.* 2011;127:189-194
19. Beaupre GS. Radiation exposure in bone measurements. *J Bone Miner Res.* 2006;21:803; author reply 804
20. Genant H, Wu C, vanKuijk C, et al. Vertebral fracture assessment using a semiquantitative technique. *J Bone Miner Res.* 1993;8:1137-1148
21. Nguyen TV. Contributions of Genetics and Environmental Factors to the Determinants of Osteoporosis Fractures. PhD Thesis. Garvan University of Medicine, Department of Community Medicine, Faculty of Medicine, The University of New South Wales, Sydney, Australia.1998; 388
22. Pocock NA, Eisman JA, Hopper JL, et al. Genetic determinants of bone mass in adults. A twin study. *J Clin Invest.* 1987;80:706-710
23. Young D, Hopper JL, Nowson CA, et al. Determinants of bone mass in 10- to 26-year-old females: a twin study. *J Bone Miner Res.* 1995;10:558-567
24. Cummings SR, Nevitt MC, Browner WS, et al. Risk factors for hip fracture in white women. Study of Osteoporotic Fractures Research Group. *N Engl J Med.* 1995;332:767-773
25. Gilsanz V, Nelson DA. Childhood and adolescence. In: Favus MJ, ed. *Primer on the Metabolic Bone Diseases and Disorders of Mineral Metabolism.* Washington, DC: American Society for Bone and Mineral Research; 2003: 71-80
26. Gilsanz V, Skaggs DL, Kovanlikaya A, et al. Differential effect of race on the axial and appendicular skeletons of children. *J Clin Endocrinol Metab.* 1998;83:1420-1427

27. Lloyd T, Andon MB, Rollings N, et al. Calcium supplementation and bone mineral density in adolescent girls. *JAMA*. 1993;270:841-844
28. Wyshak G. Teenaged girls, carbonated beverage consumption, and bone fractures. *Arch Pediatr Adolesc Med*. 2000;154:610-613
29. Bachrach LK, Katzman DK, Litt IF, et al. Recovery from osteopenia in adolescent girls with anorexia nervosa. *J Clin Endocrinol Metab*. 1991;72:602-606
30. Sillence DO, Senn A, Danks DM. Genetic heterogeneity in osteogenesis imperfecta. *J Med Genet*. 1979;16:101-116
31. van Dijk F, Byers P, Dalgleish R, et al. EMQN best practice guidelines for the laboratory diagnosis of osteogenesis imperfecta. *Eur J Hum Genet*. 2012;20:1-9
32. Dent CE. Osteoporosis in childhood. *Postgrad Med J*. 1977;53:450-457
33. Rauch F, Bishop N. Juvenile osteoporosis. In: Favus MJ, ed. *Primer on the Metabolic Bone Diseases and Disorders of Mineral Metabolism*. Washington, DC: American Society for Bone and Mineral Research; 2007:293-302
34. Soyka LA, Grinspoon S, Levitsky LL, et al. The effects of anorexia nervosa on bone metabolism in female adolescents. *J Clin Endocrinol Metab*. 1999;84:4489-4496
35. Grinspoon S, Thomas E, Pitts S, et al. Prevalence and predictive factors for regional osteopenia in women with anorexia nervosa. *Ann Intern Med*. 2000;133:790-794
36. Golden NH, Lanzkowsky L, Schebendach J, et al. The effect of estrogen-progestin treatment on bone mineral density in anorexia nervosa. *J Pediatr Adolesc Gynecol*. 2002;15:135-143
37. Soyka LA, Misra M, Frenchman A, et al. Abnormal bone mineral accrual in adolescent girls with anorexia nervosa. *J Clin Endocrinol Metab*. 2002;87:4177-4185
38. Misra M, Aggarwal A, Miller KK, et al. Effects of anorexia nervosa on clinical, hematologic, biochemical, and bone density parameters in community-dwelling adolescent girls. *Pediatrics*. 2004;114:1574-1583
39. Misra M, Katzman DK, Cord J, et al. Bone metabolism in adolescent boys with anorexia nervosa. *J Clin Endocrinol Metab*. 2008;93:3029-3036
40. Lucas AR, Melton LJ 3rd, Crowson CS, et al. Long-term fracture risk among women with anorexia nervosa: a population-based cohort study. *Mayo Clin Proc*. 1999;74:972-977
41. Vestergaard P, Emborg C, Stoving RK, et al. Fractures in patients with anorexia nervosa, bulimia nervosa, and other eating disorders—a nationwide register study. *Int J Eat Disord*. 2002;32:301-308
42. Miller KK, Lee EE, Lawson EA, et al. Determinants of skeletal loss and recovery in anorexia nervosa. *J Clin Endocrinol Metab*. 2006;91:2931-2937
43. Naessen S, Carlstrom K, Glant R, et al. Bone mineral density in bulimic women—influence of endocrine factors and previous anorexia. *Eur J Endocrinol*. 2006;155:245-251
44. Rigotti NA, Neer RM, Skates SJ, et al. The clinical course of osteoporosis in anorexia nervosa. A longitudinal study of cortical bone mass. *JAMA*. 1991;265:1133-1138
45. Misra M, Prabhakaran R, Miller KK, et al. Weight gain and restoration of menses as predictors of bone mineral density change in adolescent girls with anorexia nervosa. *J Clin Endocrinol Metab*. 2008;93:1231-1237
46. Klibanski A, Biller BM, Schoenfeld DA, et al. The effects of estrogen administration on trabecular bone loss in young women with anorexia nervosa. *J Clin Endocrinol Metab*. 1995;80:898-904
47. Strokosch GR, Friedman AJ, Wu SC, et al. Effects of an oral contraceptive (norgestimate/ethinyl estradiol) on bone mineral density in adolescent females with anorexia nervosa: a double-blind, placebo-controlled study. *J Adolesc Health*. 2006;39:819-827
48. Misra M, Katzman D, Miller KK, et al. Physiologic estrogen replacement increases bone density in adolescent girls with anorexia nervosa. *J Bone Miner Res*. 2011;26:2430-2438
49. Nattiv A, Loucks AB, Manore MM, et al. American College of Sports Medicine position stand. The female athlete triad. *Med Sci Sports Exerc*. 2007;39:1867-1882
50. Pollock N, Grogan C, Perry M, et al. Bone-mineral density and other features of the female athlete triad in elite endurance runners: a longitudinal and cross-sectional observational study. *Int J Sport Nutr Exerc Metab*. 2010;20:418-426

51. Nichols JF, Rauh MJ, Lawson MJ, et al. Prevalence of the female athlete triad syndrome among high school athletes. *Arch Pediatr Adolesc Med.* 2006;160:137-142
52. Barrack MT, Gibbs JC, De Souza MJ, et al. Higher incidence of bone stress injuries with increasing female athlete triad-related risk factors: a prospective multisite study of exercising girls and women. *Am J Sports Med.* 2014;42:949-958
53. Cromer BA, Stager M, Bonny A, et al. Depot medroxyprogesterone acetate, oral contraceptives and bone mineral density in a cohort of adolescent girls. *J Adolesc Health.* 2004;35:434-441
54. Scholes D, LaCroix AZ, Ichikawa LE, et al. Change in bone mineral density among adolescent women using and discontinuing depot medroxyprogesterone acetate contraception. *Arch Pediatr Adolesc Med.* 2005;159:139-144
55. Cromer BA, Scholes D, Berenson A et al. Depot medroxyprogesterone acetate and bone mineral density in adolescents—the Black Box Warning: a Position Paper of the Society for Adolescent Medicine. *J Adolesc Health.* 2006;39:296-301
56. American College of Obstetricians and Gynecologists Committee on Adolescent Health Care and Committee on Gynecologic Practice. ACOG Committee Opinion No. 415: Depot medroxyprogesterone acetate and bone effects. *Obstet Gynecol.* 2008;112:727-730
57. Cibula D, Skrenkova J, Hill M, et al. Low-dose estrogen combined oral contraceptives may negatively influence physiological bone mineral density acquisition during adolescence. *Eur J Endocrinol.* 2012;166:1003-1011
58. Scholes D, Hubbard RA, Ichikawa LE, et al. Oral contraceptive use and bone density change in adolescent and young adult women: a prospective study of age, hormone dose, and discontinuation. *J Clin Endocrinol Metab.* 2011;96:E1380-1387
59. Lopez LM, Chen M, Mullins S, et al. Steroidal contraceptives and bone fractures in women: evidence from observational studies. *Cochrane Database Syst Rev.* 2012;8:CD009849
60. Liu D, Ahmet A, Ward L, et al. A practical guide to the monitoring and management of the complications of systemic corticosteroid therapy. *Allergy Asthma Clin Immunol.* 2013;9:30-54
61. Weinstein RS, Jilka RL, Parfitt AM, et al. Inhibition of osteoblastogenesis and promotion of apoptosis of osteoblasts and osteocytes by glucocorticoids. Potential mechanisms of their deleterious effects on bone. *J Clin Invest.* 1998;102:274-282
62. Yao W, Cheng Z, Busse C, et al. Glucocorticoid excess in mice results in early activation of osteoclastogenesis and adipogenesis and prolonged suppression of osteogenesis: a longitudinal study of gene expression in bone tissue from glucocorticoid-treated mice. *Arthritis Rheum.* 2008;58:1674-1686
63. Manolagas SC. Corticosteroids and fractures: a close encounter of the third cell kind. *J Bone Miner Res.* 2000;15:1001-1005
64. Canalis E, Bilezikian JP, Angeli A, et al. Perspectives on glucocorticoid-induced osteoporosis. *Bone.* 2004;34:593-598
65. van Staa TP, Leufkens HG, Cooper C. The epidemiology of corticosteroid-induced osteoporosis: a meta-analysis. *Osteoporos Int.* 2002;13:777-787
66. Sambrook PN. Glucocorticoid-induced osteoporosis. In: Favus MJ, ed. *Primer on the Metabolic Bone Diseases and Disorders of Mineral Metabolism.* Washington, DC: American Society for Bone and Mineral Research; 2006:296-302
67. Pappa H, Thayu M, Sylvester F, et al. A clinical report on skeletal health of children and adolescents with inflammatory bowel disease. *J Pediatr Gastroenterol Nutr.* 2011;53:11-25
68. Loftus EV Jr, Crowson CS, Sandborn WJ, et al. Long-term fracture risk in patients with Crohn's disease: a population-based study in Olmsted County, Minnesota. *Gastroenterology.* 2002;123:468-475
69. Loftus EV Jr, Achenbach SJ, Sandborn WJ, et al. Risk of fracture in ulcerative colitis: a population-based study from Olmsted County, Minnesota. *Clin Gastroenterol Hepatol.* 2003;1:465-473
70. Siffledeen JS, Siminoski K, Jen H, et al. Vertebral fractures and role of low bone mineral density in Crohn's disease. *Clin Gastroenterol Hepatol.* 2007;5:721-728
71. Fasano A, Berti I, Gerarduzzi T, et al. Prevalence of celiac disease in at-risk and not-at-risk groups in United States: a large multicenter study. *Arch Inter Med.* 2003;163:286-292

72. Bennett TI, Hunter D, Vaugham JM. Idiopathic steatorrhea. A nutritional disturbance associated with tetany, osteomalacia and anaemia. Q J Med. 1932;1:603-677
73. Holms WH, Starr P. A nutritional disturbance in adults resembling coeliac disease and sprue: emaciation, anemia, tetany, chronic diarrhea and malabsorption of fat. JAMA. 1929;92:975-980
74. Salvesen HA, Boe J. Osteomalacia in sprue. Acta M Scan. 1953;146:290-299
75. Kemppainen T, Kroger H, Janatuinen E, et al. Osteoporosis in adult patients with celiac disease. Bone. 1999;24:249-255
76. Meyer D, Stavropolous S, Diamond B, et al. Osteoporosis in a North American adult population with celiac disease. Am J Gastroenterol. 2001;96:112-119
77. Turner J, Pellerin G, Mager D. Prevalence of metabolic bone disease in children with celiac disease is independent of symptoms at diagnosis. J Pediatr Gastroenterol Nutr. 2009;49:589-593
78. Fouda MA, Khan AA, Sultan M, et al. Evaluation and management of skeletal health in celiac disease: Position statement. Can J Gastroenterol. 2012;26(11):819-829
79. Ludvigsson JF, Michaelsson K, Ekbom A, et al. Coeliac disease and the risk of fractures: a general population-based cohort study. Aliment Pharmacol Ther. 2007;25:273-285
80. Lewiecki EM, Watts NB, McClung MR, et al. Official positions of the international society for clinical densitometry. J Clin Endocrinol Metab. 2004;89:3651-3655
81. Henderson RC, Madsen CD. Bone mineral content and body composition in children and young adults with cystic fibrosis. Pediatr Pulmonol. 1999;27:80-84
82. Aris RM, Merkel PA, Bachrach LK, et al. Guide to bone health and disease in cystic fibrosis. J Clin Endocrinol Metab. 2005;90:1888-1896
83. Hecker TM, Aris RM. Management of osteoporosis in adults with cystic fibrosis. Drugs. 2004;64:133-147
84. Haworth CS, Selby PL, Webb AK, et al. Inflammatory related changes in bone mineral content in adults with cystic fibrosis. Thorax. 2004;59:613-617
85. Ionescu AA, Nixon LS, Evans WD, et al. Bone density, body composition, and inflammatory status in cystic fibrosis. Am J Respir Crit Care Med. 2000;162:789-794
86. Papaioannou A, Kennedy CC, Freitag A, et al. Longitudinal analysis of vertebral fracture and BMD in a Canadian cohort of adult cystic fibrosis patients. BMC Musculoskelet Disord. 2008;9:125
87. Hardin DS, Ahn C, Prestidge C, et al. Growth hormone improves bone mineral content in children with cystic fibrosis. J Pediatr Endocrinol Metab. 2005;18:589-595
88. Almeida M, Han L, Ambrogini E, et al. Glucocorticoids and tumor necrosis factor alpha increase oxidative stress and suppress Wnt protein signaling in osteoblasts. J Biol Chem. 2011;286:44326-44335
89. Okamoto K, Takayanagi H. Regulation of bone by the adaptive immune system in arthritis. Arthritis Res Ther. 2011;13:219
90. Henderson CJ, Cawkwell GD, Specker BL, et al. Predictors of total body bone mineral density in non-corticosteroid-treated prepubertal children with juvenile rheumatoid arthritis. Arthritis Rheum. 1997;40:1967-1975
91. Huber AM, Gaboury I, Cabral DA, et al. Canadian Steroid-Associated Osteoporosis in the Pediatric Population (STOPP) Consortium. Prevalent vertebral fractures among children initiating glucocorticoid therapy for the treatment of rheumatic disorders. Arthritis Care Res. 2010;62:516-526
92. Rodd C, Lang B, Ramsay T, et al. Incident vertebral fractures among children with rheumatic disorders 12 months after glucocorticoid initiation: a national observational study. Arthritis Care Res. 2012;64:122-131
93. LeBlanc C, Ma J, Scuccimarri R, et al. Glucocorticoid therapy and the risk of incident vertebral fractures in children with rheumatic disorders. Arthritis Rheumatol. 2014;66(Suppl 3):S199-S200
94. Winkel ML, Pieters R, Hop WCJ, et al. Bone mineral density at diagnosis determines fracture rate in children with acute lymphoblastic leukemia treated according to the DCOG-ALL9 protocol. Bone. 2014;59:223-228
95. Haddy TB, Mosher RB, Reaman GH. Osteoporosis in survivors of acute lymphoblastic leukemia. Oncologist. 2001;6:278-285

96. Mostoufi-Moab S, Brodsky J, Isaacoff E, et al. Longitudinal assessment of bone density and structure in childhood survivors of acute lymphoblastic leukemia without cranial radiation. *J Clin Endocrinol Metab.* 212:97;3584-3592
97. Bakalov VK, Chen ML, Baron J, et al. Bone mineral density and fractures in Turner syndrome. *Am J Med.* 2003;115:259-264
98. Bakalov VK, Axelrod L, Baron J, et al. Selective reduction in cortical bone mineral density in Turner syndrome independent of ovarian hormone deficiency. *J Clin Endocrinol Metab.* 2003;88:5717-5722
99. Rubin K. Turner syndrome and osteoporosis: mechanisms and prognosis. *Pediatrics.* 1998;102(2 Pt 3):481-485
100. Hough JP, Boyd RN, Keating JL. Systematic review of interventions for low bone mineral density in children with cerebral palsy. *Pediatrics.* 2010;125(3):e670-e678
101. Mergler S, Evenhuis HM, Boot AM. Epidemiology of low bone mineral density and fractures in children with severe cerebral palsy: a systematic review. *Dev Med Child Neurol.* 2009:51;773-778
102. Henderson RC, Lark RK, Gurka MJ, et al. Bone density and metabolism in children and adolescents with moderate to severe cerebral palsy. *Pediatrics.* 2002;110(1 Pt 1):e5
103. Henderson RC. Bone density and other possible predictors of fracture risk in children and adolescents with spastic quadriplegia. *Dev Med Child Neurol.* 1997;39:224-227
104. Golden NH, Abrams SA; American Academy of Pediatrics Committee On Nutrition. Optimizing bone health in children and adolescents. *Pediatrics.* 2014;134:e1229-e1243
105. US Department of Agriculture, Agricultural Research Service. Data tables: results from USDA's 1994–96 Continuing Survey of Food Intakes by Individuals and 1994–96 Diet and Knowledge Survey.1999. Available at: www.ars.usda.gov/services/docs.htm?docid=7760. Accessed April 7, 2013
106. Suitor CW, Gleason PM. Using dietary reference intake-based methods to estimate the prevalence of inadequate nutrient intake among school-aged children. *J Am Diet Assoc.* 2002:102:530-536
107. Matkovic V, Ilich JZ. Calcium requirements for growth: are current recommendations adequate? *Nutr Rev.*1993;51:171-180
108. Jackman LA, Millane SS, Martin BR, et al. Calcium retention in relation to calcium intake and postmenarcheal age in adolescent females. *Am J Clin Nutr.* 1997;66:327-333
109. Holick MF. Vitamin D deficiency. *N Engl J Med.* 2007;357:266-281
110. Institute of Medicine. *2011 Dietary Reference Intakes for Calcium and Vitamin D.* Washington DC: The National Academies Press; 2011
111. Misra M, Pacaud D, Petryk A, et al. Vitamin D deficiency in children and its management: review of current knowledge and recommendations. *Pediatrics.* 2008;122:398-417
112. Holick MF, Binkley NC, Bischoff-Ferrari HA, et al. Evaluation, treatment, and prevention of vitamin D deficiency: an Endocrine Society clinical practice guideline. *J Clin Endocrinol Metab.* 2011;96:1911-1930
113. Gallagher JC, Riggs BL, Eisman J, et al. Intestinal calcium absorption and serum vitamin D metabolites in normal subjects and osteoporotic patients: effect of age and dietary calcium. *J Clin Invest.* 1979;64:729-736
114. Boucher-Berry C, Speiser PW, Carey DE, et al. Vitamin D, osteocalcin, and risk for adiposity as comorbidities in middle school children. *J Bone Mineral Res.* 2012;27:283-293
115. Bedner M, Lippa KA, Tai SS. An assessment of 25-hydroxyvitamin D measurements in comparability studies conducted by the Vitamin D Metabolites Quality Assurance Program. *Clin Chim Acta.* 2013;426:6-11
116. Fraser WD, Milan AM. Vitamin D assays: past and present debates, difficulties, and developments. *Calcif Tissue Int.* 2013;92:118-127
117. Wyness SP, Straseski JA. Performance characteristics of six automated 25-hydroxyvitamin D assays: mind your 3's and 2's. Poster session presented at the Endocrine Society's 96th Annual Meeting (ENDO), Chicago, Illionois, 2014

118. He CS, Gleeson M, Fraser WD. Measurement of circulating 25-hydroxy vitamin D using three commercial enzyme-linked immunosorbent assay kits with comparison to liquid chromatography: tandem mass spectrometry method. *ISRN Nutr.* 2013;13:723139
119. Heaney RP1, Recker RR, Grote J, et al. Vitamin D(3) is more potent than vitamin D(2) in humans. *J Clin Endocrinol Metab.* 2011;96:E447-E452
120. Holick MF, Biancuzzo RM, Chen TC, et al. Vitamin D2 is as effective as vitamin D3 in maintaining circulating concentrations of 25-hydroxyvitamin D. *J Clin Endocrinol Metab.* 2008;93:677-681
121. MacKelvie KJ, Khan KM, Petit MA, et al. A school-based exercise intervention elicits substantial bone health benefits: a 2-year randomized controlled trial in girls. *Pediatrics.* 2003;112(6 Pt 1):e447
122. McKay H, MacLean L, Petit MA, et al. "Bounce at the Bell": a novel program of short bouts of exercise improves proximal femur bone mass in early pubertal children. *Br J Sports Med.* 2005;39:521-526
123. Snow-Harter C, Bouxsein ML, Lewis BT, et al. Effects of resistance and endurance exercise on bone mineral status of young women: a randomized exercise intervention trial. *J Bone Miner Res.* 1992;7:761-769
124. Tangpricha V, Kelly A, Stephenson A, et al. An update on the screening, diagnosis, management, and treatment of vitamin D deficiency in individuals with cystic fibrosis: evidence-based recommendations from the Cystic Fibrosis Foundation. *J Clin Endocrinol Metab.* 2012;97:1082-1093
125. Sonneville KR, Gordon CM, Kocher MS, et al. Vitamin D, calcium, and dairy intakes and stress fractures among female adolescents. *Arch Pediatr Adolesc Med.* 2012;166:595-600
126. Lapatsanis D, Moulas A, Cholevas V, et al. Vitamin D: a necessity for children and adolescents in Greece. *Calcif Tissue Int.* 2005;77:348-355
127. Dong Y, Pollock N, Stallmann-Jorgensen IS, et al. Low 25-hydroxyvitamin D levels in adolescents: race, season, adiposity, physical activity, and fitness. *Pediatrics.* 2010;125:1104-1111
128. Harkness LS, Cromer BA. Vitamin D deficiency in adolescent females. *J Adolesc Health.* 2005;37:75
129. Gordon CM, DePeter KC, Feldman HA, et al. Prevalence of vitamin D deficiency among healthy adolescents. *Arch Pediatr Adolesc Med.* 2004;158:531-537
130. Looker AC, Dawson-Hughes B, Calvo MS, et al. Serum 25-hydroxyvitamin D status of adolescents and adults in two seasonal subpopulations from NHANES III. *Bone.* 2002;30:771-777
131. Powe CE, Evans MK, Wenger J, et al. Vitamin D-binding protein and vitamin D status of black Americans and white Americans. *N Engl J Med.* 2013;369:1991-2000
132. Harel Z, Flanagan P, Forcier M, et al. Low vitamin D status among obese adolescents: prevalence and response to treatment. *J Adolesc Health.* 2011;48:448-452
133. Turer CB, Lin H, Flores G. Prevalence of vitamin D deficiency among overweight and obese US children. *Pediatrics.* 2013;131:e152-e161
134. Wortsman J, Matsuoka LY, Chen TC, et al. Decreased bioavailability of vitamin D in obesity. *Am J Clin Nutr.* 2000;72:690-693
135. Kremer R, Campbell RP, Reinhardt T, et al. Vitamin D status and its relationship to body fat, final height, and peak bone mass in young women. *J Clin Endocrinol Metab.* 2009;94:67-73
136. Lenders CM, Feldman HA, Von Scheven E, et al; Elizabeth Glaser Pediatric Research Network Obesity Study Group. Relation of body fat indexes to vitamin D status and deficiency among obese adolescents. *Am J Clin Nutr.* 2009;90:459-467
137. Root AW, Diamond FB. Disorders of mineral homeostasis the newborn, infant, child and adolescent. In: Sperling MA, ed. *Pediatric Endocrinology.* 3rd ed. Philadelphia, PA: Saunders Elsevier; 2008:686-769
138. Pettifor JM. Nutritional rickets. In: Glorieux FH, Pettifor JM, Juppner H, eds. *Pediatric Bone: Biology & Diseases.* San Diego, CA: Academic Press; 2003:541-566
139. Pappa HM, Mitchell PD, Jiang H, et al. Treatment of vitamin D insufficiency in children and adolescents with inflammatory bowel disease: a randomized clinical trial comparing three regimens. *J Clin Endocrinol Metab.* 2012;97:2134-2142

140. Lorenzo J, ed. How much calcium and vitamin D? The American Society for Bone and Mineral Research. March 27, 2013. Available at: community.asbmr.org/index.php?/topic/1188-how-much-calcium-and-vitamin-d/. Accessed May 13, 2015
141. Jackson RD, LaCroix AZ, Gass M, et al. Calcium plus vitamin D supplementation and the risk of fractures. *N Engl J Med.* 2006:354;669-683
142. US Preventive Services Task Force. Final Recommendation Statement: Vitamin D and Calcium to Prevent Fractures: Preventive Medication, February 2013. Available at: http://www.uspreventiveservicestaskforce.org/Page/Topic/recommendation-summary/vitamin-d-and-calcium-to-prevent-fractures-preventive-medication?ds=1&s=vitamin%20d%20and%20calcium. Accessed April 7, 2013
143. Bertelloni S, Baroncelli GI, Ferdeghini M, et al. Normal volumetric bone mineral density and bone turnover in young men with histories of constitutional delay of puberty. *J Clin Endocrinol Metab.* 1998;83:4280-4283
144. Speiser PW, Clarson CL, Eugster EA, et al. Bisphosphonate treatment of pediatric bone disease. *Pediatr Endocrinol Rev.* 2005;3:87-96
145. Glorieux FH, Bishop NJ, Plotkin H, et al. Cyclic administration of pamidronate in children with severe osteogenesis imperfecta. *N Engl J Med.* 1998;339:947-952
146. Rauch F, Cornibert S, Cheung M, et al. Long-bone changes after pamidronate discontinuation in children and adolescents with osteogenesis imperfecta. *Bone.* 2007;40:821-827
147. Shapiro JR, McCarthy EF, Rossiter K, et al. The effect of intravenous pamidronate on bone mineral density, bone histomorphometry and parameters of bone turnover in adults with type IA osteogenesis imperfecta. *Calcif Tissue Int.* 2003;27:103-112
148. Ward LM, Rauch F, Whyte MP, et al. Alendronate for the treatment of pediatric osteogenesis imperfecta: a randomized placebo-controlled study. *J Clin Endocrinol Metab.* 2011;96:355-364
149. Bishop N, Adami S, Ahmed S, et al. Risedronate in children with osteogenesis imperfecta: a randomised, double-blind, placebo-controlled trial. *Lancet.* 2013;382:1424-1432
150. Ward L, Rauch F. Oral bisphosphonates for paediatric osteogenesis imperfecta? *Lancet.* 2013;382:1388-1389
151. Steelman J, Zeitler P. Treatment of symptomatic pediatric osteoporosis with cyclic single-day intravenous pamidronate infusions. *J Pediatr.* 2003;142:417-423
152. Ward L, Tricco AC, Phuong P, et al. Bisphosphonate therapy for children and adolescents with secondary osteoporosis. *Cochrane Database Syst Rev.* 2007;4:CD005324
153. Bachrach LK, Ward LM. Clinical review 1: bisphosphonate use in childhood osteoporosis. *J Clin Endocrinol Metab.* 2009;94:400-409
154. Reid DM, Devogelaer JP, Saag K, et al. Zoledronic acid and risedronate in the prevention and treatment of glucocorticoid-induced osteoporosis (HORIZON): a multicentre, double-blind, double-dummy, randomised controlled trial. *Lancet.* 2009;373:1253-1263
155. Golden NH, Iglesias EA, Jacobson MS, et al. Alendronate for the treatment of osteopenia in anorexia nervosa: a randomized, double-blind, placebo-controlled trial. *J Clin Endocrinol Metab.* 2005;90:3179-3185
156. Miller KK, Meenaghan E, Lawson EA, et al. Effects of risedronate and low-dose transdermal testosterone on bone mineral density in women with anorexia nervosa: a randomized, placebo-controlled study. *J Clin Endocrinol Metab.* 2011;96:2081-2088
157. Henderson RC, Lark RK, Kecskemethy HH, et al. Bisphosphonates to treat osteopenia in children with quadriplegic cerebral palsy: a randomized, placebo-controlled clinical trial. *J Pediatr.* 2002;141:644-651
158. Ward KA, Adams JE, Freemont TJ, et al. Can bisphosphonate treatment be stopped in a growing child with skeletal fragility? *Osteoporos Int.* 2007;18:1137-1140
159. Black D, Rosen CJ. Bisphosphonates for prevention and Treatment of Osteoporosis. Favus MJ, ed. *Primer on the Metabolic Bone Diseases and Disorders of Mineral Metabolism.* Washington, DC: American Society for Bone and Mineral Research; 2006:277-282
160. Graepel P, Bentley P, Fritz H, et al. Reproduction toxicity studies with pamidronate. *Arzneimittelforschung.* 1992;42:654-667

161. Brumsen C, Hamdy T, Neveen A, et al. Long-term effects of bisphosphonates on the growing skeleton: studies of young patients with severe osteoporosis. *Medicine.* 1997;76:266-283
162. Djokanovic N, Klieger-Grossmann C, Koren G. Does treatment with bisphosphonates endanger the human pregnancy? *J Obstet Gynaecol Can.* 2008;30:1146-1148
163. Kauffman RP, Overton TH, Shiflett M, et al. Osteoporosis in children and adolescent girls: case report of idiopathic juvenile osteoporosis and review of the literature. *Obstet Gynecol Surv.* 2001;56:492-504
164. Whyte MP, Wenkert D, Clements KL, et al. Bisphosphonate-induced osteopetrosis. *N Engl J Med.* 2003;349:457-463
165. Munns CF, Rauch F, Zeitlin L, et al. Delayed osteotomy but not fracture healing in pediatric osteogenesis imperfecta patients receiving pamidronate. *J Bone Miner Res.* 2004;19:1779-1786
166. Bilezikian JP. Osteonecrosis of the jaw—do bisphosphonates pose a risk? *N Engl J Med.* 2006;355:2278-2281
167. Brown JJ, Ramalingam L, Zacharin MR. Bisphosphonate-associated osteonecrosis of the jaw: does it occur in children? *Clin Endocrinol (Oxf).* 2008;68:863-867
168. Neer RM, Arnaud CD. Effect of parathyroid hormone (1-34) on fractures and bone mineral density in postmenopausal women with osteoporosis. *N Engl J Med.* 2001;344:1434-1441
169. Riggs BL, Parfitt AM. Drugs used to treat osteoporosis: the critical need for a uniform nomenclature based on their action on bone remodeling. *J Bone Miner Res.* 2005;20:177-184
170. Brown J, Prince R, Deal C, et al. Comparison of the effect of denosumab and alendronate on BMD and biochemical markers of bone turnover in postmenopausal women with low bone mass: a randomized, blinded, phase 3 trial. *J Bone Miner Res.* 2009;24;153-161
171. Costa A, Bilezikian J. Sclerostin: therapeutic horizons based upon its actions. *Curr Osteoporos Rep.* 2012;10:64-72

Polycystic Ovarian Syndrome

Jason Klein, MD; Meghan Craven, MD; Patricia M. Vuguin, MD, MSc*

Division of Pediatric Endocrinology, Cohen Children's Medical Center of New York, North Shore–Long Island Jewish Health System, New Hyde Park, New York; Hofstra–North Shore LIJ School of Medicine, Hempstead, New York

INTRODUCTION

First described by Stein and Leventhal[1] in 1935, polycystic ovarian syndrome (PCOS) is the most common endocrine disorder of women of reproductive age, affecting 6% to 15% of such women[2] and accounting for 72% to 84% of adult hyperandrogenism.[3-5] The cause of PCOS is unknown, but evidence suggests that it is a polygenic condition exacerbated by prenatal and postnatal environmental factors.[6] There is a strong link between genetics and PCOS, seen in the context of family clusters, as well as concordance of symptoms in identical compared with nonidentical twin pairs.[7,8] In addition, evidence from animal studies shows that exposure to androgen excess during key developmental windows results in features of PCOS in adult women.[9] Girls who were exposed to an adverse intrauterine environment and were born small or large for gestational age are at risk of developing features of PCOS.[10,11] Similarly, a high prevalence of hyperandrogenism among obese peripubertal adolescents suggests that excessive weight gain and body mass index (BMI) greater or equal to the 95th percentile for age is a risk for development of the syndrome.[12]

Clinical features of PCOS include chronic anovulation, polycystic ovaries, and clinical hyperandrogenism, which can be accounted for by ovarian or adrenal dysfunction.[13-16] These abnormalities are intrinsic to dysfunctional ovarian steroidogenesis[17] and can also be caused or exacerbated by the associated metabolic abnormalities seen in obesity and insulin resistance.

---

*Corresponding author
E-mail address: pvuguin@nshs.edu

The syndrome is clinically and biochemically heterogeneous. Three international conferences have developed diagnostic criteria for adult women: The National Institutes of Health conference (1992),[18] the Rotterdam consensus (2004),[19] and the Androgen Excess-PCOS Society consensus (2006) (Table 1).[20] A 2012 international evidence-based workshop suggested that the Rotterdam criteria be used with specification of different phenotypes based on the severity of the condition.[21]

Polycystic ovarian syndrome is a complex reproductive and metabolic disorder that increases the lifetime risk of type 2 diabetes, cardiovascular disease, and endometrial cancer.[22-27] Although PCOS presents clinically during adolescence in most females, some features can manifest during earlier stages of development, such as pubic hair and androgen excess in girls before 8 years of age.[11,28,29] Because anovulatory or irregular periods may occur after menarche and clinical evidence suggesting androgen excess (eg, acne) is common during pubertal development, one needs to be cautious about making the diagnosis of PCOS during or immediately after puberty.[30-35]

PATHOGENESIS

The pathogenesis of PCOS is still unknown. Theories have suggested a dysregulation of ovarian hormone production triggered by puberty in females who are genetically predisposed to hypersecretion of ovarian androgens. Polycystic ovaries have a thickened thecal layer, and thecal cells derived from these ovaries secrete excessive androgens in response to luteinizing hormone (LH) stimulation.[36] This hyperandrogenism then results in an elevated LH level and a low follicle-stimulating hormone (FSH) level. In addition, by comparison, polycystic ovaries have 2 to 5 times more primary and secondary follicles. Studies have reported a positive correlation between follicle number and both serum testosterone and androstenedione concentrations.[37] This finding is supported by the

Table 1

Diagnostic criteria for polycystic ovarian syndrome

Diagnostic criteria	Hyperandrogenism (clinical or biochemical)	Oligo- or anovulation	Ultrasonographic evidence of polycystic ovaries
NIH (1992)	Required	Required	Not included
Rotterdam (2003): 2 of 3 required	Required (2/3)	Required (2/3)	Required (2/3)
AE-PCOS Society (2006): hyperandrogenism with at least 1 of the other 2	Required	Required (1/2)	Required (1/2)

AE-PCOS, Androgen Excess–Polycystic Ovarian Syndrome; NIH, National Institutes of Health.

fact that 60% to 80% of women with PCOS have high concentrations of circulating testosterone, and 25% have high concentrations of dehydroepiandrosterone sulfate (DHEAS).[38-40] However, the mechanism leading to increased follicle numbers is unknown. Some suggest the increase in follicle numbers is the result of a trophic effect of androgens, whereas others postulate that the follicles of a polycystic ovary grow at a slower rate, either because of deficient growth signals from the oocyte or the inhibitory effect of excess antimüllerian hormone.[37,41,42]

In addition, it has been proposed that insulin resistance may initiate or augment this process, leading to abnormal androgen production, similar to the hyperandrogenism–insulin resistance–acanthosis nigricans (HAIR-AN) syndrome.[43] Insulin resistance in these disorders is characterized by tissue-selective insulin sensitivity, in which some tissues (eg, skeletal muscle) seem highly resistant and others (eg, adrenal and ovarian tissue) highly sensitive.[44] Insulin acts with LH to increase androgen production and promotes LH binding to the receptors via insulin-like growth factor-1 (IGF-1) in ovarian theca cells.[45] High concentrations of insulin also reduce circulating sex hormone-binding globulin (SHBG), thereby increasing free testosterone, resulting in stimulation of adrenal and ovarian androgen synthesis.[46,47] This same pathway is also suspected in premature adrenarche, in which decreased IGF-1 binding protein leads to increased free IGF-1, producing increased adrenal and ovarian androgens. Longitudinal studies are needed to determine whether children with premature adrenarche are at increased risk for developing PCOS.[28,48]

Genetic studies of the families of affected women have shown a high incidence of affected relatives, but chromosomal studies to date have not shown any consistent abnormality. Recent studies have focused on the genes that encode for enzymes involved in androgen synthesis, including serine hyperphosphorylation, protein transducers of insulin signals, and insulin receptors.[49-51]

CLINICAL PRESENTATION

Irregular Menses

Ovulatory dysfunction can be subclinical with no obvious disruption in the regularity of vaginal bleeding, or it may present with disruption of the menstrual flow pattern, such as oligomenorrhea (vaginal bleeding episodes at >35-day intervals or <10 bleeds per year), polymenorrhea (<25 days between bleeds), amenorrhea (lack of menstrual bleeding for more than 3-6 months), or abnormal uterine bleeding.[52] During the first 2 years after menarche, anovulatory cycles are common, affecting approximately 50% of cycles while the hypothalamic–pituitary–ovarian (HPO) axis matures.[53] Maturation of the HPO axis occurs as FSH secretion rises and pulsatility of LH is established.[54] Approximately 95% of ovulatory cycles reach the 21- to 45-day range, with periods lasting 2 to 7 days, in the third year after menarche.[52,55]

Between 75% and 85% of adult women have clinical evidence of menstrual dysfunction, characterized by infrequent or absent menstrual bleeding. Interestingly, almost 20% to 30% of women with PCOS present with a history of eumenorrhea despite evidence of oligo- or anovulation; the remainder present with overt oligo- or amenorrhea, and less than 2% of the patients present with polymenorrhea. Primary amenorrhea is an uncommon manifestation of PCOS, ranging from 1.4% to 14% according to the different cohorts.[31,56-58] In adolescents, the prevalence of irregular menses is variable and depends on the cohort. Some studies have reported irregular menses in 50% to 85% of adolescent females.[59,60] It has been suggested that adolescents with primary amenorrhea secondary to PCOS exhibit a greater degree of hyperandrogenism and metabolic disturbances.[57] Menstrual irregularity can start at menarche and may change with age, tending to decrease as the patient approaches menopause.[61] Some patients give a history of regular cycles for a short period of time after menarche, followed by the onset of oligomenorrhea.[20] In a recent study by West et al,[62] menstrual irregularity at 16 years of age was associated with an increased risk of menstrual irregularity (adjusted odds ratio [OR] 1.37, 95% confidence interval [CI] 1.00-1.88, $P = .050$), PCOS (adjusted OR 2.91, 95% CI 1.74-4.84, $P <.001$), and infertility problems (adjusted OR 2.07, 95% CI 1.16-3.76, $P = .013$) at 26 years of age.

Clinical and Biochemical Features of Hyperandrogenism: Hirsutism, Acne, Androgenic Alopecia, and Elevated Testosterone Levels

Hirsutism is considered "the evidence for clinical hyperandrogenism" according to all adult criteria. It is defined as excessive terminal hair that develops in androgen-dependent ("male-pattern") regions.[63-65] Because hair growth becomes thick and coarse with increasing duration of androgen exposure, the prevalence of hirsutism is often less prominent during the early adolescent period, tends to have a gradual onset over time, and is dependent on the patient's ethnicity, BMI, and other factors.[53,66-68] Hirsutism is common among women with hyperandrogenism and may be suggestive of PCOS in adolescents.[69] It is described as the major symptom in 60% of adolescent patients.[50,70] Despite this finding, it is important to remember that hyperandrogenism can occur in the absence of hirsutism,[2,3] and hirsutism may occur without hyperandrogenism. Interestingly, hirsutism in white girls may be an uncommon finding, suggesting that hirsutism may take longer to develop in the presence of increased androgens in this ethnic group.[30,71-73]

As opposed to hirsutism, acne vulgaris is normal in pubertal girls and has not been considered as clinical evidence of hyperandrogenism in existing adult PCOS criteria. Despite this, acne may be the only manifestation of hyperandrogenism.[74] However, an expert consensus panel has recommended that hormonal therapy be considered in moderate (>20 inflammatory lesions and >20 comedones) and severe (extensive inflammatory lesions with nodules or scarring) acne that does not respond adequately to topical agents.[75,76] Such therapy, if undertaken as a matter of routine, has the potential to mask hyperandrogenism.

Little information is available on the prevalence of androgenic alopecia in women with PCOS and even less in the adolescent population. Thus, alopecia should not be considered a clinical feature associated with the diagnosis.

Biochemical Hyperandrogenism

Testosterone is the major circulating androgen.[65] Serum testosterone determination has several pitfalls. Diurnal patterning and cyclic changes in levels, as well as issues with the assay itself (limited accurate and sensitive assays commercially available),[65,77] have made its determination problematic. Assays are available that measure "child and female" testosterone levels and are indicated in investigation of this condition. In addition, both ethnic and BMI differences have been associated with variations in androgen levels in women.[50,78] In adult women, hyperandrogenism is diagnosed when testosterone or free testosterone levels are elevated, as documented by a reliable assay. Elevated testosterone levels are observed in approximately 70% of adult and 25% of adolescent patients with PCOS.[20,31] Testosterone levels increase as adolescent anovulatory cycles lengthen in both asymptomatic and symptomatically anovulatory schoolgirls.[53,79]

In adolescents, adult androgen levels are attained within a few years after menarche.[80,81] Despite the uncertainty about mild hyperandrogenism as a normal perimenarchal phenomenon, it has been shown that higher free androgen index quartiles at 16 years of age are associated with a higher prevalence of PCOS at 26 years of age.[82] Similarly, a cohort of healthy adolescent volunteers followed for 12 years showed that adolescent serum androgen levels were preserved into adulthood and that above-average levels in adolescence were significantly associated with lower fertility, suggesting PCOS.[83,84]

Polycystic Ovaries on Ultrasound

Until recently, 3 features have generally been assessed to define polycystic ovarian morphology (PCOM) in adult females: (1) ovarian size and volume (OV); (2) stromal volume; and (3) follicle size and number (FNPO) by transvaginal ultrasound (TV).

The Rotterdam criteria define PCOM as the presence of 12 or more follicles throughout the ovary measuring 2 to 9 mm in diameter or increased OV greater than 10 mL in at least 1 ovary. With the new available ultrasound technology (ie, transducer frequency 8 MHz), a task force report from the Androgen Excess and Polycystic Ovarian Syndrome Society recommended using FNPO for the definition of PCOM, setting the threshold at 25 or more follicles. If such technology is not available, the recommendation is to use OV for the diagnosis of PCOM.[85]

In adolescents, the use of ultrasound has been challenged by 2 recent guidelines, both of which are in support of the fact that PCOM are nonspecific and transient findings during adolescence.[5,83,86] Furthermore, TV is not routinely performed on presexually active adolescents, and transabdominal ultrasound (TA) results in lower resolution and less accurate observation of ovarian morphology. Based on these observations and in the absence of a true consensus, various ultrasound criteria have been used to define adolescent PCOM. It has been suggested that the defining OV be 11.8 mL (instead of 10 mL as in adults), with a normal upper limit for adolescent FNPO of 17 follicles. A recent study using the old ultrasound criteria for the diagnosis of PCOM in adolescents has found that TA ultrasound is a useful diagnostic tool to determine OV greater than 10 mL and follicle number more than 10 in both lean and obese adolescents. Mortensen et al[87] showed that a significant number of asymptomatic adolescents with PCOM have evidence of abnormal steroidogenesis, although these findings were not found in a study performed by Codner et al.[88] Thus, the question that remains is whether adolescent PCOM is associated with clinically significant abnormalities or even increases the risk of developing PCOS. The studies to date have been inconclusive.

DIAGNOSIS

We suggest that the diagnosis of PCOS in an adolescent girl be made based on the presence of clinical or biochemical evidence of hyperandrogenism in the presence of persistent oligomenorrhea. A PCOM morphology is not sufficient to make a diagnosis in adolescents. Thus, consideration should be given to evaluating any girl with an abnormal degree of hirsutism or menstrual abnormality or any girl with features suggestive of PCOS, such as obesity or hirsutism, particularly if associated with menstrual abnormalities. It is imperative to exclude other causes of hyperandrogenism, such as 21-hydroxylase deficiency (nonclassic congenital adrenal hyperplasia), androgen-secreting neoplasms, androgenic/anabolic drug use, Cushing syndrome, HAIR-AN syndrome, thyroid dysfunction, and hyperprolactinemia. The clinical presentation should be followed by laboratory testing for androgen excess, measuring total or free testosterone via a reliable assay.

Testosterone is the main circulating active androgen, and total serum testosterone concentration is the first-line recommendation for assessing androgen excess in women. The present recommendation is to measure free testosterone concentration directly by equilibrium dialysis or to calculate free testosterone based on the total testosterone measured accurately (eg, by radioimmunoassay using column chromatography or liquid or gas chromatography–mass spectrometry [LC-MS or GC-MS]) and SHBG (eg, measured using competitive binding or a high-quality immune-based assay). There has not been any evidence that measuring androstenedione, the immediate precursor of testosterone, offers better specificity or sensitivity. Similarly, measurement of DHEAS, an androgen precursor produced in the adrenal gland, is not required in routine practice.[3] In addition, recent research has focused on measurements of antimüllerian hormone, which has been shown to be elevated in adolescents and adults with PCOS compared with control groups.[30]

TREATMENT

When approaching the adolescent patient with PCOS, considerations should be given to the multiple aspects of the disease, including (1) menstrual dysfunction, (2) hyperandrogenism, (3) risk of subfertility, (4) metabolic dysfunction/risk of abnormal glucose metabolism, and (5) psychosocial concerns related to the condition itself or the treatment.

Menstrual Dysfunction

Because menstrual dysfunction in adolescent patients with PCOS may present in varying fashions, it is important to recognize that amenorrhea, oligomenorrhea, or menorrhagia/prolonged bleeding all may be consistent with the diagnosis. Patients with menorrhagia or menometrorrhagia may be at risk for anemia as a result of heavy menstrual bleeding and therefore may need iron replacement or even blood transfusion. Nearly 20% of all adolescents and adult women with abnormal uterine bleeding have a bleeding disorder, most commonly von Willebrand disease. Patients with severe abnormal and excessive bleeding should undergo an evaluation for bleeding dyscrasias before starting hormonal treatment.

After correcting any hemodynamic instability, the primary management goal is to regulate the menstrual cycle. Hormonal contraceptives (HCs) remain the first-line treatment of menstrual dysfunction in adolescent patients with PCOS.[5] Combined estrogen/progestin HCs inhibit folliculogenesis; decrease albumin levels and in turn decrease DHEAS; inhibit 5-alpha-reductase; increase SHBG, thereby decreasing bioactive testosterone (by function of the estrogen component); inhibit LH, thereby decreasing thecal cell production of androgens; increase hepatic clearance of testosterone; and compete with androgens at the receptor level (by function of the progestin component).[89,90]

In addition to helping to regulate amenorrhea, oligomenorrhea, and menorrhagia, certain HCs function to improve the signs and symptoms of hyperandrogenism (eg, acne, hirsutism).[5] When choosing an oral HC for use in PCOS patients, consideration should be made toward using a progestin with low or antiandrogenic effects (Table 2). The estrogen component of HCs should be started at a low to moderate dose (20-35 μg).

Table 2

Common progestins and their androgenic effects

Generation	Progestin	Androgenic effect
First	Norgestrel	+++
	Ethynodiol diacetate	+
	Norethindrone	++
Second	Levonorgestrel	++++
Third	Norgestimate	++
Fourth	Drospirenone	-

Complications of oral HC treatment include headache, nausea, breast tenderness, mood changes, weight gain, decreased libido, decreased insulin sensitivity, and increased cholesterol and triglyceride levels. Contraindications to use include pregnancy, prior venous thromboembolism, liver or gallbladder disease, hypertension, migraine with aura, major surgery with prolonged immobilization, severe dyslipidemia/hypertriglyceridemia, or thrombophilia. A careful social history should be taken in all adolescents before an oral HC is prescribed, including family, sexual, and smoking histories. In April 2012, the United States Food and Drug Administration (FDA) announced that the combination HCs containing the 4th-generation synthetic progestin drospirenone (contained in Yaz, Yazmin, and others) may be associated with a 1.7 times higher risk of thrombosis, although other studies have not replicated this difference.[91,92] This progestin in particular has antiandrogenic activity, approximating that of 25 mg of spironolactone, and is efficacious in the treatment of the signs and symptoms of hyperandrogenism (eg, hirsutism). When prescribing this agent as a part of combined HCs, a complete history should be taken and the patient closely monitored for signs or symptoms of thrombosis and other adverse events. (For comparison, though, it is important to remember that the thrombosis risk with any HC is much lower than that of pregnancy.)

Although clinical practice guidelines do not recommend a particular agent (oral contraceptive pill, transdermal patch, vaginal hormonal ring), it is imperative for the provider to take the patient's medical history, risk factors, and personal preferences into consideration when determining a treatment plan.

Hyperandrogenism

The physical effects of hyperandrogenism may manifest in adolescent PCOS patients as acne and hirsutism, both of which may be upsetting to the patient and cause psychosocial distress. Severe acne should be treated by a dermatologist and may involve both topical and oral agents, including retinoids such as isotretinoin.

When assessing hirsutism, it is important to recognize the distribution of hair growth. Familial excessive hair or hypertrichosis, fine vellus hair growth, is not under the influence of androgens and will not improve with antiandrogenic directed treatment. For the adolescent patient, the simplest and safest approach is cosmetic removal of unwanted hair (ie, waxing, plucking, threading, laser treatment). Treatment with HCs can reduce androgen production and thereby improve hirsutism. For refractory cases necessitating frequent unwanted hair removal, spironolactone, an aldosterone-antagonist, potassium-sparing diuretic may be used, starting at a dose of 50 mg twice daily (maximum dose 100 mg twice daily). This medication can cause hyperkalemia, and patients should be cautioned to not take potassium supplements, to have a diet rich in potassium, and to remain well hydrated. In addition, providers should take caution if prescribing both spironolactone and drospirenone together, because this effect can be potentiated. Terminal hair turnover is a slow process, and patients should be told that results may not be visible for at least 6 months.

Fertility Concerns

Although it is true that patients with PCOS may have a more difficult time conceiving, adolescent girls with PCOS must clearly understand that unprotected sex may still lead to unwanted pregnancy, even for those on hormonal contraception. This is especially a concern for adolescents being treated with metformin, which has been the treatment of choice to improve ovulation in PCOS patients. Patients with PCOS are also at increased risk for developing high-risk pregnancy, including gestational diabetes, preterm labor, and preeclampsia.[93,94] These risks are reduced at a normal BMI percentile; therefore, regulation of weight is crucial when these patients are ready to conceive.

Metabolic Dysfunction

Polycystic ovarian syndrome is associated with a number of dysmetabolic concerns, including obesity, hypertension, dyslipidemia, liver dysfunction (nonalcoholic fatty liver disease [NAFLD] and nonalcoholic steatohepatitis [NASH]), abnormal fasting glucose and glucose intolerance, metabolic syndrome, insulin resistance, and type 2 diabetes mellitus,[95] ultimately increasing the risk of early cardiovascular disease. Adolescents with PCOS have an approximately 50% reduction in insulin sensitivity and disproportionately elevated increases in serum insulin levels.[96] Patients with severe hyperandrogenism seem to be at the highest risk for insulin resistance and metabolic inflammation.[97] Although the role of hyperandrogenism itself as a causative factor in the development of metabolic dysfunction has been both implicated as well as called into question, even normal-BMI patients, especially those with insulin resistance, are at elevated risk for cardiometabolic disease compared with normal-BMI non-PCOS controls.[98-101]

Adolescents with a diagnosis of PCOS should be routinely evaluated with measurement of BMI, based on age and gender normative data. Lifestyle interventions, including nutritional education, increased physical activity, and behavioral therapy, have long been regarded as the treatment of choice for weight loss, and patients with a calculated BMI greater than or equal to the 85th percentile (overweight) or greater than or equal to the 95th percentile (obese) must be educated regarding these changes starting from their first medical encounter. Activity should be geared toward aerobic exercise, with a goal of 30 minutes per day, 5 days per week. Other nonaerobic activities, such as yoga, may also be effective in modifying the metabolic profile, although not through weight loss.[102] Dietary changes should be made in concert with a registered dietitian and should be focused on decreasing excessive caloric intake (eg, elimination of sugared beverages such as juice, soda, and sports drink), reducing total calories from carbohydrates, and increasing fruit and vegetable intake.

Weight loss goals in overweight or obese adolescent patients with PCOS should be personalized. Even small reductions of 5% to 10% of body weight can result in striking improvements in both the metabolic and androgen profiles, as well as intima-media thickness, a noninvasive marker of early atherosclerotic disease.[103-105] Adolescents of normal weight who have PCOS may still be at risk for insulin resistance, although monitoring with homeostatic model assessment (HOMA) testing may miss these patients.[106] Normal screening fasting insulin levels, especially in patients with BMI in the normal range, should not be exclusionary for determining the need for medical treatment.

The insulin sensitizer metformin, both in mono- and combination therapy, has been used frequently to help with the metabolic complications of PCOS.[107] Metformin increases insulin sensitivity in the liver, increases peripheral glucose uptake, decreases fatty acid oxidation, and decreases gastrointestinal glucose absorption.[108] A retrospective review showed that patients with PCOS treated with metformin had a reduced conversion rate from normal glucose tolerance to impaired glucose tolerance of 1.4% compared with the expected rate of 16% to 19%. In addition, none of the patients taking metformin progressed to develop frank type 2 diabetes mellitus.[109] A dose of 1500 to 2000 mg daily in 2 divided doses seems to improve insulin resistance, assist with weight loss, improve the lipid panel, and decrease androgens, helping to regulate menses. The main adverse effects of treatment with metformin are gastrointestinal upset, nausea, and vomiting; a gradual increase in the dose may temporize these issues. Metformin could be considered the first-line treatment for those with significant insulin resistance, especially for patients with contraindications for HC use.

Improvement and possible reversal of hyperinsulinism confers improved hyperandrogenism and therefore regulation of menses. Although lifestyle modifications are first line (and should be continued despite any treatment plan), weight loss and maintenance of weight loss are difficult. Patients taking metformin seem to have better success with weight loss and reduction of BMI compared to those using only lifestyle modifications.[96,110] In addition, some evidence supports an improvement in dyslipidemia with metformin as monotherapy compared with metformin plus HC in overweight and obese adolescents with PCOS, although differences between measures of glucose metabolism were similar in both groups.[111] Additionally, early treatment of girls with precocious pubarche and a history of low birth weight (a subgroup notable for an increased incidence of PCOS[11]) with metformin starting between the ages of 8 and 12 years may provide a protective effect with respect to the development of PCOS. Girls treated later with metformin (older than 12 years) were noted to be 2 to 8 times more likely to be diagnosed with PCOS in a 7-year longitudinal study.[112]

For those who cannot or are unable to lose weight, surgical weight loss procedures such as gastric bypass are becoming more popular. What once was exclusively reserved for adult patients is now being used for an increasing number of adolescents. In adult studies, bariatric surgery has resulted in reduction of hyperandrogenism, resumption of menses, and improvement in hirsutism.[113] Adolescent-specific data are not yet available; therefore, bariatric surgery should be reserved only for the most severe cases and performed by a well-trained and experienced surgeon.

Nonalcoholic fatty liver disease, a condition classified as the hepatic manifestation of the metabolic syndrome, is common in PCOS, and its manifestations may be absent or subtle. It may only first be diagnosed upon the finding of abnormally elevated aminotransferase (AST and ALT) levels. Although NAFLD tends to be a clinical diagnosis, ultrasonography is the modality of choice to confirm fatty infiltration of the liver, as imaging does not usually change the treatment plan. Lifestyle modifications, including weight loss, dietary changes, and exercise, are the first-line treatment, with referral to a pediatric gastroenterologist or hepatologist for more complicated or refractory cases.

Psychosocial Concerns

Weight loss, dietary modifications, and increased exercise are the most effective treatments for adolescents with PCOS, but they also are the most difficult to both initiate and maintain. It is important to recognize that making these changes during the adolescent years can result in improved behaviors that continue into adulthood. Education regarding the complications of obesity and PCOS is crucial, along with providing emotional support, nutritionist/dietitian referral, and counseling/mental health referrals as needed, as part of creating independent and health-conscious adolescent patients.

Other Considerations

Overweight and obese adolescents with PCOS are at increased risk for obstructive sleep apnea. Compared with both normal-BMI patients with PCOS as well as BMI-matched non-PCOS patients, they have altered self-reported symptoms (increased sleep-disordered breathing and excessive daytime sleepiness) as well as positive findings on somnography.[114] Studies of adults with PCOS have shown associations between obstructive sleep apnea and insulin resistance, although this finding has not been replicated in pediatric and adolescent studies.[115]

CONCLUSION

A common condition with a variable presentation, PCOS provides a complex set of symptoms for the medical professional. In addition to addressing and managing hyperandrogenism, hirsutism, acne, menstrual dysfunction, and metabolic concerns such as insulin resistance, hypertension, dyslipidemia, and type 2 diabetes mellitus, the physician must meet the patient's psychosocial needs as well. Each feature of PCOS can affect the mental health and well-being of the adolescent patient. Therefore, a multidisciplinary approach involving the primary physician, endocrinologist, gynecologist, dermatologist, nutritionist, social worker, mental health professional, patient, and family will lead to the best chances of success.

References

1. Stein IF, Leventhal ML. Amenorrhea associated with bilateral polycystic ovaries. *Am J Obstet Gynecol.* 1935;29:181-191
2. Fauser BC, Tarlatzis RW, Rebar RS, et al. Consensus on women's health aspects of polycystic ovary syndrome (PCOS): the Amsterdam ESHRE/ASRM-Sponsored 3rd PCOS Consensus Workshop Group. *Fertil Steril.* 2012;97:28-38.e25
3. Azziz R, Sanchez LA, Knochenhauer ES, et al. Androgen excess in women: experience with over 1000 consecutive patients. *J Clin Endocrinol Metab.* 2004;89:453-462
4. Carmina E, Rosato F, Janni A, et al. Extensive clinical experience: relative prevalence of different androgen excess disorders in 950 women referred because of clinical hyperandrogenism. *J Clin Endocrinol Metab.* 2006;91:2-6
5. Legro RS, Arslanian SA, Ehrmann DA, et al. Diagnosis and treatment of polycystic ovary syndrome: an Endocrine Society clinical practice guideline. *J Clin Endocrinol Metab.* 2013;98:4565-4592
6. Bremer AA. Polycystic ovary syndrome in the pediatric population. *Metab Syndr Relat Disord.* 2010;8:375-394
7. Legro RS, Driscoll D, Strauss JF 3rd, et al. Evidence for a genetic basis for hyperandrogenemia in polycystic ovary syndrome. *Proc Natl Acad Sci U S A.* 1998;95:14956-14960
8. Vink JM, Sadrzadeh S, Lambalk CB, et al. Heritability of polycystic ovary syndrome (PCOS) in a Dutch twin-family study. *J Clin Endocrinol Metab.* 2006;91:2100-2104
9. Franks S, Berga S. A Debate: Does PCOS have developmental origins? *Fertil Steril.* 2012;97:2-6
10. Melo AS, Vieira CS, Barbieri MA, et al. High prevalence of polycystic ovary syndrome in women born small for gestational age. *Hum Reprod.* 2010;25:2124-2131

11. Ibañez L, de Zegher F, Potau N. Premature pubarche, ovarian hyperandrogenism, hyperinsulinism and the polycystic ovary syndrome: from a complex constellation to a simple sequence of prenatal onset. *J Endocrinol Invest.* 1998;21:558-566
12. Anderson A, Solorzano CM, McCartney CR. Childhood obesity and its impact on the development of adolescent PCOS. *Semin Reprod Med.* 2014;32:202-213
13. Ehrmann DA, Barnes RB, Rosenfield RL. Polycystic ovary syndrome as a form of functional ovarian hyperandrogenism due to dysregulation of androgen secretion. *Endocrin Rev.* 1995;16:322-353
14. Ibañez, L, Hall J, Potau N, et al. Ovarian 17-hydroxyprogesterone hyperresponsiveness to gonadotropin-releasing hormone (GnRH) agonist challenge in women with polycystic ovary syndrome is not mediated by luteinizing hormone hypersecretion: evidence from GnRH agonist and human chorionic gonadotropin stimulation testing. *J Clin Endocrinol Metab.* 1996;81:4103-4107
15. Jonard S, Dewailly D. The follicular excess in polycystic ovaries, due to intra-ovarian hyperandrogenism, may be the main culprit for the follicular arrest. *Hum Reprod Update.* 2004;10:107-117
16. Rosenfield RL, Mortensen M, Wroblewski K, et al. Determination of the source of androgen excess in functionally atypical polycystic ovary syndrome by a short dexamethasone androgen-suppression test and a low-dose ACTH test. *Hum Reprod.* 2011;26:3138-3146
17. Nelson VL, Legro RS, Strauss JF 3rd, et al. Augmented androgen production is a stable steroidogenic phenotype of propagated theca cells from polycystic ovaries. *Mol Endocrinol.* 1999;13:946-957
18. Zawadzki J, Dunaif A. Diagnostic criteria for polycystic ovary syndrome: towards a rational approach. In: Dunaif A, Givens J, Haseltine F, et al, eds. *Polycystic Ovary Syndrome.* Cambridge, MA: Blackwell Scientific Publications; 1992:377-384
19. Rotterdam ESHRE/ASRM-Sponsored PCOS Consensus Workshop Group. Revised 2003 consensus on diagnostic criteria and long-term health risks related to polycystic ovary syndrome. *Fertil Steril.* 2004;81:19-25
20. Azziz RE, Carmina D, Dewailly E, et al. The Androgen Excess and PCOS Society criteria for the polycystic ovary syndrome: the complete task force report. *Fertil Steril.* 2009;91:456-488
21. Johnson T, Kaplan L, Ouyang P, et al. National Institutes of Health evidence-based methodology workshop on polycystic ovary syndrome (PCOS). Available at: prevention.nih.gov/docs/programs/pcos/FinalReport.pdf. Published December 3-5, 2012. Accessed November 11, 2014
22. Azziz R, Marin C, Hoq L, Badamgarav E, et al. Health care-related economic burden of the polycystic ovary syndrome during the reproductive life span. *J Clin Endocrinol Metab.* 2005;90:4650-4658
23. Carmina E, Chu MC, Longo RA, et al. Phenotypic variation in hyperandrogenic women influences the findings of abnormal metabolic and cardiovascular risk parameters. *J Clin Endocrinol Metab.* 2005;90:2545-2549
24. Coviello A, Legro R, Dunaif A. Adolescent girls with polycystic ovary syndrome have an increased risk of the metabolic syndrome associated with increasing androgen levels independent of obesity and insulin resistance. *J Clin Endocrinol Metab.* 2006;91:492-497
25. Cussons AJ, Watts GF, Burke V, et al. Cardiometabolic risk in polycystic ovary syndrome: a comparison of different approaches to defining the metabolic syndrome. *Hum Reprod.* 2008;23:2352-2358
26. Ehrmann DA, Liljenquist DR, Dasza K, et al. Prevalence and predictors of the metabolic syndrome in women with polycystic ovary syndrome. *J Clin Endocrinol Metab.* 2006;91:48-53
27. Balen A. Polycystic ovary syndrome and cancer. *Hum Reprod Update.* 2001;7:522-525
28. Vuguin P, Linder B, Rosenfeld RG, et al. The roles of insulin sensitivity, insulin-like growth factor I (IGF-I), and IGF-binding protein-1 and -3 in the hyperandrogenism of African-American and Caribbean Hispanic girls with premature adrenarche. *J Clin Endocrinol Metab.* 1999;84:2037-2042
29. Vuguin P, Grinstein G, Freeman K, et al. Prediction models for insulin resistance in girls with premature adrenarche. The premature adrenarche insulin resistance score: PAIR score. *Horm Res.* 2006;65:185-191
30. Franks S. Polycystic ovary syndrome in adolescents. *Int J Obes.* 2008;32:1035-1041

31. van Hooff MH, Voorhorst FJ, Kaptein MB, et al. Endocrine features of polycystic ovary syndrome in a random population sample of 14–16 year old adolescents. *Hum Reprod.* 1999;14:2223-2229
32. Dramusic V, Rajan U, Chan P, et al. Adolescent polycystic ovary syndrome. *Ann NY Acad Sci.* 1997;816:194-208
33. Witchel SF. Puberty and polycystic ovary syndrome. *Mol Cell Endocrinol.* 2006;254-255:146-153
34. Sultan C, Paris F. Clinical expression of polycystic ovary syndrome in adolescent girls. *Fertil Steril.* 2006;86(Suppl 1):S6
35. Agapova SE, Cameo T, Sopher AB, et al. Diagnosis and challenges of polycystic ovary syndrome in adolescence. *Semin Reprod Med.* 2014;32:194-201
36. Gilling-Smith C, Willis DS, Beard RW, et al. Hypersecretion of androstenedione by isolated thecal cells from polycystic ovaries. *J Clin Endocrinol Metab.* 1994;79:1158-1165
37. Maciel GA, Baracat EC, Benda JA, et al. Stockpiling of transitional and classic primary follicles in ovaries of women with polycystic ovary syndrome. *J Clin Endocrinol Metab.* 2004;89:5321-5327
38. Balen AH, Conway GS, Kaltsas G, et al. Polycystic ovary syndrome: the spectrum of the disorder in 1741 patients. *Hum Reprod.* 1995;10:2107-2111
39. Chang WY, Knochenhauer ES, Bartolucci AA, et al. Phenotypic spectrum of polycystic ovary syndrome: clinical and biochemical characterization of the three major clinical subgroups. *Fertil Steril.* 2005;83:1717-1723
40. Kumar A, Woods KS, Bartolucci AA, et al. Prevalence of adrenal androgen excess in patients with the polycystic ovary syndrome (PCOS). *Clin Endocrinol.* 2005;62:644-649
41. Siow Y, Kives S, Hertweck P, et al. Serum Müllerian-inhibiting substance levels in adolescent girls with normal menstrual cycles or with polycystic ovary syndrome. *Fertil Steril.* 2005;84:938-944
42. Ueno S, Kuroda T, MacLaughlin DT, et al. Müllerian-inhibiting substance in the adult rat ovary during various stages of the estrous cycle. *Endocrinology.* 1989;125:1060-1066
43. Omar HA, Logsdon S, Richards J. Clinical profiles, occurrence, and management of adolescent patients with HAIR-AN syndrome. *Sci World J.* 2004;4:507-511
44. Diamanti-Kandarakis E, Papavassiliou AG. Molecular mechanisms of insulin resistance in polycystic ovary syndrome. *Trends Mol Med.* 2006;12:324-332
45. Willis DS, Watson H, Mason HD, et al. Premature response to luteinizing hormone of granulosa cells from anovulatory women with polycystic ovary syndrome: relevance to mechanism of anovulation. *J Clin Endocrinol Metab.* 1998;83:3984-3991
46. Nestler JE, Powers LP, Matt DW, et al. A direct effect of hyperinsulinemia on serum sex hormone-binding globulin levels in obese women with the polycystic ovary syndrome. *J Clin Endocrinol Metab.* 1991;72:83-89
47. Pugeat M, Crave JC, Elmidani M, et al. Pathophysiology of sex hormone binding globulin (SHBG): relation to insulin. *J Steroid Biochem Mol Biol.* 1991;40:841-849
48. Oberfield SE, Sopher AB, Gerken AT. Approach to the girl with early onset of pubic hair. *J Clin Endocrinol Metab.* 2011;96:1610-1622
49. Siegel S, Futterweit W, Davies TF, et al. A C/T single nucleotide polymorphism at the tyrosine kinase domain of the insulin receptor gene is associated with polycystic ovary syndrome. *Fertil Steril.* 2002;78:1240-1243
50. Barber TM, Bennett AJ, Gloyn AL, et al. Relationship between E23K (an established type II diabetes-susceptibility variant within KCNJ11), polycystic ovary syndrome and androgen levels. *Eur J Hum Genet.* 2007;15:679-684
51. Ehrmann DA, Sturis J, Byrne MM, et al. Insulin secretory defects in polycystic ovary syndrome: relationship to insulin sensitivity and family history of non-insulin-dependent diabetes mellitus. *J Clin Invest.* 1995;96:520-527
52. Rosenfield RL. Clinical review: adolescent anovulation: maturational mechanisms and implications. *J Clin Endocrinol Metab.* 2013;98:3572-3583
53. Apter D, Vihko R. Serum pregnenolone, progesterone, 17-hydroxyprogesterone, testosterone and 5 alpha-dihydrotestosterone during female puberty. *J Clin Endocrinol Metab.* 1977;45:1039-1048

54. Apter D, Butzow TL, Laughlin GA, et al. Gonadotropin-releasing hormone pulse generator activity during pubertal transition in girls: pulsatile and diurnal patterns of circulating gonadotropins. *J Clin Endocrinol Metab.* 1993;76:940-949
55. Hardy TS, Norman RJ. Diagnosis of adolescent polycystic ovary syndrome. *Steroids.* 2013;78:751-754
56. Practice Committee of the American Society for Reproductive Medicine. Current evaluation of amenorrhea. *Fertil Steril.* 2004;82:S33-S39
57. Franks S. Adult polycystic ovary syndrome begins in childhood. *Best Pract Res Clin Endocrinol Metab.* 2002;16:263-272
58. Rachmiel M, Kives S, Atenafu E, et al. Primary amenorrhea as a manifestation of polycystic ovarian syndrome in adolescents: a unique subgroup? *Arch Pediatr Adolesc Med.* 2008;162:521-525
59. McManus SS, Levitsky LL, Misra M. Polycystic ovary syndrome: clinical presentation in normal-weight compared with overweight adolescents. *Endocr Pract.* 2013;19:471-478
60. Nair MK, Pappachan P, Balakrishnan S, et al. Menstrual irregularity and polycystic ovarian syndrome among adolescent girls: a 2 year follow-up study. *Indian J Pediatr.* 2012;79(Suppl 1):S69-S73
61. Winters SJ, Talbott E, Guzick DS, et al. Serum testosterone levels decrease in middle age in women with the polycystic ovary syndrome. *Fertil Steril.* 2000;73:724-729
62. West S, Lashen H, Bloigu A, et al. Irregular menstruation and hyperandrogenaemia in adolescence are associated with polycystic ovary syndrome and infertility in later life: Northern Finland Birth Cohort 1986 study. *Hum Reprod.* 2014;29:2339-2351
63. DeUgarte CM, Woods KS, Bartolucci AA, et al. Degree of facial and body terminal hair growth in unselected black and white women: toward a populational definition of hirsutism. *J Clin Endocrinol Metab.* 2006;91:1345-1350
64. Deplewski D, Rosenfield RL. Role of hormones in pilosebaceous unit development. *Endocr Rev.* 2000;21:363-392
65. Martin KA, Chang RJ, Ehrmann DA, et al. Evaluation and treatment of hirsutism in premenopausal women: an endocrine society clinical practice guideline. *J Clin Endocrinol Metab.* 2008;93:1105-1120
66. Farid-ur-Rehman, Sohail I, Hayat Z, et al. Etiology of hirsutism. Is there a correlation between menstrual regularity, body mass index and severity of hirsutism with the cause? *J Pak Assoc Dermatol.* 2010; 20:4-9
67. Saxena P, Prakash A, Nigam A, et al. Polycystic ovary syndrome: Is obesity a sine qua non? A clinical, hormonal, and metabolic assessment in relation to body mass index. *Indian J Endocrinol Metab.* 2012;16:996-999
68. Wijeyaratne CN, Balen AH, Barth JH, et al. Clinical manifestations and insulin resistance (IR) in polycystic ovary syndrome (PCOS) among South Asians and Caucasians: is there a difference? *Clin Endocrinol.* 2002;57:343-350
69. Bekx MT, Connor EC, Allen DB. Characteristics of adolescents presenting to a multidisciplinary clinic for polycystic ovarian syndrome. *J Pediatr Adolesc Gynecol.* 2010;23:7-10
70. Pfeifer SM, Kives S. Polycystic ovary syndrome in the adolescent. *Obstet Gynecol Clin North Am.* 2009;36:129-152
71. Hickey M, Doherty DA, Atkinson H, et al. Clinical, ultrasound and biochemical features of polycystic ovary syndrome in adolescents: implications for diagnosis. *Hum Reprod.* 2011;26:1469-1477
72. Lucky AW, Biro FM, Daniels SR, et al. The prevalence of upper lip hair in black and white girls during puberty: a new standard. *J Pediatr Endocrinol Metab.* 2001;138:134-136
73. van Hooff MH, Voorhorst FJ, Kaptein MB, et al. Predictive values of menstrual cycle pattern, body mass index, hormone levels and polycystic ovaries at aged 15 years for oligo-amenorrhoea at aged 18 years. *Hum Reprod.* 2004;19:383-392
74. Lucky AW, McGuire J, Rosenfield RL, et al. Plasma androgens in women with acne vulgaris. *J Invest Dermatol.* 1983;81:70-74
75. Lucky AW, Koltun W, Thiboutot D, et al. A combined oral contraceptive containing 3mg drospirenone/20µg ethinyl estradiol in the treatment of acne vulgaris: a randomized, double-

blind, placebo-controlled study evaluating lesion counts and participant self-assessment. *Cutis.* 2008;82:143-150
76. Eichenfield LF, Krakowski AC, Piggott C, et al. Evidence-based recommendations for the diagnosis and treatment of pediatric acne. *Pediatrics.* 2013;131:S163-S186
77. Rosner W, Vesper H. Toward excellence in testosterone testing: a consensus statement. *J Clin Endocrinol Metab.* 2010;95:4542-4548
78. Glintborg D, Mumm H, Hougaard D, et al. Ethnic differences in Rotterdam criteria and metabolic risk factors in a multiethnic group of women with PCOS studied in Denmark. *Clin Endocrinol.* 2010;73:732-738
79. Venturoli S, Orsiru LF, Paradisi R, et al. Human urinary follicle stimulating hormone and menopausal gonadotropin in induction of multiple follicle growth and ovulation. *Fertil Steril.* 1986;45:30-35
80. Van Hooff MH, Voorhorst FJ, Kaptein MB, et al. Polycystic ovaries in adolescents and the relationship with menstrual cycle patterns, luteinizing hormone, androgens, and insulin. *Fertil Steril.* 2000;74:49-58
81. Mortensen M, Ehrmann DA, Littlejohn E, et al. Asymptomatic volunteers with a polycystic ovary are a functionally distinct but heterogeneous population. *J Clin Endocrinol Metab.* 2009;94:1579-1586
82. West S, Lashen H, Bloigu A, et al. Irregular menstruation and hyperandrogenaemia in adolescence are associated with polycystic ovary syndrome and infertility in later life: Northern Finland Birth Cohort 1986 study. *Hum Reprod.* 2014;29:2339-2351
83. Venturoli S, Porcu E, Fabbri R, et al. Longitudinal change of sonographic ovarian aspects and endocrine parameters in irregular cycles of adolescence. *Pediatr Res.* 1995;38:974-980
84. Apter D, Vihko R. Endocrine determinants of fertility: serum androgen concentrations during follow-up of adolescents into the third decade of life. *J Clin Endocrinol Metab.* 1990;71:970-974
85. Dewailly D, Lujan ME, Carmina E, et al. Definition and significance of polycystic ovarian morphology: a task force from the Androgen Excess and Polycystic Ovary Syndrome Society. *Hum Reprod Update.* 2014;20:334-352
86. Boyle J, Teede HJ. Polycystic ovary syndrome: an update. *Aust Fam Physician.* 2012;41:752-756
87. Mortensen M, Rosenfield RL, Littlejohn E. Functional significance of polycystic-size ovaries in healthy adolescents. *J Clin Endocrinol Metab.* 2006;9:3786
88. Codner E, Villarroel C, Eyzaguirre FC, et al. Polycystic ovarian morphology in postmenarchal adolescents. *Fertil Steril.* 2011;95:702
89. Cassidenti DL, Paulson RJ, Serafini P, et al. Effects of sex steroids on skin 5 alpha-reductase activity in vitro. *Obstet Gynecol.* 1991;78:103-107
90. Weigratz I, Kutschera E, Lee JH, et al. Effect of four different oral contraceptives on various sex hormones and serum-binding globulins. *Contraception.* 2003;67:25-32
91. United States Food and Drug Administration (FDA). Combined hormonal contraceptives (CHCs) and the risk of cardiovascular disease endpoints. Available at: www.fda.gov/downloads/Drugs/DrugSafety/ucm277384. Accessed December 9, 2014
92. Manzoli L, De Vito C, Marzuillo C, et al. Oral contraceptives and venous thromboembolism: a systematic review and meta-analysis. *Drug Saf.* 2012;35:191-205
93. Boomsma CM, Eijkemans MJ, Hughes EG, et al. A meta-analysis of pregnancy outcomes in women with polycystic ovary syndrome. *Hum Reprod Update.* 2006;12:673-683
94. Haakova L, Cibula D, Rezabek K, et al. Pregnancy outcome in women with PCOS and in controls matched by age and weight. *Hum Reprod.* 2003;18:1438-1441
95. Barfield E, Liu Y, Kessler M, et al. The prevalence of abnormal liver enzymes and metabolic syndrome in obese adolescent females with polycystic ovary syndrome. *J Pediatr Adolesc Gynecol.* 2009;22:318-322
96. Lewy VD, Danadian K, Witchel SF, et al. Early metabolic abnormalities in adolescent girls with polycystic ovarian syndrome. *J Pediatr.* 2001;138:38-44

97. Alemzadeh R, Kichler J, Calhoun M. Spectrum of metabolic dysfunction in relationship with hyperandrogenemia in obese adolescent girls with polycystic ovary syndrome. *Eur J Endocr.* 2010;162:1093-1099
98. Hart R, Doherty DA, Mori T, et al. Extent of metabolic risk in adolescent girls with features of polycystic ovary syndrome. *Fertil Steril.* 2011;95:2347-2353
99. Fruzzetti F, Perini D, Lazzarini V, et al. Hyperandrogenemia influences the prevalence of the metabolic syndrome abnormalities in adolescents with the polycystic ovary syndrome. *Gynecol Endocrinol.* 2009;25:335-343
100. Forrester-Dumont K, Galescu O, Kolenikov A, et al. Hyperandrogenism does not influence metabolic parameters in adolescent girls with PCOS. *Int J Endocrinol.* 2012;2012:434830
101. Flannery CA, Rackow B, Cong X, et al. Polycystic ovary syndrome in adolescence: impaired glucose tolerance occurs across the spectrum of BMI. *Pediatric Diabetes.* 2013;14:42-49
102. Nidhi R, Padmalatha V, Nagarathna R, et al. Effect of a yoga program on glucose metabolism and blood lipid levels in adolescent girls with polycystic ovary syndrome. *Int J Gynaecol Obstet.* 2012;118:37-41
103. Hoeger KM. Role of lifestyle modification in the management of polycystic ovary syndrome. *Best Pract Res Clin Endocrinol Metab.* 2006;20:293
104. Hoeger K, Davidson K, Kochman L, et al. The impact of metformin, oral contraceptives, and lifestyle modification on polycystic ovary syndrome in obese adolescent women in two randomized, placebo-controlled clinical trials. *J Clin Endocrinol Metab.* 2008;93:4299-4306
105. Lass N, Kleber M, Winkel K, et al. Effect of lifestyle intervention on features of polycystic ovarian syndrome, metabolic syndrome, and intima-media thickness in obese adolescent girls. *J Clin Endocrinol Metab.* 2011;96:3533-3540
106. Fulghesu AM, Angioni S, Portoghese E, et al. Failure of the homeostatic model assessment calculation score for detecting metabolic deterioration in young patients with polycystic ovary syndrome. *Fertil Steril.* 2006;86:398-404
107. Geller DH, Pacaud D, Gordon CM, et al. State of the art review: emerging therapies: the use of insulin sensitizers in the treatment of adolescents with polycystic ovary syndrome (PCOS). *Int J Pediatr Endocrinol.* 2011;2011:9
108. Foretz M, Guigas B, Bertrand L, et al. Metformin: from mechanisms of action to therapies. *Cell Metab.* 2014;20:953-966
109. Sharma ST, Wickman EP III, Nestler JE. Changes in glucose tolerance with metformin treatment in polycystic ovary syndrome: a retrospective analysis. *Endocr Pract.* 2007;13:373
110. Palomba S, Materazzo C, Falbo A, et al. Metformin, oral contraceptives or both to manage oligoamenorrhea in adolescents with polycystic ovary syndrome? A clinical review. *Gynecol Endocrinol.* 2014;30:335-340
111. Bredella MA, McManus S, Misra M. Impact of metformin monotherapy versus metformin with oestrogen-progesterone on lipids in adolescent girls with polycystic ovarian syndrome. *Clin Endocrinol (Oxf).* 2013;79:199-203
112. Ibáñez L, López-Bermejo A, Díaz M, et al. Early metformin therapy (age 8-12 years) in girls with precocious pubarche to reduce hirsutism, androgen excess, and oligomenorrhea in adolescence. *J Clin Endocrinol Metab.* 2011;96:E1262-E1267
113. Escobar-Morreale HF, Botella-Carretero JI, Alvarez-Blasco F, et al. The polycystic ovary syndrome associated with morbid obesity may resolve after weight loss induced by bariatric surgery. *J Clin Endocrinol Metab.* 2005;90:6364-6369
114. Nandalike K, Strauss T, Agarwal C, et al. Screening for sleep-disordered breathing and excessive daytime sleepiness in adolescent girls with polycystic ovarian syndrome. *J Pediatr.* 2011;159:591-596
115. De Sousa G, Schluter B, Menke T, et al. Relationships between polysomnographic variables, parameters of glucose metabolism, and serum androgens in obese adolescents with polycystic ovarian syndrome. *J Sleep Res.* 2011;20:472-478

Adrenal Dysfunction

Phyllis W. Speiser, MD

Chief, Division of Pediatric Endocrinology, Cohen Children's Medical Center of New York, Professor of Pediatrics, North Shore-Long Island Jewish Health System, Hofstra–North Shore LIJ School of Medicine, Hempstead, New York

Adrenal cortical disease, especially adrenal insufficiency, is more common than adrenal medullary disease and often goes unrecognized for extended periods. Physicians should consider the diagnosis of adrenal insufficiency in any patient with nonspecific unexplained signs or symptoms, including hypoglycemia, growth failure, weight loss, vomiting, or lethargy. The clinical features may be mistaken for, and should be differentiated from, infection, malnutrition, gastrointestinal disease, inborn errors of metabolism, anorexia nervosa, chronic fatigue syndrome, and depression.

ANATOMY AND PHYSIOLOGY

The adrenal glands each weighs about 4 g in full-term infants at birth, which is equivalent to that of adult glands. However, adrenal size decreases by about 50% to 60% within the first week of life and then enlarges in mid-childhood at the time of adrenarche. There is an inner medulla and an outer cortex, linked by vascular supply and hormonal influence. Within the mature adrenal cortex are 3 functionally distinct zones: (1) the glomerulosa, comprising about 15% of the gland; (2) the fasciculata, the largest zone, comprising about 75% of the gland; and (3) the reticularis, comprising about 10% of the gland.

The adrenal medulla is regulated by the sympathetic nervous system and secretes catecholamines, whereas the 3 zones of the cortex secrete steroid hormones, categorized as mineralocorticoids, glucocorticoids, and sex steroids, respectively. Mineralocorticoid production, exemplified by aldosterone, is principally regulated by the renin-angiotensin axis and by ambient potassium levels. Mineralocorticoids govern sodium and potassium homeostasis, and deficiencies in their production or action cause hyponatremia, hyperkalemia, and dehydration. Glu-

E-mail address: pspeiser@NSHS.edu

cocorticoid and adrenal sex steroid production are primarily regulated by pituitary corticotrophin (adrenocorticotropic hormone [ACTH]) and hypothalamic corticotrophin-releasing hormone, secreted mainly in the early morning hours (0400-0800 hours) or in response to stress. Cortisol is the main glucocorticoid, and dehydroepiandrosterone (DHEA) is the main adrenal sex hormone. The latter is only a weak androgen, but it may be converted via androstenedione to either estrogens or androgens. The placenta uses fetal adrenal DHEA to produce estrogens, especially estriol, a marker hormone of fetal viability. Rising levels of DHEA and its sulfate later in childhood signal adrenarche, which usually precedes the development of body hair and apocrine odor at puberty.[1]

Glucocorticoids promote protein and lipid breakdown and inhibit protein synthesis. The effects of cortisol counterregulate those of insulin, increasing the concentration of glucose by stimulating gluconeogenesis and by decreasing glucose utilization in muscle. The net effect is increased production and conservation of glucose for use by essential tissues, such as the brain and red blood cells, at the expense of less essential tissues during times of stress or starvation. Physicians should be aware that therapeutic doses of glucocorticoids are almost always supraphysiologic and may suppress growth by antagonizing the production and action of growth hormones (GHs). Susceptibility to these effects is quite variable and may be based in part on polymorphism in the glucocorticoid receptors.[2]

Cortisol contributes to the maintenance of normal blood pressure through several mechanisms, notably by increasing vascular sensitivity to pressors. At high concentrations, cortisol acts as a mineralocorticoid agonist, causing sodium and water retention. Cortisol and aldosterone deficiencies often result in shock if unrecognized and untreated.[3]

ADRENAL INSUFFICIENCY

History and Physical Examination

The symptoms of cortisol deficiency include lethargy, fatigue, weakness, dizziness, and anorexia. Signs detected at physical examination include hyperpigmentation, orthostatic hypotension, tachycardia, and weight loss. These findings are nonspecific and gradual in onset, and they may be mistaken for infection, malnutrition, gastrointestinal disease, inborn errors of metabolism, anorexia, chronic fatigue syndrome, or depression. In some patients, gastrointestinal symptoms such as abdominal cramps, nausea, vomiting, and diarrhea are prominent. In adolescents and adults, sexual or reproductive dysfunction with decreased libido, potency, or amenorrhea may accompany either primary or secondary adrenal insufficiency. Orthostatic hypotension is more marked in primary than secondary adrenal insufficiency. This is because primary adrenal insufficiency is often associated with a combination of cortisol, aldosterone, and, in some cases, catecholamine deficiencies.

The most commonly recognized screening laboratory findings are hypoglycemia and low early morning plasma cortisol. Such patients should be referred to a pediatric endocrinologist for further evaluation.

Patients with chronic primary adrenal insufficiency often have hyperpigmentation of the non–sun-exposed skin and mucosal surfaces. This is the result of high plasma corticotrophin (ACTH) and accompanying melanocyte-stimulating hormone secretion because of absent cortisol feedback. Skin pigment changes may be difficult to appreciate in dark-skinned individuals. In contrast, patients with secondary adrenal insufficiency tend to be pale. Another symptom of primary adrenal insufficiency is a craving for salt, which is a result of aldosterone deficiency and resultant sodium wasting. Weight loss and failure to thrive may also be observed. Loss of axillary or pubic hair is common among hypoadrenal patients, who have low levels of adrenal androgens.

Individuals with secondary adrenal insufficiency might have delayed growth and puberty, manifestations of multiple anterior pituitary hormone deficiencies including GH, and gonadotropin deficiencies in addition to ACTH deficiency. Polyuria and polydipsia indicative of diabetes insipidus may also be seen in pituitary disorders affecting the neurohypophysis. Chronic unexplained signs or symptoms such as those already described should prompt consultation with a pediatric endocrinologist to determine whether further testing is required. Patients in hypotensive crisis or shock at the time they seek care should be treated urgently in the office or transferred immediately by ambulance to the nearest emergency center.

Pathology

Primary adrenal disease may be associated with either glandular hypoplasia or hyperplasia. The most common forms of adrenal pathology involve either deficient or excessive cortisol production. Table 1 lists various causes of adrenal insufficiency. Only the most commonly encountered disorders will be reviewed in detail in this article. Online Mendelian Inheritance in Man (OMIM) should be consulted for a more detailed discussion of rarer diseases; OMIM catalog numbers for each adrenal disease are listed in Table 1.

Causes Primary of Adrenal Failure

Congenital adrenal hyperplasia (CAH) is the most common inborn error in adrenal function and the most common cause of adrenal insufficiency in the pediatric age group. It is most often caused by deficiency of steroid 21-hydroxy-

Table 1
Causes of adrenal cortical insufficiency

Primary

Disorders Associated with Adrenal Gland Hyperplasia
21-Hydroxylase deficiency (gene *CYP21A2*, OMIM 210910)
3β-Hydroxysteroid dehydrogenase deficiency (gene *HSD3B2*, OMIM 201810)
Cholesterol desmolase deficiency (gene *CYP11A*, OMIM 201710, 118485)
Lipoid hyperplasia (gene *STAR*, OMIM 201710)
Glucocorticoid resistance (gene *GCCR*, OMIM 138040)
Wolman disease (gene *LIPA*, OMIM 278000)

Disorders Associated with Adrenal Gland Hypoplasia
Adrenal hypoplasia congenita (gene *NR0B1[DAX-1]*, OMIM 300200)
Adrenocortical insufficiency with or without ovarian defect (gene *NR5A1 [SF-1]*, OMIM 184757)
Familial glucocorticoid deficiency (ACTH resistance) (gene *MC2R/MRAP*, OMIM 202200)
Triple A (ACTH resistance, achalasia, alacrima) (gene *AAAS*, OMIM 231550)
IMAGe (intrauterine growth retardation, metaphyseal dysplasia, adrenal hypoplasia congenital and genital anomalies) syndrome (X-linked, OMIM 300290)

Metabolic Diseases
Adrenoleukodystrophy (X-linked) (gene *ABCD1*, OMIM 300100)
Smith-Lemli-Opitz syndrome (gene *DCHR7*, OMIM 270400)
Kearns-Sayre syndrome (gene *mitochondrial DNA deletions*, OMIM 530000)

Disorders Associated with Isolated Aldosterone Deficiency
Pseudohypoaldosteronism, type 1 (AR) (gene *ENaC*, OMIM 264350)
Pseudohypoaldosteronism, type 1 (AD) (gene *MR*, OMIM 177735)
Pseudohypoaldosteronism, type 2 (AR) (gene *WNK4; WNK1*, OMIM 145260)
Corticosterone methyl oxidase deficiency I (gene *CYP11B2*, OMIM 124080)
Corticosterone methyl oxidase deficiency I (gene *CYP11B2*, OMIM 610600)

Acquired
Autoimmune adrenalitis, isolated
Autoimmune polyendocrine syndrome type 1 (gene *AIRE*, OMIM 240300)
Autoimmune polyendocrine syndrome type 2 (gene *MICA5.1 and HLA-DR3/DQ2*, OMIM 269200)
Hemorrhage or infarction resulting from
    Trauma
    Waterhouse-Friderichsen syndrome
    Anticoagulation
    Drug effects (aminoglutethimide, mitotane, ketoconazole, metyrapone, medroxyprogesterone, megestrol, etomidate, rifampin, phenytoin, barbiturates)
    Infection
    Virus (human immunodeficiency virus, cytomegalovirus)
    Fungus (coccidiomycosis, histoplasmosis, blastomycosis, cryptococcosis)
    Mycobacterium (tuberculosis)
    Amebic
    Infiltrative
        Hemochromatosis, histiocytosis, sarcoidosis, amyloidosis
        Neoplasm

Secondary

Hypothalamus
Congenital
Septo-optic dysplasia (gene *HESX1*, OMIM 182230)

Corticotropin releasing hormone deficiency (gene *CRH*, OMIM 122560)
Maternal hypercortisolemia
Acquired
Inflammatory disorders
Trauma
Radiotherapy
Surgery
Tumors
Infiltrative disease (sarcoidosis, histiocytosis X)
Steroid withdrawal after prolonged administration

Pituitary
Congenital
Pituitary hormone deficiency, combined (gene *POU1F1/PIT1*, OMIM 173110, gene *PROP-1*, OMIM 601538)
Proopiomelanocortin deficiency (gene *POMC*, OMIM 609734)
Proconvertase 1 (gene *PCSK1*, OMIM 600955)
Isolated ACTH deficiency (gene *TBX19/TPIT*, OMIM 604614)
Acquired
Trauma
Tumor (craniopharyngioma)
Radiotherapy
Lymphocytic hypophysitis
Steroid withdrawal after prolonged administration

lase.[4] In classic severe salt-wasting CAH, both cortisol and aldosterone production are impaired, whereas adrenal androgen production is excessive. As a result of the lack of the vital hormones cortisol and aldosterone, patients are susceptible to potentially lethal adrenal insufficiency if untreated; this is also true of other forms of CAH that interrupt synthesis of these hormones (eg, the rarer 3β-hydroxysteroid dehydrogenase deficiency and cholesterol desmolase deficiency). Excess androgen production, a side effect of 21-hydroxylase deficiency, causes genital ambiguity in newborn girls. In contrast, boys affected with severe 21-hydroxylase deficiency have no overt genital anomalies. To prevent mortality from adrenal crisis, among other reasons, the United States and many other countries perform newborn screening for this disease. Prompt treatment with glucocorticoids and mineralocorticoids is lifesaving. About one-fourth of patients with classic CAH produce enough aldosterone to avoid salt-wasting crises and are termed *simple virilizers*.

A milder, nonclassic form of CAH not associated with genital ambiguity or adrenal insufficiency may be missed by newborn screening programs. Because nonclassic CAH is characterized by less marked adrenal androgen excess, symptoms and signs do not often develop before middle childhood. These often include early growth of pubic hair or rapid advances in height in both sexes. In many cases, nonclassic CAH in these individuals either goes undetected or is diagnosed in adolescent girls or women with hirsutism, oligomenorrhea, or acne.

The mild form of CAH may be mistaken in girls for polycystic ovarian syndrome.[5]

Not all persons with nonclassic 21-hydroxylase deficiency are symptomatic. Boys in particular are much less likely to be troubled by this mild adrenal hormone imbalance. Even some girls and women remain asymptomatic. Thus, in the absence of precocious pubarche or other symptoms of androgen excess, treatment may not be needed.

Laboratory Evaluation
The diagnosis of CAH rests on both the clinical manifestations and specific hormone measurements. The gold standard test is a corticotropin-stimulated serum 17-hydroxyprogesterone, although analysis of serum levels of this hormone taken before 0800 hours may also be diagnostic. This is true because of the natural circadian pattern of endogenous ACTH secretion, which is highest between 0400 and 0800. It is important to measure adrenal hormones by the method of tandem mass spectrometry in an endocrine specialty laboratory that follows strict quality-control standards to avoid false-positive high levels generated by other nonspecific assays that capture cross-reacting hormones.

Genetics
Phenotypic variability among classic and nonclassic forms of CAH is attributable to allelic variation in the gene encoding active steroid 21-hydroxylase, *CYP21A2*. The disease is inherited as an autosomal recessive trait. There are more than 150 known disease-causing mutations, but approximately 10 mutations comprise about 90% of disease alleles in most populations. The spectrum of disease ranges from severe to mild, depending on which *CYP21A2* mutations are carried by the patient. Genotyping can be useful in verifying an equivocal hormonal diagnosis and is particularly valuable in prenatal diagnosis and genetic counseling.[6]

Management and Long-Term Follow-up
Congenital adrenal hyperplasia is treatable with oral corticosteroid medications. In its classic form, CAH requires lifelong medical management. Salt-wasting patients require both glucocorticoids and mineralocorticoids in early life. However, increasing dietary salt consumption may permit mineralocorticoids to be tapered and in some cases discontinued. Infants who consume very little dietary sodium, patients in tropical climates, and those who engage in intense exercise with excessive sweat sodium losses may require supplemental sodium chloride. Poorly controlled simple virilizing patients also benefit from mineralocorticoid therapy because it spares the use of high-dose glucocorticoids in some cases. Symptomatic nonclassic patients require low-dose glucocorticoids therapy only.[6] The preferred drugs are hydrocortisone for its lower potential for adverse side effects and fludrocortisone as the only available oral mineralocorticoid. Table 2 lists approximate relative glucocorticoids potencies.

Table 2

Glucocorticoid potencies

Drug	Potency relative to cortisol	Equivalent cortisol dose	Mineralocorticoid activity
Cortisol (hydrocortisone)	1	100	+
Cortisone	0.8	125	+
Prednisone	5	20	−
Prednisolone	5	20	−
Methylprednisolone	6	17	−
Dexamethasone	50	2	−

+ indicates present; − indicates absent.

Dosing should be titrated to maintain the levels of adrenal androgen precursors in the normal to mildly increased range. The assay should consist of 17-hydroxyprogesterone, androstenedione, and testosterone; plasma renin activity is added to this profile in patients requiring mineralocorticoid replacement. Blood pressure should be monitored regularly in all patients. Attempts to suppress 17-hydroxyprogesterone to the normal range usually require excessively high glucocorticoids doses and have the undesirable consequence of growth suppression and iatrogenic Cushing syndrome. Measurement of ACTH is not helpful; this hormone seldom is completely suppressible in treated CAH patients. It is important to recognize that testosterone is not as useful a hormonal marker of adequate therapy in adolescent boys and men, although it is helpful in managing prepubertal children of both sexes as well as adolescent girls and women.

Other aspects of CAH treatment include ensuring that adolescent females with severe forms of CAH undergo gynecologic examination in anticipation of sexual activity. Vaginoplasty may be necessary, depending on whether and which genital surgical procedures were performed in the past.[7] Psychological counseling should be provided to these young women by a professional experienced in treating this type of disorder.[8]

Adolescent boys should undergo careful testicular palpation and sonography to exclude testicular adrenal rests that can compromise fertility. Strict control of adrenal hormone levels can shrink such benign tumors in many cases.[9]

Other Causes of Adrenal Failure

Primary adrenal insufficiency is estimated to affect about 100 per million people.[10] The syndrome, originally described by English physician Thomas Addison, included wasting, hyperpigmentation, and adrenal gland atrophy. In adults, more than 80% of cases are caused by autoimmune adrenal destruction, which is most prevalent in women aged 25 to 45 years but is observed in both sexes at any age. The female-to-male ratio is about 3:1. Autoimmune adrenalitis may be isolated or found in association with other autoimmune syndromes. Autoimmune polyendocrine syndrome 1 (APECED; caused by defects in the AIRE autoimmune regulator gene) is associated with autoimmune polyendocrinopathy, candidiasis, and ectodermal dystrophy. Addison disease and autoimmune hypoparathyroidism may be accompanied by autoimmune pernicious anemia, hepatitis, thyroiditis, and diabetes. The age at onset and severity of each of these problems are variable. Autoimmune polyendocrine syndrome 2, also termed *Schmidt syndrome*, is associated with Addison disease, autoimmune thyroiditis, and diabetes; no specific gene defect has been identified to date. Table 1 lists other rare diseases associated with adrenal insufficiency.

Adrenal infiltration by tuberculosis is the second most common cause worldwide. Infection by human immunodeficiency virus is another potential infectious cause of adrenalitis.[10] Both of these infections tend to cause insidious progression to hypoadrenalism. In contrast, catastrophic adrenal hemorrhage during overwhelming bacterial sepsis causes the abrupt onset of adrenal failure, from which patients may eventually recover.[11]

Perhaps because of its rarity in children and adolescents or the nonspecific symptoms, the diagnosis of adrenal insufficiency is frequently delayed or missed. If unrecognized, adrenal insufficiency may present as a life-threatening crisis with acute cardiovascular collapse.

History and Physical Examination
As noted earlier, signs and symptoms of adrenal insufficiency may include abdominal pain, headache, anorexia, weight loss, lethargy, postural hypotension or shock, proneness to dehydration, salt craving, and hyperpigmentation. Patients with adrenal insufficiency with and without GH deficiency may have hypoglycemia, but this is seldom severe enough to cause seizures.

Laboratory Evaluation
Primary adrenal insufficiency can be detected on the basis of low early morning (0800 hours) cortisol accompanied by increased ACTH. If zona glomerulosa function is affected, hyponatremia and hyperkalemia will be accompanied by high plasma renin activity and low serum aldosterone. In adrenal insufficiency as a result of pituitary or hypothalamic dysfunction, ACTH levels will be inappropriately low in comparison with a low cortisol measurement. The diagnosis can be confirmed by absence of at least a 2-fold increment in serum cortisol 60 minutes after stimulation with a standard dose of intravenous cosyntropin (ACTH 1–24). A low dose of cosyntropin can be used to test ACTH reserve in cases of suspected secondary adrenal insufficiency. The threshold for a normal cortisol response is variably 16 to 18 μg/dL.[10]

Imaging Studies
Adrenal hemorrhage, if suspected, can be detected by ultrasonography or computed tomographic (CT) scan.

Management
Once the diagnosis of adrenal insufficiency is established, continuing reminders to patients, families, and medical personnel regarding the need for higher doses of glucocorticoid replacement therapy during intercurrent illnesses and surgery are required. Failure to increase glucocorticoid supplementation during physical stress remains a significant cause of morbidity and mortality in these patients. Patients should be given letters explaining their condition and appropriate emergency management. Sample letters may be found at the Web sites of the National Adrenal Diseases Foundation (www.nadf.us/tools/Addison's_Disease_Alert_Flyer.pdf) for patients with Addison disease and the Congenital Adrenal Hyperplasia Research Education & Support Foundation (www.caresfoundation.org/dosing/illness-and-emergency) for patients with CAH. The latter Web site provides a link to an instructional video on emergency intramuscular hydrocortisone injection.

SECONDARY ADRENAL INSUFFICIENCY

Secondary adrenal insufficiency is more common than primary adrenal insufficiency. The estimated prevalence is 150 to 280 per million people.[12] Abrupt discontinuation of glucocorticoid therapy exacerbated by stress is the most frequent cause of secondary adrenal insufficiency. This results from the widespread chronic treatment of inflammatory and neoplastic conditions with glucocorticoids. Acute hypoglycemia as a symptom of adrenal insufficiency has even been reported after the use of inhaled glucocorticoids.[13] It is important to recognize that normal statural growth does not preclude adrenal suppression during treatment with inhaled glucocorticoids.[14]

Administration of steroids orally, intramuscularly, intranasally, inhaled, transdermally, or intraorbitally may result in suppression of the hypothalamic-pituitary-adrenal axis. As few as 2 weeks of high-dose glucocorticoid treatment may result in suppression of endogenous cortisol production for up to a year.[15] In children being treated for leukemia, a 4-week course of glucocorticoids has been shown to suppress the hypothalamic-pituitary axis for up to 8 weeks after discontinuation.[16] Suppression of the axis cannot reliably be predicted by either the dose or the duration of therapy.[17]

Laboratory Evaluation

Documentation of an intact hypothalamic-pituitary-adrenal axis should be obtained before a patient with a known history of glucocorticoid treatment undergoes surgery. This may be accomplished by documenting plasma cortisol level taken at 0800 hours of more than 10 μg/dL or by performing a cosyntropin (ACTH 1–24) challenge test and observing blood cortisol levels greater than 15 μg/dL after 30 to 60 minutes. Another robust test of ACTH reserve is insulin-induced hypoglycemia; however, many physicians are reluctant to use this test because of the danger of potential hypoglycemic seizures. If such documentation cannot be obtained in time, it is safest to treat patients with supplemental stress corticosteroid coverage in the perioperative period within 1 year of withdrawal of therapy.[18]

Most secondary adrenal insufficiency that is unrelated to withdrawal of glucocorticoid therapy occurs in association with other pituitary hormone deficiencies. *Panhypopituitarism,* or deficiency of 2 or more pituitary hormones, may be either congenital or acquired. Anatomic abnormalities in the pituitary or stalk may be detected on magnetic resonance imaging (MRI). A history of head trauma or cranial surgery should raise suspicion of potential pituitary dysfunction.[19] Aside from these causes of secondary adrenal insufficiency, there are several other rare syndromes, including ACTH resistance associated with triple A syndrome (ACTH resistance, alacrima, and achalasia). This clinical picture is caused by mutations in the *AAAS* gene encoding a protein of uncertain function.[20] In contrast, an isolated form of ACTH resistance is caused by a different genetic defect in the gene encoding the ACTH receptor *MC2R*, as well as several more recently identified genetic causes. This syndrome is characterized by a familial form of glucocorticoid deficiency associated with hyperpigmentation and hypoglycemia without accompanying systemic abnormalities.[21] In the category of inflammatory and immune disorders, granulomatous diseases such as sarcoid, which is rare in the age group younger than 20 years,[22] or histiocytosis[23] can cause pituitary failure leading to secondary adrenal insufficiency.

The risk of adrenal crisis in adults with primary adrenal insufficiency is slightly higher (3.8 admissions per 100 patient-years) compared with those having secondary adrenal insufficiency (2.5 per 100 patient-years).[12] Information concerning mortality in secondary adrenal insufficiency mostly comes from follow-up of individuals treated with pituitary GH. Up to a 4-fold increase in mortality has been observed compared with the general population in children treated with pituitary GH.[24-27] This is presumably because patients with 1 pituitary hormone deficiency are more likely to develop other hormone deficiencies over time. Deaths were often attributed to hypoglycemia or secondary adrenal insufficiency.

Management of secondary adrenal deficiency is similar to that of primary adrenal insufficiency. It usually is not helpful to measure ACTH or cortisol levels in plasma to gauge the efficacy of treatment with corticosteroids. Rather, the patient's growth, weight gain, vital signs, and her own sense of well-being should guide therapy.

Relative Adrenal Insufficiency in the Intensive Care Unit

Among critically ill children and adolescents, a low incremental cortisol response to ACTH does not predict mortality.[28] Much controversy exists regarding how to best look for adrenal insufficiency in hospitalized patients, as well as whether and when to treat.[29] Glucocorticoid treatment of shock remains controversial because most of the published trials had methodologic flaws, varied endpoints, and conflicting outcomes.[30] Thus, the decision to treat a critically ill patient with glucocorticoids must be made on a case-by-case basis until further definitive evidence is available from prospective randomized trials.

Management of Acute Adrenal Insufficiency

Hypotension and lethargy are common signs at presentation of acute adrenal insufficiency. Patients and family members should be taught to recognize a change in energy level or demeanor as potential warning signs in patients with an established diagnosis. Acute adrenal insufficiency may occur during febrile illness, especially one accompanied by dehydration, vomiting, or diarrhea. Supplemental stress dosing is required in such circumstances, and families must be instructed as to proper management. Individuals who are unable to tolerate oral fluids or medications or stress doses during an illness require parenteral isotonic fluids and glucocorticoid administration. In the absence of diarrhea, a temporizing option is to administer rectal hydrocortisone suppositories.[31]

Once the patient is seen in the emergency department, a large-bore intravenous catheter should be inserted for repletion of intravascular volume with saline solutions containing at least 5% dextrose because of the risk of hypoglycemia in adrenal crisis. If the patient's adrenal status is unknown, blood should be drawn for cortisol, electrolytes, glucose, ACTH, plasma renin activity, and aldosterone, preferably before exogenous steroids are administered. If acute and severe adrenal insufficiency is suspected, however, treatment should not by delayed while awaiting results of diagnostic testing. Simultaneous with the administration of fluids, stress doses of glucocorticoids should be given parenterally. Hydrocortisone is the treatment of choice because of its quick onset of action and mineralocorticoid activity.[32]

Prednisone and dexamethasone are long-acting glucocorticoids with a slower onset of biologic action; neither has mineralocorticoid activity. Table 2 lists the relative potencies of various steroid medications. Prednisone is not an ideal choice for treating acute adrenal crisis because it must be converted to prednisolone to be effective. Dexamethasone does not cross-react in cortisol assays, so a diagnostic ACTH stimulation test may be performed right after its administration.

Liberal quantities of intravenous sodium chloride accompanied by large doses of hydrocortisone usually will restore normotension and correct electrolyte abnormalities, obviating mineralocorticoid treatment or pressor agents in adrenal crisis. As vital signs stabilize, glucocorticoids and fluid infusions are tapered over several days. Once the patient is able to eat and take oral medications, oral glucocorticoids may be substituted at regular maintenance doses, generally about 10 mg/m^2/day. Fludrocortisone is given in primary adrenal insufficiency if aldosterone production is inadequate. Supplemental sodium chloride may be provided if dietary salt intake is low.

Chronic Replacement Therapy

Maintenance glucocorticoid replacement therapy is based on estimated normal cortisol secretion rates.[33] Glucocorticoid dosing must be individually adjusted to prevent signs and symptoms of adrenal insufficiency while also preventing the growth retardation and cushingoid features that can accompany overtreatment. Once growth is complete, longer-acting glucocorticoids such as prednisone or dexamethasone may be considered to enhance adherence. In general, lower doses of glucocorticoids are required to treat Addison disease compared with CAH. It is not usually helpful to measure plasma cortisol or ACTH levels in titrating the glucocorticoid dose. Patients with low serum sodium, high potassium, or increased plasma renin activity should receive daily oral fludrocortisone and sodium chloride supplements, adjusted to normalize these analytes. The patient's own sense of well-being, energy level, and blood pressure can help guide the adequacy of therapy in patients with Addison disease. Frequent headaches, lethargy, nausea, vomiting, or abdominal pain may indicate inadequate treatment. Objective signs of inadequate replacement therapy are orthostatic pulse and blood pressure changes. If skin hyperpigmentation becomes more prominent in primary adrenal insufficiency, plasma ACTH levels may be helpful in guiding therapy. Dehydroepiandrosterone is not recommended for treatment of adolescent girls or older women with adrenal insufficiency, low energy, or loss of libido.[34]

Stress Dosing

Patients with adrenal insufficiency (primary or secondary, and patients with CAH) must be informed about the need to increase their glucocorticoid dose during stress to prevent a potentially lethal adrenal crisis. All such patients should wear a medical alert tag and carry an emergency medical information card, letter or diagnosis, and contact information on their mobile phone to ensure that medical professionals know about their underlying disorder.

Mild physical stresses such as immunizations, uncomplicated viral illnesses, and low-grade fever (temperature <101.3°F [38.5°C]) do not require stress doses of glucocorticoids. Athletic activity and emotional stress also do not usually require a boost in glucocorticoid dose. In 1 study, adolescents with CAH who received an additional morning dose of hydrocortisone causing a 100% increase in serum cortisol level did not show any improvement in athletic performance.[35] More severe stresses such as illness accompanied by higher fever (temperature ≥101.3°F [38.5°C]), surgery, and major trauma should be accompanied by tripling of oral hydrocortisone maintenance doses (distributed every 8 hours) to prevent hypoglycemia, hypotension, and cardiovascular collapse.

Supplemental parenteral hydrocortisone is suggested before general anesthesia and surgery. Doses are empiric and are not determined by evidence-based guidelines.[36] Stress doses should not be excessive and should be tapered rapidly until the patient is able to resume oral maintenance doses.

ADRENOCORTICAL HYPERFUNCTION

The spectrum of disorders causing adrenal hyperfunction is more limited compared with those causing hypofunction (Table 3).

Premature Adrenarche, Obesity, and Polycystic Ovarian Syndrome

Adrenal androgen excess is most commonly observed in children with early onset of pubic and body hair growth. The traditional age limit has been 8 years for the onset of pubic hair in girls and 9 years in boys. The lowest age limit for girls has been contested after a large cross-sectional study revealed the relatively common occurrence of either early pubic hair or breast enlargement in healthy black girls after age 6 years and in white girls after age 7 years.[37]

Definition

The early onset of adrenal androgen secretion accompanied by pubic hair (*pubarche*) is termed *premature adrenarche*.

Table 3
Causes of adrenal cortical hyperfunction

Iatrogenic
    Glucocorticoid or mineralocorticoid treatment
    Adrenocorticotropic hormone treatment
    Pituitary
Pituitary tumors
Adrenal tumors
    Carcinoma
    Adenoma
Adrenal nodular hyperplasia
    Carney complex (AD) (gene *PRKAR1A*, OMIM 160980)
    McCune-Albright syndrome (gene *GNAS1*, OMIM 174800)
Ectopic ACTH-producing tumors
Apparent mineralocorticoid excess (gene *HSD11B2*, OMIM 218030)
Glucocorticoid remediable hyperaldosteronism (AD) (gene chimeric *CYP11B1/B2*, OMIM 103900)

Laboratory Evaluation

Premature adrenarche is heralded by mildly increased levels of DHEA and DHEA-sulfate. These hormone levels tend to be consistent with the child's Tanner stage of pubic hair. Dehydroepiandrosterone, a weak androgen, is the most abundantly produced adrenal steroid. The sulfated form has a longer half-life in the circulation and thus is not subject to circadian variability, making it a robust screening tool. Premature adrenarche is generally considered a benign condition that does not warrant treatment with glucocorticoid suppression. Presence of isolated pubic hair or axillary hair with or without apocrine body odor before age 8 does not necessarily presage early breast development and menstruation in girls. In most cases, children with premature adrenarche do not manifest rapid statural growth or advanced bone age. An exception is cases of obesity or rapid weight gain, in whom statural growth and bone age are often inappropriate for chronologic age. With the high prevalence of obesity, bone age cannot be used as a guide for determining the need for medical treatment to suppress puberty.

Endocrine evaluation should be reserved for those children who manifest unusually early and rapidly progressive signs of puberty, including crossing centiles for statural growth, breast or testicular enlargement, or nonisosexual puberty (eg, a girl with hirsutism or other signs of virilization, or a prepubertal boy with gynecomastia).

Obese children and adolescents secrete more adrenal sex hormones than do lean children[38] and can metabolize these weak adrenal sex hormones in fat to more active sex hormones. Consequently, they may develop secondary sexual characteristics at an earlier-than-average age. In contrast to nonobese children with premature adrenarche, obese children often show advanced bone ages but usually are not short.[39]

Most overweight and obese individuals who are growing in height at a normal pace do not have a causal underlying endocrine disease. Thus, the primary care provider should not embark on an extensive evaluation in search of hormonal abnormalities without due cause. Rather, they should advise and institute dietary counseling and propose a rigorous exercise program to determine whether weight gain can be controlled before obesity becomes severe and difficult to reverse. Telephone consultation with a pediatric endocrinologist is advised if in doubt.

Obese adolescent females are hard to differentiate on clinical grounds from those with adrenal hyperplasia or polycystic ovarian syndrome with respect to the cardinal signs of oligomenorrhea, hirsutism, and acne. Measuring an early morning (before 0800) serum 17-hydroxyprogesterone by liquid chromatography tandem mass spectrometry (LC/MS/MS) is an excellent screening test, which can largely exclude nonclassic CAH (NCAH). However, there are no specific diagnostic tests to prove the diagnosis of polycystic ovarian syndrome, especially among adolescents. Measurements of total testosterone, sex hormone binding globulin, and DHEA-sulfate are useful, as are other endocrine tests, such as follicle-stimulating hormone, luteinizing hormone, estradiol, prolactin, and thyroid functions in oligomenorrhea or amenorrhea. Because weight management is beneficial in both cases, lifestyle changes should be encouraged before medical treatment is considered, after excluding nonclassic CAH and other pathologic causes of androgenic symptoms.[40]

Cushing Syndrome

Cushing syndrome refers to any form of glucocorticoid excess, whereas *Cushing disease* refers to glucocorticoid excess as a result of ACTH hypersecretion. Although Cushing disease is rare, it is the most frequently identified noniatrogenic etiology for glucocorticoid excess in adolescents, estimated at about 0.5 per million persons per year.[41] Table 3 lists causes of glucocorticoid excess.

History and Physical Examination
Prominent clinical features of adrenocortical hyperfunction in adolescents are excess central body weight gain with stunted statural growth. It should be emphasized that most obese individuals do not have Cushing syndrome and do not require screening, unless growth arrest or other suspicious signs are observed. An obese adolescent with statural growth arrest should be referred to a pediatric endocrinologist for more complete evaluation. Examination of annual school photographs can often help reveal subtle changes in physiognomy and habitus over time. Other characteristic findings are easy bruisability, broad, purplish striae over the abdomen and flanks, a prominent dorsal fat pad, hyperglycemia, and hypertension.

Therapeutic glucocorticoids are in widespread use the treatment of a variety of inflammatory and neoplastic diseases. Exogenous administration of relatively high doses of these drugs over long periods of time by any route is the most common cause of Cushing syndrome as well as secondary adrenal insufficiency. Although the relative safety of alternate-day oral and inhaled glucocorticoids has been demonstrated, individual differences in drug metabolism or sensitivity may cause cushingoid effects. Therefore, it is important to obtain a thorough medication history in children treated with these drugs. If possible, exogenous glucocorticoids should be tapered as soon as practical while substituting other therapeutic agents. In some patients, attenuation of cushingoid features and improvement of statural growth may take months to years.[42]

Laboratory Evaluation
Clinical suspicion of Cushing syndrome in the absence of administration of exogenous glucocorticoids should prompt appropriate screening diagnostic

studies, primarily measurement of midnight salivary cortisol, which is easier and outperforms 24-hour urine free cortisol.[43] The diagnosis may be confirmed by finding a nonsuppressed morning cortisol after dexamethasone administration. The latter test has been refined by the post-dexamethasone administration of corticotrophin-releasing hormone.[44] An inappropriately brisk rise in plasma ACTH after corticotrophin-releasing hormone suggests an ACTH-producing pituitary tumor, and MRI with attention to this portion of the brain is indicated. If the tumor cannot be localized by imaging, selective catheterization of the inferior petrosal sinuses with measurement of ACTH level on both sides should be performed at a specialized center. Ancillary laboratory studies frequently reveal impaired glucose tolerance and low bone density on radiographs or dual V-ray absorptiometry.[44]

Adrenal carcinomas (but not typically adenomas) secrete cortisol as well as mineralocorticoids and androgens. Adrenal tumors are the most common cause of endogenous steroid excess in young children. The typical case is a round-faced, ruddy child with rapidly advancing premature pubarche, hypertension, and an abdominal mass. If adrenal carcinoma is suspected on the basis of ACTH-independent (ie, nonsuppressible) cortisol excess, the patient should undergo additional hormone measurements of aldosterone and plasma renin activity, as well as DHEA-sulfate and androgens.

Imaging Studies
Thin-slice CT or MRI of the abdomen including the adrenal glands should be performed if preliminary hormonal test results implicate an adrenal source for excess secretion of cortisol or other steroid hormones. Carcinoma often shows a necrotic center and calcification and irregular borders, whereas benign nonfunctioning adenomas typically are more similar in density to normal adrenal tissue and homogeneous. Ectopic ACTH production by carcinomas is almost never seen in the pediatric age group.

Management
Cushing disease has traditionally been treated primarily with transsphenoidal pituitary tumor resection. Surgical success largely depends on the skill of the surgeon and the nature of the lesion. In 1 recent large series, the cure rate for periadolescents was 86% to 93%.[45] Data show that directed radiotherapy, such as gamma knife[46] and linear accelerator[47] techniques, can also induce gradual remission of ACTH hypersecretion in recurrent or refractory cases. Patients who cannot undergo surgery or newer radiotherapies may benefit from several drugs that inhibit glucocorticoid synthesis or action.[48] Once ACTH levels have decreased, the patient needs chronic glucocorticoid replacement therapy.

ADRENAL MEDULLARY DISEASES

Neuroblastoma

In young children, neuroblastoma is the most common tumor encountered. The incidence is about 1 in 100,000 children younger than age 15 per year. The average age at diagnosis in North America is 2 years.[49] Mass screening of infants has been attempted, but this practice per se has not led to improved outcomes.[50]

Relevant Findings
Common presenting signs include abdominal mass, fever of unknown origin, hematuria, spinal cord compression, pathologic fracture, and hypertension. Metastases to liver and bone occur in more than 50% of cases by the time of tumor detection. Biochemical markers include plasma and urinary dopamine, vanillylmandelic acid, and homovanillic acid.

Metaiodobenzylguanidine (mIBG) with iodine-123 plays an important role in the diagnosis and staging of neuroblastoma, allowing whole-body disease assessment. This modality is highly sensitive and specific for neuroblastoma, with the isotope concentrated in more than 90% of tumors.[51] The medical and surgical management of such tumors depends on staging risk; there is a possibility of spontaneous regression in low-grade tumors.[52]

Pheochromocytoma

In adolescents, medullary disease is most often caused by a pheochromocytoma, although only about 20% of all pheochromocytomas occur in this age group.

History and Physical Examination
This rare tumor may cause either episodic or chronic hypertension, usually accompanied by tachycardia, headaches, anxiety, sweating, or flushing. Weight loss may also be observed. The differential diagnosis in adolescents includes panic attacks, thyrotoxicosis, and renovascular disease. Use of sympathomimetic drugs, such as cocaine, amphetamines, phencyclidine, epinephrine, phenylephrine, terbutaline, or the combination of a monoamine oxidase inhibitor and the ingestion of tyramine-containing foods all may lead to symptoms suggestive of pheochromocytoma.

Laboratory Evaluation
Other screening tests may include 24-hour ambulatory blood pressure monitoring. The chemistry profile may demonstrate hyperglycemia or glycosuria. Such findings should prompt referral to appropriate specialists with subsequent mea-

surement of plasma free metanephrines.[53] Extreme hypertension should prompt immediate emergency referral and hospitalization.

Imaging Studies
Confirmatory imaging may be done by mIBG scan.[54] This imaging test is particularly helpful in cases in which either thin-slice contrast-enhanced CT or MRI fails to show a mass, yet biochemical tests and the clinical scenario are suspicious for pheochromocytoma. Other imaging options include positron emission tomography and the use of somatostatin analogs.[55]

A careful family history should be obtained from those with endocrine tumors (especially medullary thyroid carcinoma and hyperparathyroidism) because multiple endocrine neoplasia type 2 may be associated with pheochromocytoma. Transmission is autosomal dominant. Genotyping for the RET oncogene should be performed in the proband, and, if positive, other family members should be tested.[56] Other syndromes prone to adrenal tumors or pheochromocytomas include von Hippel Lindau disease, neurofibromatosis type 1, paraganglioma, and tuberous sclerosis.[57] About 30% of young patients with pheochromocytoma have 1 of these familial disorders and therefore should be genotyped. Familial cases are more often bilateral.[58]

Children with a family history of familial tumor syndromes should be referred to the appropriate specialists for evaluation because early detection of affected genetic status may dictate intervention before tumors develop.

Management
Calcium channel–blocking drugs such as nifedipine are primarily used to control hypertension because calcium is needed for catechol secretion. In preparation for surgery, the patient should be treated for at least 1 week with a drug with both alpha-adrenergic blocking (eg, phenoxybenzamine) and beta-adrenergic blocking (eg, labetalol) properties. Unopposed alpha-blockade would precipitate a hypotensive crisis at surgery, whereas unopposed beta-blockade would exacerbate the hypertension from endogenous epinephrine, a potent vasoconstrictor. In addition, alpha-methyl-L-tyrosine (Demser) is used to inhibit the rate-limiting step of catechol synthesis. Because 10% of pheochromocytomas are bilateral, both adrenals should be explored at surgery. If both adrenals are removed, substitution therapy will be required for primary adrenal insufficiency. Malignancy and recurrence may occur in about 10% to 15% of cases. Careful long-term follow-up of patients with regular checks of blood pressure and catechol measurements is crucial.[59]

References

1. Auchus RJ, Rainey WE. Adrenarche: physiology, biochemistry and human disease. *Clin Endocrinol (Oxf)*. 2004;60(3):288-296
2. Huizenga NA, Koper JW, De Lange P, et al. A polymorphism in the glucocorticoid receptor gene may be associated with and increased sensitivity to glucocorticoids in vivo. *J Clin Endocrinol Metab*. 1998;83(1):144-151
3. Whitworth JA, Kelly JJ, Brown MA, Williamson PM, Lawson JA. Glucocorticoids and hypertension in man. *Clin Exp Hypertens*. 1997;19:871-884
4. Speiser PW, White PC. Congenital adrenal hyperplasia. *N Engl J Med*. 2003;349:776-788
5. Speiser PW, Knochenhauer ES, Dewailly D, et al. A multicenter study of women with nonclassical congenital adrenal hyperplasia: relationship between genotype and phenotype. *Mol Genet Metab*. 2000;71:527-534
6. Speiser PW, Azziz R, Baskin LS, et al. Congenital adrenal hyperplasia due to steroid 21-hydroxylase deficiency: an Endocrine Society clinical practice guideline. *J Clin Endocrinol Metab*. 2010;95:4133-4160
7. Merke DP, Poppas DP. Management of adolescents with congenital adrenal hyperplasia. *Lancet Diabetes Endocrinol*. 2013;1:341-352
8. Berenbaum SA, Korman BK, Duck SC, Resnick SM. Psychological adjustment in children and adults with congenital adrenal hyperplasia. *J Pediatr*. 2004;144:741-746
9. Claahsen-van der Grinten HL, Sweep FC, Blickman JG, Hermus AR, Otten BJ. Prevalence of testicular adrenal rest tumours in male children with congenital adrenal hyperplasia due to 21-hydroxylase deficiency. *Eur J Endocrinol*. 2007;157:339-344
10. Charmandari E, Nicolaides NC, Chrousos GP. Adrenal insufficiency. *Lancet*. 2014;383:2152-2167
11. Jahangir-Hekmat M, Taylor HC, Levin H, Wilbur M, Llerena LA. Adrenal insufficiency attributable to adrenal hemorrhage: long-term follow-up with reference to glucocorticoid and mineralocorticoid function and replacement. *Endocr Pract*. 2004;10:55-61
12. Arlt W, Allolio B. Adrenal insufficiency. *Lancet*. 2003;361:1881-1893
13. Todd GR, Acerini CL, Ross-Russell R, et al. Survey of adrenal crisis associated with inhaled corticosteroids in the United Kingdom. *Arch Dis Child*. 2002;87:457-461
14. Dunlop KA, Carson DJ, Steen HJ, et al. Monitoring growth in asthmatic children treated with high dose inhaled glucocorticoids does not predict adrenal suppression. *Arch Dis Child*. 2004;89:713-716
15. Lamberts SW, Bruining HA, de Jong FH. Corticosteroid therapy in severe illness. *N Engl J Med*. 1997;337:1285-1292
16. Felner EI, Thompson MT, Ratliff AF, White PC, Dickson BA. Time course of recovery of adrenal function in children treated for leukemia. *J Pediatr*. 2000;137:21-24
17. Schlaghecke R, Kornely E, Santen RT, Ridderskamp P. The effect of long-term glucocorticoid therapy on pituitary-adrenal responses to exogenous corticotropin-releasing hormone. *N Engl J Med*. 1992;326:226-230
18. Oelkers W. Adrenal insufficiency. *N Engl J Med*. 1996;335:1206-1212
19. Rose SR, Auble BA. Endocrine changes after pediatric traumatic brain injury. *Pituitary*. 2012;15:267-275
20. Brooks BP, Kleta R, Stuart C, et al. Genotypic heterogeneity and clinical phenotype in triple A syndrome: a review of the NIH experience 2000-2005. *Clin Genet*. 2005;68:215-221
21. Charmandari E, Kino T, Chrousos GP. Primary generalized familial and sporadic glucocorticoid resistance (Chrousos syndrome) and hypersensitivity. *Endocr Dev*. 2013;24:67-85

22. Krumholz A, Stern BJ. Neurologic manifestations of sarcoidosis. *Handb Clin Neurol.* 2014;119: 305-333
23. Kurtulmus N, Mert M, Tanakol R, Yarman S. The pituitary gland in patients with Langerhans cell histiocytosis: a clinical and radiological evaluation. *Endocrine.* 2015:48:949-956
24. Bell J, Parker KL, Swinford RD, et al. Long-term safety of recombinant human growth hormone in children. *J Clin Endocrinol Metab.* 2010;95:167-177
25. Buchanan CR, Preece MA, Milner RD. Mortality, neoplasia, and Creutzfeldt-Jakob disease in patients treated with human pituitary growth hormone in the United Kingdom. *BMJ.* 1991;302:824-828
26. Mills JL, Schonberger LB, Wysowski DK, et al. Long-term mortality in the United States cohort of pituitary-derived growth hormone recipients. *J Pediatr.* 2004;144:430-436
27. Taback SP, Dean HJ. Mortality in Canadian children with growth hormone (GH) deficiency receiving GH therapy 1967-1992. The Canadian Growth Hormone Advisory Committee. *J Clin Endocrinol Metab.* 1996;81:1693-1696
28. Pizarro CF, Troster EJ, Damiani D, Carcillo JA. Absolute and relative adrenal insufficiency in children with septic shock. *Crit Care Med.* 2005;33:855-859
29. Levy-Shraga Y, Pinhas-Hamiel O. Critical illness-related corticosteroid insufficiency in children. *Horm Res Paediatr.* 2013;80:309-317
30. Menon K, McNally D, Choong K, Sampson M. A systematic review and meta-analysis on the effect of steroids in pediatric shock. *Pediatr Crit Care Med.* 2013;14:474-480
31. Ni CM, Fallon M, Kenny D, et al. Rectal hydrocortisone during vomiting in children with adrenal insufficiency. *J Pediatr Endocrinol Metab.* 2003;16:1101-1104
32. Charmandari E, Lichtarowicz-Krynska EJ, Hindmarsh PC, et al. Congenital adrenal hyperplasia: management during critical illness. *Arch Dis Child.* 2001;85:26-28
33. Kerrigan JR, Veldhuis JD, Leyo SA, Iranmanesh A, Rogol AD. Estimation of daily cortisol production and clearance rates in normal pubertal males by deconvolution analysis. *J Clin Endocrinol Metab.* 1993;76:1505-1510
34. Wierman ME, Arlt W, Basson R, et al. Androgen therapy in women: a reappraisal: an Endocrine Society clinical practice guideline. *J Clin Endocrinol Metab.* 2014;99:3489-3510
35. Weise M, Drinkard B, Mehlinger SL, et al. Stress dose of hydrocortisone is not beneficial in patients with classic congenital adrenal hyperplasia undergoing short-term, high-intensity exercise. *J Clin Endocrinol Metab.* 2004;89:3679-3684
36. Taylor LK, Auchus RJ, Baskin LS, Miller WL. Cortisol response to operative stress with anesthesia in healthy children. *J Clin Endocrinol Metab.* 2013;98:3687-3693
37. Herman-Giddens ME, Slora EJ, Wasserman RC, et al. Secondary sexual characteristics and menses in young girls seen in office practice: a study from the Pediatric Research in Office Settings network. *Pediatrics.* 1997;99:505-512
38. Reinehr T, Kulle A, Wolters B, et al. Steroid hormone profiles in prepubertal obese children before and after weight loss. *J Clin Endocrinol Metab.* 2013;98:E1022-E1030
39. Sopher AB, Jean AM, Zwany SK, et al. Bone age advancement in prepubertal children with obesity and premature adrenarche: possible potentiating factors. *Obesity (Silver Spring).* 2011;19:1259-1264
40. Legro RS, Arslanian SA, Ehrmann DA, et al. Diagnosis and treatment of polycystic ovary syndrome: an Endocrine Society clinical practice guideline. *J Clin Endocrinol Metab.* 2013;98:4565-4592
41. Lindholm J, Juul S, Jorgensen JO, et al. Incidence and late prognosis of Cushing's syndrome: a population-based study. *J Clin Endocrinol Metab.* 2001;86:117-123
42. Lai HC, FitzSimmons SC, Allen DB, et al. Risk of persistent growth impairment after alternate-day prednisone treatment in children with cystic fibrosis. *N Engl J Med.* 2000;342:851-859
43. Elias PC, Martinez EZ, Barone BF, Mermejo LM, Castro M, Moreira AC. Late-night salivary cortisol has a better performance than urinary free cortisol in the diagnosis of Cushing's syndrome. *J Clin Endocrinol Metab.* 2014;99:2045-2051

44. Raff H. Salivary cortisol and the diagnosis of Cushing's syndrome: a coming of age. *Endocrine.* 2012;41:353-354
45. Libuit LG, Karageorgiadis AS, Sina N, et al. A gender-dependent analysis of Cushing's disease in childhood: pre- and post-operative follow-up. *Clin Endocrinol (Oxf).* 2014;[Epub ahead of print] doi: 10.1111/cen.12644
46. Sheehan JP, Xu Z, Salvetti DJ, Schmitt PJ, Vance ML. Results of gamma knife surgery for Cushing's disease. *J Neurosurg.* 2013;119:1486-1492
47. Wilson PJ, Williams JR, Smee RI. Single-centre experience of stereotactic radiosurgery and fractionated stereotactic radiotherapy for prolactinomas with the linear accelerator. *J Med Imaging Radiat Oncol.* 2014;[Epub ahead of print] doi: 10.1111/1754-9485.12257
48. Gadelha MR, Vieira NL. Efficacy of medical treatment in Cushing's disease: a systematic review. *Clin Endocrinol (Oxf).* 2014;80:1-12
49. Perkins SM, Shinohara ET, DeWees T, Frangoul H. Outcome for children with metastatic solid tumors over the last four decades. *PLoS One.* 2014;9:e100396
50. Tsubono Y, Hisamichi S. A halt to neuroblastoma screening in Japan. *N Engl J Med.* 2004;350:2010-2011
51. Sharp SE, Gelfand MJ, Shulkin BL. Pediatrics: diagnosis of neuroblastoma. *Semin Nucl Med.* 2011;41:345-353
52. Kim S, Chung DH. Pediatric solid malignancies: neuroblastoma and Wilms' tumor. *Surg Clin North Am.* 2006;86:469-487, xi
53. Lenders JW, Pacak K, Walther MM, et al. Biochemical diagnosis of pheochromocytoma: which test is best? *JAMA.* 2002;287:1427-1434
54. Guller U, Turek J, Eubanks S, et al. Detecting pheochromocytoma: defining the most sensitive test. *Ann Surg.* 2006;243:102-107
55. Rufini V, Calcagni ML, Baum RP. Imaging of neuroendocrine tumors. *Semin Nucl Med.* 2006;36:228-247
56. Krampitz GW, Norton JA. RET gene mutations (genotype and phenotype) of multiple endocrine neoplasia type 2 and familial medullary thyroid carcinoma. *Cancer.* 2014;120:1920-1931
57. King KS, Prodanov T, Kantorovich V, et al. Metastatic pheochromocytoma/paraganglioma related to primary tumor development in childhood or adolescence: significant link to SDHB mutations. *J Clin Oncol.* 2011;29:4137-4142
58. Amar L, Bertherat J, Baudin E, et al. Genetic testing in pheochromocytoma or functional paraganglioma. *J Clin Oncol.* 2005;23:8812-8818
59. Pham TH, Moir C, Thompson GB, et al. Pheochromocytoma and paraganglioma in children: a review of medical and surgical management at a tertiary care center. *Pediatrics.* 2006;118:1109-1117

Screening and Treatment of Common Lipid Disorders in Adolescents

Shara R. Bialo, MD[a] and Charlotte M. Boney, MD, MS[b]*

[a]*Division of Pediatric Endocrinology, Rhode Island Hospital and Alpert Medical School of Brown University, Providence, Rhode Island;* [b]*Division of Pediatric Endocrinology, Baystate Medical Center and Tufts University School of Medicine, Springfield, Massachusetts*

INTRODUCTION

Among adolescents aged 12 to 19 years, the prevalence of abnormal lipid levels is as high as 20.3%.[1] This statistic comprises genetic and secondary dyslipidemias. Familial hypercholesterolemia (FH) has a prevalence of 1 in 500 individuals in western populations, causes increased low-density lipoprotein (LDL) cholesterol from birth, and leads to early cardiovascular events.[2] The most common cause of secondary dyslipidemia is obesity, and the incidence continues to increase in the setting of the current obesity epidemic. Multiple large, prospective epidemiologic studies have demonstrated that cardiovascular disease (CVD) risk factors in children and adolescents, notably elevated LDL cholesterol and obesity, predict clinical manifestations of atherosclerosis in young adults.[3-6] Cardiovascular disease continues to be a leading cause of mortality in the adult population, with coronary heart disease alone causing 1 of every 6 deaths in the United States.[7]

Such data form the basis of the pediatric cholesterol screening guidelines, which were updated in 2011 by the National Heart, Lung, and Blood Institute (NHLBI) to include universal screening of all children and adolescents. This substantial and controversial addition greatly affects clinical practice by pediatricians and adolescent specialists. In this article, we will review basic lipid metabolism, describe common dyslipidemias affecting children and adolescents, and discuss the 2011 screening and treatment guidelines for childhood lipid disorders. Based

---

*Corresponding author
E-mail address: charlotte.boneymd@baystatehealth.org

Copyright © 2015 American Academy of Pediatrics. All rights reserved. ISSN 1934-4287

on our own evidence-based practice in a multidisciplinary lipid clinic, we have included "clinical tips" as useful principles for the practitioner.

OVERVIEW OF LIPID METABOLISM

A basic understanding of normal lipid metabolism is paramount for appropriate diagnostic and therapeutic decision-making in patients at risk for developing CVD. Plasma lipoproteins are determined by 3 interrelated pathways: transport of dietary (exogenous) fat, transport of hepatic (endogenous) fat, and reverse cholesterol transport.

In the exogenous or dietary pathway, chylomicrons (CM) are synthesized in the intestine from dietary fat and hydrolyzed by lipoprotein lipase (LPL), thus releasing free fatty acids (FFA) for uptake by peripheral and adipose tissue (Figure 1). The CM remnants contain apolipoprotein E (ApoE), which binds remnant receptors to deliver triglycerides (TG) to the liver for repackaging as very-low-density lipoprotein (VLDL) particles. Lipoprotein lipase activity and clearance by ApoE-binding remnant receptors are the major regulators of postprandial TG levels.

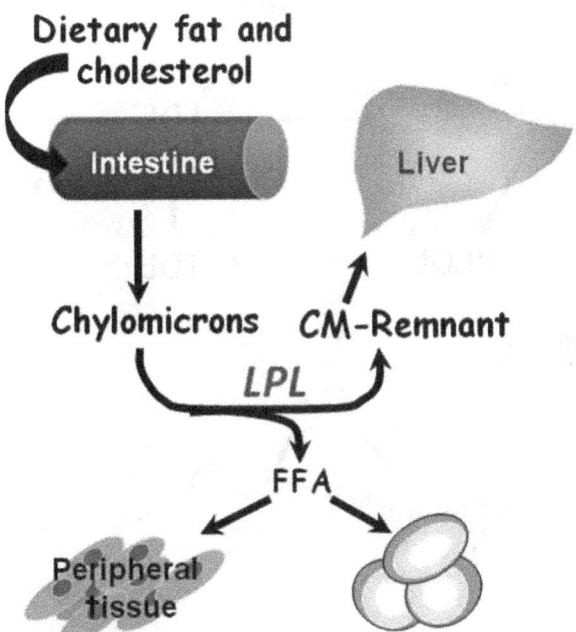

Fig 1. Dietary (exogenous) fat pathway. CM, chylomicron; FFA, free fatty acid; LPL, lipoprotein lipase.

In the endogenous or hepatic fat pathway, VLDLs are synthesized and secreted from the liver, hydrolyzed by LPL, and ultimately converted to LDLs (Figure 2). Very-low-density lipoprotein contains approximately 80% TG, 20% cholesterol ester (CE), and the apolipoprotein ApoB100. It undergoes hydrolysis by LPL and picks up CE from high-density lipoprotein (HDL) by cholesterol ester transport protein (CETP) to become intermediate-density lipoprotein (IDL). The IDL is further hydrolyzed by LPL and hepatic lipase (HL) and accepts transfer of more CE from HDL by CETP to become LDL particles. Low-density lipoprotein is removed from the blood by binding of ApoB100 to the LDL receptor (LDLR) on tissues, particularly the liver. Hepatic cholesterol stores originate from 3 sources: endocytosis of LDL bound to its receptor, de novo cholesterol synthesis, of which HMG co-A reductase is the rate-limiting step and the target of cholesterol-lowering therapy known as statins, and dietary CE delivered by CM remnants. Regulation of this pathway includes insulin activation of LPL to promote lipolysis of VLDL-containing TG and clearance of LDL by binding the LDLR. Fasting TG levels reflect VLDL synthesis and metabolism, and LDL levels are determined by its synthesis from IDL and uptake into cells after binding to

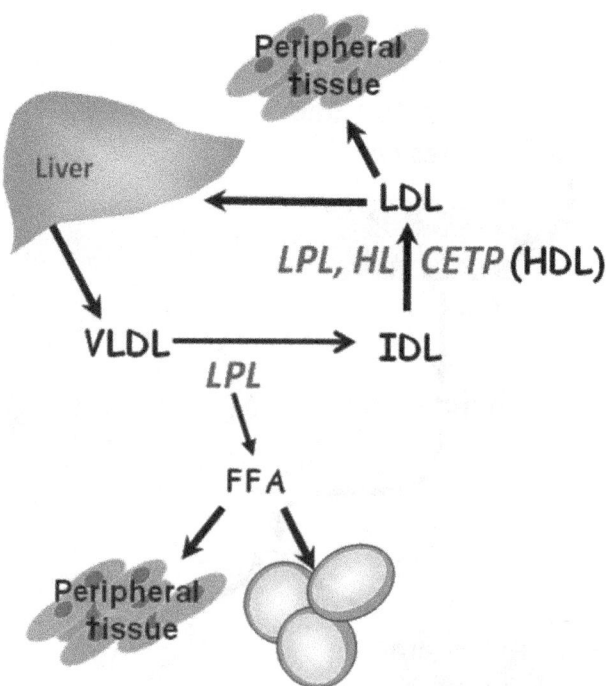

Fig 2. Hepatic (endogenous) fat pathway. CETP, cholesterol ester transport protein; FFA, free fatty acid; HDL, high-density lipoprotein; HL, hepatic lipase; IDL, intermediate-density lipoprotein; LDL, low-density lipoprotein; LPL, lipoprotein lipase; VLDL, very-low-density lipoprotein.

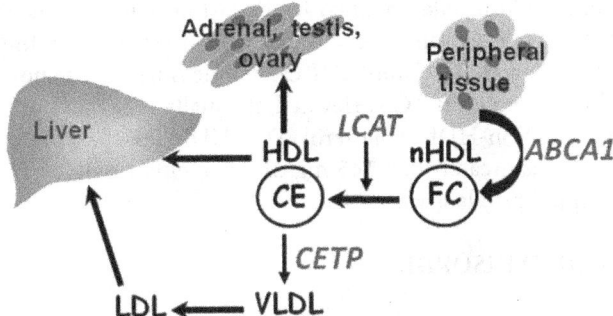

Fig 3. Reverse cholesterol transport. ABCA1, ATP binding cassette transporter A1; CE, cholesterol ester; CETP, cholesterol ester transport protein; FC, free cholesterol; HDL, high-density lipoprotein; LCAT, lecithin cholesterol acyltransferase; LDL, low-density lipoprotein; nHDL, nascent high-density lipoprotein particle; VLDL, very-low-density lipoprotein.

its receptor. Clearance of LDL is increased by upregulation of LDLR when dietary cholesterol and de novo synthesis are limited.

In reverse cholesterol transport, nascent high-density lipoprotein (nHDL) particles are synthesized in the liver and intestines and acquire free cholesterol (FC) from cells via the cholesterol transport protein ATP binding cassette transporter A1 (ABCA1) (Figure 3). Lecithin cholesterol acyltransferase converts FC to CE to form a stable, mature HDL, which delivers CE back to the liver (reverse cholesterol transport) or to cholesterol-requiring tissues via its specific receptor, which binds its major apolipoprotein, ApoA1. HDL also transfers CE via CETP to VLDL and IDL particles to form LDL. Levels of HDL are determined by its synthesis and clearance: insulin increases HDL levels by reducing clearance through its action on HL.

INTERPRETATION OF LIPID PROFILES

Plasma lipoproteins contain CE, some FC, and TG in precise proportions with specific apolipoproteins that confer structure and function. A serum lipid profile reflects the lipoproteins carrying cholesterol and TG.

Total cholesterol (TC) largely reflects LDL and HDL. The LDL level can be measured directly or estimated by the Friedewalk equation (LDL = TC − HDL − TG/5), which is accurate only when TG is less than 400 mg/dL. The HDL level is measured directly; fasting has no effect on TC and HDL levels.

The TG level measured in the fasting state largely reflects VLDL. In the nonfasting state, TG reflects dietary fat in CM. The TG carried in CM can take 8 to 10 hours to return to baseline after eating. Lipoprotein(a) is not measured in a lipid profile but is a modified LDL particle that is an independent risk factor for CVD.

Clinical Tip: A lipid profile obtained in the fasting state reflects TG in VLDL particles. If the TG is elevated, be sure the patient was truly fasting before the blood draw. The levels of TC and HDL can be measured in the nonfasting state (random blood sample). If TC is elevated, it usually is because of high LDL or HDL cholesterol. Non-HDL cholesterol (TC – HDL) less than 145 mg/dL is normal; if the value is greater than 145 mg/dL, then either LDL or TG is elevated and a fasting lipid profile is warranted.

COMMON LIPID DISORDERS

Hyperlipidemias can be classified as primary or secondary.[8] Primary dyslipidemias are caused by genetic abnormalities that alter normal metabolic pathways. The defects can be single or polygenic and occur at any step of metabolism (Table 1). Secondary causes of dyslipidemia include obesity, diabetes mellitus, chronic kidney disease, hypothyroidism, cholestatic liver disease, alcohol overuse, and use of a variety of medications (Table 2). This review focuses on several common causes of dyslipidemia in the adolescent population.

Table 1

Primary causes of dyslipidemia

Elevated low-density lipoprotein (LDL) cholesterol and normal triglycerides	Low LDL cholesterol
Familial hypercholesterolemia (FH)	Familial hypobetalipoproteinemia (FHB)
Familial defective ApoB-100 (FDB)	PCSK9 deficiency
Autosomal dominant hypercholesterolemia resulting from mutations in PCSK9	Abetalipoproteinemia
Autosomal recessive hypercholesterolemia	
Sitosterolemia	
Polygenic hypercholesterolemia	
Elevated plasma levels of lipoprotein(a)	
Low HDL cholesterol	Elevated high-density lipoprotein (HDL) cholesterol
Tangier disease (ABCA1 deficiency)	CETP deficiency
Lecithin cholesterol acyltransferase deficiency	Familial hyperalphalipoproteinemia
Primary hypoalphalipoproteinemia	
Gene deletions and coding mutations in APOA-1	
Elevated triglycerides	
Familial chylomicronemia syndrome	
ApoA-V deficiency	
GPIHBP1 deficiency	
Hepatic lipase deficiency	
Familial dysbetalipoproteinemia	
Familial hypertriglyceridemia	

Derived from Rader DJ, Hobbs HH. Disorders of lipoprotein metabolism. In: Longo DL, Fauci AS, Kasper DL, et al, eds. *Harrison's Principles of Internal Medicine.* 18th ed. New York: McGraw-Hill; 2012.

Table 2
Causes of secondary dyslipidemia

Exogenous	Other
Alcohol	Kawasaki disease
Drug Therapy	Anorexia nervosa
Corticosteroids	After solid organ transplantation
Isotretinoin	Childhood cancer survivor
Beta-blockers	Progeria
Select oral contraceptives	Idiopathic hypercalcemia
Select chemotherapeutic agents	Klinefelter syndrome
Select antiretroviral agents	Werner syndrome
Endocrine/Metabolic	Storage Disease
Hypothyroidism/hypopituitarism	Glycogen storage disease
Type 1 diabetes mellitus, type 2 diabetes mellitus	Gaucher disease
Pregnancy	Cystine storage disease
Polycystic ovarian syndrome	Juvenile Tay-Sachs disease
Lipodystrophy	Niemann-Pick disease
Acute intermittent porphyria	
Renal	Inflammatory Disease
Chronic renal disease	Systemic lupus erythematosus
Hemolytic uremic syndrome	Juvenile rheumatoid arthritis
Nephrotic syndrome	
Hepatic	Infectious
Obstructive liver disease/cholestatic conditions	Acute viral/bacterial infection
Biliary cirrhosis	Human immunodeficiency virus
Alagille syndrome	Hepatitis

Adapted from Expert Panel on Integrated Guidelines for Cardiovascular Health and Risk Reduction in Children and Adolescents, National Heart, Lung, and Blood Institute. Expert panel on integrated guidelines for cardiovascular health and risk reduction in children and adolescents: summary report. *Pediatrics.* 2011;128(Suppl 5):S213-S256.

Familial Hypercholesterolemia

Familial hypercholesterolemia is the result of mutations of LDLR or a component affecting LDLR activity.[9] It is a monogenic, autosomal dominant disorder that results in markedly elevated LDL cholesterol levels. More than 1500 mutations of this gene have been detected and account for more than 80% of cases of monogenetic FH.[2]

Homozygous mutations occur in approximately 1 in 1,000,000 persons and cause rapidly progressive atherosclerosis, cardiovascular events, and early mortality.[10] Most patients with homozygous FH present in childhood with cutaneous xanthomas on the elbows, knees, heels, wrists, or buttocks. The LDL levels are greater than 300 mg/dL, with TC levels greater than 425 mg/dL in children and greater than 500 mg/dL in adults.[11] Children with homozygous FH frequently develop coronary atherosclerosis before puberty and rarely survive beyond the second decade. Homozygous FH can be confirmed by measurement of LDLR activity in cultured skin fibroblasts from a skin biopsy or by quantifying the number of LDLRs on the surfaces of lymphocytes using cell sorting technology.[8] Molecular assays are also available to define the mutations in LDLRs by DNA sequencing.

Heterozygous FH usually is caused by the inheritance of 1 mutant LDLR allele and is much more common, estimated to affect between 1 in 500 to 1 in 200 people worldwide.[10] Plasma levels of LDL cholesterol usually are 180 to 300 mg/dL, with TC levels of 250 to 500 mg/dL. Patients with heterozygous FH have hypercholesterolemia from birth, leading to cardiovascular events such as stroke and myocardial infarction before age 50. However, LDL levels do not directly predict CVD severity or age of onset.

Having a first-degree relative with characteristic LDL levels and a family history of early CVD constitutes a clinical diagnosis of FH. Both parents of FH homozygotes usually have hypercholesterolemia given that the disease has greater than 90% penetrance. Because heterozygous FH is codominant in inheritance, usually 1 parent and approximately 50% of the patient's siblings also have hypercholesterolemia. Identifying cases of FH in childhood is challenging because a family history of premature CVD is often not known and elevated LDL cholesterol may go unrecognized if the parents are young and have not undergone assessment. Children and adolescents with heterozygous FH rarely manifest xanthomas.

Clinical Tip: LDL cholesterol greater than 180 mg/dL is FH until proven otherwise because a high intake of dietary fat alone will not cause such a significant LDL cholesterol elevation. Polygenic hypercholesterolemia is the most common cause of LDL levels of 150 to 180 mg/dL, but there is no family history of early CVD. High intake of dietary fat will increase LDL levels to 120 to 150 mg/dL, which are easily amenable to dietary restriction.

Hypertriglyceridemia

Hypertriglyceridemia can range from mild or moderate (TG >150-500 mg/dL) to severe (TG >500 mg/dL). Secondary causes of elevated TG are common and include obesity, poorly controlled diabetes, hypothyroidism, and medications.[9] Moderate to severe hypertriglyceridemia may result from familial causes but also may result from undiagnosed or uncontrolled diabetes mellitus, so a careful history and blood glucose levels should be obtained in the event of newly discovered TG greater than 500 mg/dL. Recurrent pancreatitis is a significant concern for persistently elevated TG greater than 1000 mg/dL.

Patients with TG greater than 1,000 mg/dL are more likely to have an inherited defect in the metabolism of TG-containing particles. Mutations in the LPL gene, which cause impaired or absent LPL activity, lead to reduced lipolysis of CM and elevated TG levels. Most patients present with TG greater than 10,000 mg/dL.[12]

Deficiency of LPL is prevalent in 1 in 1,000,000 persons and presents in infancy or childhood with episodes of abdominal pain, acute pancreatitis, hepatosplenomegaly, lipemia retinalis, or diffuse xanthomas. Patients often suffer from recurrent pancreatitis and premature atherosclerosis.[13]

Clinical Tip: TG greater than 500 mg/dL may reflect nonfasting dietary fat, a metabolic disorder such as undiagnosed diabetes, or dyslipidemia of obesity. A TG level greater than 1,000 mg/dL is more likely to be the result of familial causes such as familial hypertriglyceridemia, remnant receptor disease (also known as familial dysbetalipoproteinemia), or rarely LPL deficiency.

Familial Combined Hyperlipidemia

Familial combined hyperlipidemia (FCHL) involves isolated or combined hypercholesterolemia and hypertriglyceridemia (caused, in part, by VLDL overproduction) as well as a family history of premature CVD.[14] It is highly prevalent, affecting 1 in 100 persons, and is believed to be polygenic.[15] The FCHL phenotype is heterogeneous, so afflicted family members may possess different lipid abnormalities. Because FCHL in adults is frequently associated with metabolic syndrome and type 2 diabetes mellitus (T2DM), some experts suggest that FCHL is a continuum that progresses to metabolic syndrome and then to T2DM.[9]

Clinical Tip: Adolescents with abnormal TG with or without any LDL abnormality and a family history of premature CVD warrant referral to a lipid specialist because the lipid phenotype of FCHL is variable even within families.

Dyslipidemia of Obesity

The most prevalent secondary cause of hyperlipidemia in any age group is obesity and is an increasing concern in the wake of the current obesity epidemic. In the United States, 17% of youth younger than 19 years and more than 30% of adults are obese.[16] The prevalence of dyslipidemia has been shown to be directly proportional to body mass index (BMI); 14.2% of normal weight, 22.3% of overweight, and 42.9% of obese youths had at least 1 abnormal lipid level.[1] Dyslipidemia of obesity is characterized by elevated TG, low HDL, and small, dense LDL. The major mechanism is insulin resistance, which impairs VLDL metabolism and increases HDL clearance, thereby increasing TG while lowering HDL levels.[17] Some obese patients may have mildly elevated LDL concentrations because of excess dietary consumption of fat. Obesity is so common that it may also coexist with familial lipid disorders such as FH.

Analysis of data from the Bogalusa Heart Study demonstrated that 39% of children with BMI in the 95th percentile or greater and 59% of children with BMI in the 99th percentile or greater had 2 or more cardiovascular risk factors, including elevated TG or LDL levels, reduced HDL levels, or elevations in systolic and diastolic blood pressures and fasting insulin.[18] As the number of cardiovascular risk factors increases, the severity of aortic atherosclerosis in youth escalates, thus justifying early and rigorous intervention to reduce CVD.[19]

Clinical Tip: Dyslipidemia of obesity (elevated TG, low HDL) is easily modifiable with weight loss and exercise and is not treated with cholesterol-lowering drugs such as statin therapy.

GUIDELINES FOR SCREENING OF DYSLIPIDEMIA

The 2011 NHLBI guidelines for screening and management of hyperlipidemia in children and adolescents are the first to recommend universal lipid screening in this age group.[20] All children between the ages of 9 and 11 years and between 17 and 21 years should undergo either a fasting lipid profile or a nonfasting (random) calculation of non-HDL cholesterol (by measuring TC and HDL) (Table 3). If non-HDL levels are greater than 145 mg/dL, then a fasting lipid profile should be drawn to determine whether either TG or LDL levels are elevated. Persistently abnormal results are classified by LDL cholesterol, TG, and risk factors (Tables 4 and 5).

The primary focus for the addition of universal screening is early identification and treatment of children and adolescents with FH, given its high prevalence and associated early CVD.

TREATMENT OF DYSLIPIDEMIA

LDL cholesterol levels of 180 mg/dL or greater or TG levels 500 mg/dL or greater usually are the result of a primary (genetic) lipid disorder, so these patients may benefit from management by lipid specialists. Children and adolescents with LDL and TG levels below these thresholds and without associated conditions associated with a high risk of early CVD can be managed by the primary care physician as detailed in Table 6.

Dietary Cholesterol Restriction

Dietary restriction is the cornerstone of hyperlipidemia treatment, regardless of etiology. For obesity-associated dyslipidemia, diet modification is initiated with Cardiovascular Health Integrated Lifestyle Diet-1 (CHILD-1) for at least 3 months.[20] This regimen limits total fat intake to less than 30% of daily calories, saturated fat to 8% to 10%, cholesterol intake to less than 300 mg/day, and avoidance of trans fats. For patients with FH, adherence to the Cardiovascular Health Integrated Lifestyle Diet-2 (CHILD-2) is warranted, which further restricts

Table 3

Recommendations for lipid assessment

0-2 years	No lipid screening
2-8 years	No routine lipid screening
	Measure FLP twice and average results if:
	Positive family history
	Parent with TC ≥240 mg/dL or known dyslipidemia
	Patient has high-level risk factors
	Patient has moderate- or high-risk medical condition
9-11 years	Universal screening once in this time period:
	Nonfasting (random) TC and HDL: Calculate non-HDL cholesterol (TC − HDL cholesterol)
	If non-HDL-C ≥145 mg/dL ± HDL <40 mg/dL, obtain FLP twice and average the results
	OR
	Fasting lipid profile:
	If LDL cholesterol ≥130 mg/dL ± non-HDL-C 145 mg/dL ± HDL-C <40 mg/dL ± TG ≥100 mg/dL <10 years, ≥130 if ≥10 years, repeat FLP and average the results
12-16 years	No routine screening
	Measure FLP twice and average results if new knowledge of:
	Positive family history
	Parent with TC ≥240 mg/dL or known dyslipidemia
	Patient has high-level risk factors
	Patient has moderate- or high-risk medical condition
17-21 years	Universal screening once in this time period:
	17-19 years:
	Nonfasting (random) TC and HDL: Calculate non-HDL cholesterol (TC − HDL cholesterol)
	If non-HDL-C 145 mg/dL ± HDL <40 mg/dL, obtain FLP twice and average the results
	OR
	Fasting lipid profile:
	If LDL cholesterol ≥130 mg/dL ± non-HDL-C ≥145 mg/dL ± HDL-C <40 mg/dL ± TG ≥130 mg/dL, repeat FLP and average the results
	20-21 years
	Nonfasting (random) TC and HDL: Calculate non-HDL cholesterol (TC − HDL cholesterol)
	If non-HDL-C ≥190 mg/dL ± HDL <40 mg/dL, obtain FLP twice and average the results
	OR
	Fasting lipid profile:
	If LDL cholesterol ≥160 mg/dL ± non-HDL-C ≥190 mg/dL ± HDL-C <40 mg/dL ± TG ≥150 mg/dL, repeat FLP and average the results

FLP, fasting lipid profile; HDL, high-density lipoprotein; LDL, low-density lipoprotein; TC, total cholesterol; TG, triglycerides.

Adapted from Expert Panel on Integrated Guidelines for Cardiovascular Health and Risk Reduction in Children and Adolescents, National Heart, Lung, and Blood Institute. Expert panel on integrated guidelines for cardiovascular health and risk reduction in children and adolescents: summary report. Pediatrics. 2011;128(Suppl 5):S213-S256.

Table 4
Cardiovascular risk factor definitions

Positive family history: myocardial infarction, angina, coronary artery bypass graft/stent/angioplasty, sudden cardiac death in parent, grandparent, aunt, or uncle <55 years for males, <65 years for females

High-level risk factors
  Hypertension requiring drug therapy (blood pressure ≥99th percentile + 5 mm Hg)
  Current cigarette smoker
  BMI ≥97th percentile
  Presence of high-risk medical conditions: type 1 diabetes mellitus, type 2 diabetes mellitus, chronic kidney disease/end-stage renal disease/postrenal transplant, postorthotopic heart transplant, Kawasaki disease with current aneurysms

Moderate-level risk factors
  Hypertension not requiring drug therapy
  BMI between 95th-97th percentile
  High-density lipoprotein cholesterol <40 mg/dL
  Presence of moderate-risk medical conditions: Kawasaki disease with regressed coronary aneurysms, chronic inflammatory disease (systemic lupus erythematosus, juvenile rheumatoid arthritis), human immunodeficiency virus infection, nephrotic syndrome

BMI, body mass index.
Adapted from Expert Panel on Integrated Guidelines for Cardiovascular Health and Risk Reduction in Children and Adolescents, National Heart, Lung, and Blood Institute. Expert panel on integrated guidelines for cardiovascular health and risk reduction in children and adolescents: summary report. Pediatrics. 2011;128(Suppl 5):S213-S256.

Table 5
NHLBI cholesterol cutpoints for children and adolescents

Category	Age	Acceptable (mg/dL)	Borderline (mg/dL)	Abnormal (mg/dL)
Total cholesterol		<170	170-199	≥200
LDL cholesterol		<110	110-129	≥130
Non-HDL cholesterol		<20	120-144	≥145
Triglycerides	0-9 years	<75	75-99	≥100
	10-19 years	<90	90-129	≥130
HDL cholesterol		>45	40-45	<40

HDL, high-density lipoprotein; LDL, low-density protein.
Adapted from Expert Panel on Integrated Guidelines for Cardiovascular Health and Risk Reduction in Children and Adolescents, National Heart, Lung, and Blood Institute. Expert panel on integrated guidelines for cardiovascular health and risk reduction in children and adolescents: summary report. Pediatrics. 2011;128(Suppl 5):S213-S256.

Table 6

Treatment guidelines for dyslipidemia in children and adolescents

Low-density lipoprotein cholesterol level	Action
≥190 mg/dL	Diet and physical activity up to 6 months
	Consider statin therapy after age 10 years or
	after Tanner 2 in boys, postmenarche in girls
130-189 mg/dL	Diet and physical activity
	Reassess fasting lipid panel every 6-12 months
160-189 mg/dL with	Diet and physical activity for 6-12 months
Positive family history, or	Consider statin therapy after age 10 years or
1 high-level risk factor/condition, or	after Tanner 2 in boys, postmenarche in girls
≥2 moderate-level risk factors/conditions	
130-159 mg/dL with	Diet and physical activity for 6-12 months
Clinical cardiovascular disease, or	Consider statin therapy after age 10 years or
≥2 high-level risk factors/conditions, or	after Tanner 2 in boys, postmenarche in girls
1 high-level risk factor/condition and 2	
moderate-level risk factors/conditions	

Triglyceride level	Action
≥500 mg/dL	Referral to lipid specialist
	Diet and physical activity
	Omega-3 fish oil therapy
≥200-499 mg/dL	Diet and physical activity for 6-12 months
	Consider omega-3 fish oil therapy
	Consider referral to lipid specialist
≥100-200 mg/dL (<10 years old) or	Diet and physical activity for 6-12 months
≥130-200 mg/dL (>10 years old)	Increase dietary fish content
	Fasting lipid panel every 6 months
<100 mg/dL (<10 years old) or	Continue diet and physical activity
<130 mg/dL (>10 years old)	Fasting lipid panel annually

Adapted from Expert Panel on Integrated Guidelines for Cardiovascular Health and Risk Reduction in Children and Adolescents, National Heart, Lung, and Blood Institute. Expert panel on integrated guidelines for cardiovascular health and risk reduction in children and adolescents: summary report. *Pediatrics.* 2011;128(Suppl 5):S213-S256.

saturated fat to less than 7% of daily caloric intake and cholesterol intake to less than 200 mg/day. Proper adherence to these diet plans is best accomplished with the aid of a registered dietitian. Also, for any patient with BMI in the 85th percentile or greater, the addition of increased physical activity, reduced screen time, and calorie restriction are recommended.

For patients with FH, water-soluble fiber and plant sterols can be added as an adjunct to the CHILD-2 diet because they compete with cholesterol for intestinal absorption via Niemann-Pick C1-Like Protein (NPC1L1). Plant sterols are available as over-the-counter supplements and doses of up to 2 g/day may reduce LDL cholesterol by up to 15%.[9]

Patients with elevated TG also warrant the CHILD-2 diet along with a special emphasis on reduction of sugar intake.[20] Complex carbohydrates should replace simple sugars, beverages sweetened with sugar should be eliminated, and fish consumption should be increased in order to maximize omega-3 fatty acid intake.[20]

After 6 months of dietary restriction of cholesterol (CHILD-2), pharmacologic therapy should be considered in patients with FH and significant risk of CVD if LDL levels are not at target.

Clinical Tip: In our practice, all patients with either elevated LDL or TG must demonstrate adherence to dietary restriction before medical therapy is started. In patients with FH who restrict cholesterol to less than 200 mg/day, LDL cholesterol levels will decrease by 10% or more; this is accomplished by eliminating fat-containing dairy products, eggs, and red meat. Vegetarian or vegan diets (negligible cholesterol intake) decrease LDL levels by up to 15%. Patients with hypertriglyceridemia who restrict fat intake (especially long-chain fats) to less than 15% of total calories will dramatically reduce their TG levels.

Pharmacologic Therapy

The 2011 NHLBI guidelines suggest that children with a primary hyperlipidemia such as FH or a high-risk condition such as type 1 diabetes that is associated with serious CVD be considered for medical therapy. Statin therapy is approved by the US Food and Drug Administration (FDA) for boys aged 8 to 10 years or for postmenarchal girls, but there remains a paucity of long-term data in pediatric populations.[21] For patients aged 10 to 21 years, decisions regarding the need for pharmacologic therapy should be based on the average of fasting lipid profile results from at least 2 measurements after dietary restriction has failed to get LDL levels to target (Table 6).

Recommendations for medical treatment did not change with the 2011 guidelines (Table 6) and are intended for patients with FH or other hyperlipidemias that lead to early CVD. If LDL levels remain greater than 190 mg/dL after successful dietary restriction, then these patients have FH, and statin treatment should be initiated. Patients with a family history of early CVD in whom LDL levels are still greater than 160 mg/dL after dietary restriction have either FH or FCHL, so a statin should be prescribed. Statin therapy is also recommended for patients with chronic diseases such as type 1 diabetes and a high risk for early CVD in whom LDL levels remain greater than 130 mg/dL after dietary restriction.

Elevated LDL Cholesterol
HMG-CoA reductase inhibitors, or statins, and bile acid sequestrants are the 2 main classes of drugs currently used in children who have significantly elevated

LDL cholesterol. Assuming an inadequate response to dietary restriction, analysis of the most recent National Health and Nutrition Examination Survey (NHANES) data specifies a minimum of 0.85% of American children will be recommended for statin therapy under the most recent guidelines, or roughly 215,000 children aged 12 to 17 years.[20]

Statins inhibit cholesterol synthesis in hepatic cells and decrease the cholesterol pool, resulting in upregulation of LDLRs. However, without concurrent dietary restriction, statins are less effective. Therapy works to primarily lower LDL cholesterol, although a modest decrease in TG and increase in HDL cholesterol can occur. Adverse reactions include increases in hepatic enzymes and creatine kinase, as well as myopathy that can progress to rhabdomyolysis. There is robust evidence supporting the safety and efficacy of statin therapy for reduction of LDL cholesterol in children with FH. However, statins should be considered only after an appropriate trial of dietary and lifestyle interventions.[20] Statin therapy is initiated with the lowest available dose. If target LDL cholesterol levels are not met after 3 months of adherent use, the dose may be increased by 1 increment (usually 10 mg) with reassessment after 3 months and further dose titration. Hepatic transaminase and creatine kinase levels should be monitored with fasting lipid profiles as doses are increased, along with routine clinical monitoring for symptoms of muscle toxicity. Adolescent females should be counseled about the toxicity of statin use in pregnancy and contraceptive options. Oral contraceptive pills are not contraindicated with use of statin therapy.

The most common reason that LDL cholesterol goals are not met is lack of adherence to dietary restriction of cholesterol. However, some patients warrant a second agent. The newer bile acid sequestrant colesevelam (Welchol) is often used, either as monotherapy or as a second agent. Conventional bile acid sequestrants are poorly tolerated in the pediatric population because of gastrointestinal side effects of bloating, constipation, and cramps, so they are rarely used. Ezetimibe is another lipid-lowering agent that works by decreasing absorption of cholesterol in the small intestine, although it is not currently FDA-approved for use in the pediatric population.

A number of new therapies that rely on novel mechanisms to further lower LDL cholesterol are under investigation in adult patients with high risk of CVD, including patients with FH and other inherited disorders of lipid metabolism. One example is mipomersen, an antisense oligonucleotide that inhibits the production of ApoB-100, which is an essential component of all atherogenic lipoproteins.[22] The drug is subcutaneously injected once per week, and early data show that concomitant use of mipomersen and a statin can result in a 21% to 34% reduction in LDL cholesterol levels in patients with heterozygous FH, as well as substantial decreases in TC, TG, and plasma ApoB100. Studies have yet to be conducted in pediatric populations.

The recent development of monoclonal antibodies against proprotein convertase subtilisin kexin type 9 (PCSK9) is another promising treatment of familial and other types of hypercholesterolemia.[23] The PCSK9 is an intracellular protein in hepatocytes that binds LDLR and targets it for lysosomal degradation.[24] The drugs are injected every 15 to 30 days and reduce the concentration of PCSK9 in plasma.[23] By decreasing PCSK9, there is less lysosomal degradation of the LDLR, greater surface expression of LDLR, and reduced plasma LDL concentrations. Early studies in patients with heterozygous FH demonstrated a 45% to 70% reduction in LDL cholesterol, although studies have not yet been conducted in youth.

Clinical Tip: Colesevelam (Welchol) is the only bile acid sequestrant commonly used in the pediatric population and is a fairly effective alternative to statin therapy. In our practice, it is well tolerated and can reduce LDL cholesterol up to 20% in conjunction with dietary restriction. We prescribe colesevelam in young children with LDL levels greater than 190 mg/dL and a concerning family history of early CVD who are not yet candidates for statins or older children and adolescents who are reluctant to take statins.

Elevated Triglycerides

Most cases of hypertriglyceridemia diagnosed in late childhood and adolescence result from secondary causes such as obesity and diabetes. Mild to moderate hypertriglyceridemia is highly amenable to dietary restriction of fat and calories. The use of omega-3 fish oil in adults has been shown to lower TG by 30% to 40% with modest increases in HDL cholesterol without safety concerns.[20] There are limited data on use of omega-3 fish oil in children with hypertriglyceridemia, but it can be considered in pediatric patients with persistent TG 200 mg/dL or greater as an adjunct to diet and physical activity.

Other agents for reduction of TG in adults include fibrates, which decrease TG and increase HDL cholesterol, and niacin, which slightly decreases LDL cholesterol and TG while increasing HDL cholesterol.[24] For substantially elevated TG caused by inherited defects such as LPL deficiency, dietary fat is restricted to 15% of total calories. Despite this extreme reduction, diet does not always effectively prevent sequelae such as recurrent pancreatitis in this patient population. Novel treatments, including targeted gene therapy, are now available for adult patients with LPL deficiency.[25]

Clinical Tip: In our practice, we prescribe omega-3 fatty acids (900 mg twice per day) if TG remains at 500 mg/dL or greater after dietary restriction. Most of these patients have familial hypertriglyceridemia, which has a prevalence of 5% to 10% and is associated with low HDL levels and a risk of increased CVD. The dose is increased to approximately 2 g twice per day if needed. Lovaza (omega-3-acid ethyl esters) may be prescribed, or equivalent over-the-counter fish oil supplements are recommended.

Dyslipidemia of Obesity

Obesity-related lipid disorders involve derangements in multiple lipoproteins and are responsive to weight loss via diet as well as surgery. In applying the new guidelines to data obtained by the NHANES from 1999 to 2010, statin therapy may be recommended for 3.1% of obese children with dyslipidemia compared to only 0.6% of nonobese children.[26] The discrepancy is explained by the multiple lipid abnormalities, insulin resistance, and hypertension associated with increased BMI.[27] The effectiveness of weight loss and dietary cholesterol restriction alone, however, is substantial. In a retrospective review of 53 patients aged 6 to 18 years with combined dyslipidemia who underwent up to 9 months of diet composition changes and increased activity, the authors noted statistically significant improvement in all lipid parameters except for HDL cholesterol, which remained unchanged.[28] These data illustrate that lifestyle changes must be emphasized as primary therapy.

Clinical Tip: Children with obesity can have mild elevations in LDL cholesterol that are amenable to dietary restriction. An LDL level above 160 mg/dL in an obese child warrants a more detailed history to uncover a possible diagnosis of FH or FCHL.

CONTROVERSY

The 2011 NHLBI guidelines are aggressive and continue to stir significant controversy among medical clinicians. Former lipid guidelines promoted targeted screening of children with risk factors for CVD, such as family history of premature CVD or TC greater than 240 mg/dL, dyslipidemia, or obesity.[29] However, this cost-effective approach failed to identify 30% to 60% of affected patients, especially those children with FH, because parents may be young and free of CVD or unaware of their own abnormal lipid levels.[30] The current guidelines advocate targeted screening of children at risk for early CVD as well as universal screening at 2 different ages in order to identify children with FH who have no known risk factors.

The major focus of controversy stems from the concern that broad screening will result in children without FH being started on medication without first attempting diet modification, thus potentially increasing the risk and incidence of adverse effects.[31] Critics also emphasize the paucity of data on long-term outcomes of statin use in children and adolescents, although long-term use in adults has shown far more benefit than risk. Clinical trials of statins for up to 2 years in youth with FH have not demonstrated adverse effects on parameters such as pubertal development, linear growth, or cognition.[32] The 2011 guidelines did not change recommendations for statin use and include specific, evidence-based recommendations for initiation and monitoring of lipid-lowering medication while addressing the need to better identify youth with FH who are at high risk for early CVD.

SUMMARY

Cardiovascular disease remains a substantial health care burden in the adult population, the roots of which begin in childhood. Universal screening for dyslipidemia in all children and adolescents has been implemented to identify cases of FH that are otherwise missed by conventional screening because untreated FH can result in early CVD and untimely death. Recommendations for medical therapy did not change with the 2011 NHLBI guidelines. LDL levels targeted for therapy usually are elevated because of primary genetic disorders such as FH. Although these recommendations remain controversial, the benefit of universal screening and subsequent treatment of high-risk patients far outweighs the risk of not screening, although more investigation is warranted to understand the long-term outcomes of CVD risk in youth.

References

1. Centers for Disease Control and Prevention. Prevalence of abnormal lipid levels among youths—United States, 1999-2006. *Morb Mortal Wkly Rep.* 2010;59:29-33
2. Varghese MJ. Familial hypercholesterolemia: a review. *Ann Pediatr Cardiol.* 2014;7:107-117
3. Davis PH, Dawson JD, Riley WA, Lauer RM. Carotid intimal-medial thickness is related to cardiovascular risk factors measured from childhood through middle age: the Muscatine Study. *Circulation.* 2001;104:2815-2819
4. Li S, Chen W, Srinivasan SR, et al. Childhood cardiovascular risk factors and carotid vascular changes in adulthood: the Bogalusa Heart Study. *JAMA.* 2003;290:2271-2276
5. Gidding SS, McMahan CA, McGill HC, et al. Prediction of coronary artery calcium in young adults using the Pathobiological Determinants of Atherosclerosis in Youth (PDAY) risk score: the CARDIA study. *Arch Intern Med.* 2006;166:2341-2347
6. Juonala M, Viikari JS, Ronnemaa T, et al. Associations of dyslipidemias from childhood to adulthood with carotid intima-media thickness, elasticity, and brachial flow-mediated dilatation in adulthood: the Cardiovascular Risk in Young Finns Study. *ArteriosclerThromb Vasc Biol.* 2008;28:1012-1017
7. Go AS, Mozaffarian D, Roger VL, et al. Heart disease and stroke statistics—2014 update: a report from the American Heart Association. *Circulation.* 2014;129:e28-e292
8. Rader DJ, Hobbs HH. Disorders of lipoprotein metabolism. In: Longo DL, Fauci AS, Kasper DL, et al, eds. *Harrison's Principles of Internal Medicine.* 18th ed. New York: McGraw-Hill; 2012
9. Bamba V. Update on screening, etiology, and treatment of dyslipidemia in children. *J Clin Endocrinol Metab.* 2014;99:3093-3102
10. Nordestgaard BG, Chapman MJ, Humphries SE, et al. Familial hypercholesterolaemia is underdiagnosed and undertreated in the general population: guidance for clinicians to prevent coronary heart disease: consensus statement of the European Atherosclerosis Society. *Eur Heart J.* 2013;34:3478-3490
11. Nair DR, Sharifi M, Al-Rasadi K. Familial hypercholesterolaemia. *Curr Opin Cardiol.* 2014;29:381-388
12. Feoli-Fonseca JC, Levy E, Godard M, Lambert M. Familial lipoprotein lipase deficiency in infancy: clinical, biochemical, and molecular study. *J Pediatr.* 1998;133:417-423
13. Benlian P, De Gennes JL, Foubert L, et al. Premature atherosclerosis in patients with familial chylomicronemia caused by mutations in the lipoprotein lipase gene. *N Eng J Med.* 1996;335:848-854
14. Goldstein JL, Schrott HG, Hazzard WR, Bierman EL, Motulsky AG. Hyperlipidemia in coronary heart disease. II. Genetic analysis of lipid levels in 176 families and delineation of a new inherited disorder, combined hyperlipidemia. *J Clin Invest.* 1973;52:1544-1568

15. Brouwers MC, de Graaf J, van Greevenbroek MM, et al. Novel drugs in familial combined hyperlipidemia: lessons from type 2 diabetes mellitus. *Curr Opin Lipidol*. 2010;21:530-538
16. Ogden CL, Carroll MD, Kit BK, Flegal KM. Prevalence of childhood and adult obesity in the United States, 2011-2012. *JAMA*. 2014;311:806-814
17. Medina-Urrutia A, Juarez-Rojas JG, Cardoso-Saldana G, et al. Abnormal high-density lipoproteins in overweight adolescents with atherogenic dyslipidemia. *Pediatrics*. 2011;127:e1521-e1527
18. Freedman DS, Mei Z, Srinivasan SR, Berenson GS, Dietz WH. Cardiovascular risk factors and excess adiposity among overweight children and adolescents: the Bogalusa Heart Study. *J Pediatr*. 2007;150:12-17.e2
19. Berenson GS, Srinivasan SR, Bao W, et al. Association between multiple cardiovascular risk factors and atherosclerosis in children and young adults. The Bogalusa Heart Study. *N Engl J Med*. 1998;338:1650-1656
20. Expert Panel on Integrated Guidelines for Cardiovascular Health and Risk Reduction in Children and Adolescents, National Heart, Lung, and Blood Institute. Expert panel on integrated guidelines for cardiovascular health and risk reduction in children and adolescents: summary report. *Pediatrics*. 2011;128(Suppl 5):S213-S256
21. Vuorio A, Docherty KF, Humphries SE, Kuoppala J, Kovanen PT. Statin treatment of children with familial hypercholesterolemia—trying to balance incomplete evidence of long-term safety and clinical accountability: are we approaching a consensus? *Atherosclerosis*. 2013;226:315-320
22. Noto D, Cefalu AB, Averna MR. Beyond statins: new lipid lowering strategies to reduce cardiovascular risk. *Curr Atheroscler Rep*. 2014;16:414
23. Santos RD, Watts GF. Familial hypercholesterolaemia: PCSK9 inhibitors are coming. *Lancet*. 2015;385:307-310
24. Ridker PM. LDL cholesterol: controversies and future therapeutic directions. *Lancet*. 2014;384:607-617
25. Gaudet D, Methot J, Dery S, et al. Efficacy and long-term safety of alipogene tiparvovec (AAV1-LPLS447X) gene therapy for lipoprotein lipase deficiency: an open-label trial. *Gene Ther*. 2013;20:361-369
26. McCrindle BW, Tyrrell PN, Kavey RE. Will obesity increase the proportion of children and adolescents recommended for a statin? *Circulation*. 2013;128:2162-2165
27. Sinaiko AR, Steinberger J, Moran A, et al. Relation of body mass index and insulin resistance to cardiovascular risk factors, inflammatory factors, and oxidative stress during adolescence. *Circulation*. 2005;111:1985-1991
28. Pratt RE, Kavey RE, Quinzi D. Combined dyslipidemia in obese children: response to a focused lifestyle approach. *J Clin Lipidol*. 2014;8:181-186
29. American Academy of Pediatrics. National Cholesterol Education Program: Report of the Expert Panel on Blood Cholesterol Levels in Children and Adolescents. *Pediatrics*. 1992;89:525-584
30. Daniels SR, Greer FR; American Academy of Pediatrics Committee on Nutrition. Lipid screening and cardiovascular health in childhood. *Pediatrics*. 2008;122:198-208
31. McCrindle BW, Kwiterovich PO, McBride PE, Daniels SR, Kavey RE. Guidelines for lipid screening in children and adolescents: bringing evidence to the debate. *Pediatrics*. 2012;130:353-356
32. Avis HJ, Vissers MN, Stein EA, et al. A systematic review and meta-analysis of statin therapy in children with familial hypercholesterolemia. *Arterioscler Thromb Vasc Biol*. 2007;27:1803-1810

Prevention and Management of Pregnancy in Adolescents with Endocrine Disorders

Paula J. Adams Hillard, MD

Professor of Obstetrics and Gynecology, Stanford University Medical Center, Stanford University School of Medicine, Palo Alto, California

INTRODUCTION

Most adolescent pregnancies are unintended, and adolescents with chronic medical conditions are as likely as healthy teens to be sexually involved. Preventing unintended pregnancies among teens with chronic endocrine conditions, including diabetes mellitus (both types 1 and 2), polycystic ovary syndrome (PCOS), and thyroid dysfunction, is critically important. Evidence-based guidelines are available to assist with assessment of the risks versus the benefits of specific options for contraception in teens with these and other medical conditions. In most adolescents, the top-tier contraceptive methods—implants and intrauterine devices—represent the most effective, safest, and most successful contraceptive options. Prepregnancy counseling is an important tool for managing chronic endocrine conditions and lowering the risks for both mother and fetus, but it is underutilized among all women, particularly adolescents. The management of pregnancies complicated by diabetes mellitus, PCOS, and thyroid conditions is facilitated by a coordinated effort among obstetricians, endocrinologists, dietitians, and nurse educators. Primary physicians should be aware of their potential role in preventing unplanned pregnancies among all adolescents, but particularly among those with chronic medical conditions. Special care should be taken during the transition of care from pediatric subspecialists to those caring for adults.

ENDOCRINE CONDITIONS IN THE PEDIATRIC AND ADOLESCENT FEMALE: PREVENTING UNINTENDED PREGNANCIES

A number of endocrine conditions are first diagnosed during adolescence or even earlier, during childhood. These conditions include type 1 diabetes mellitus (T1DM), which has a bimodal distribution of age of diagnosis, with 1 peak at age

E-mail address: phillard@stanford.edu

6 to 8 years and a second in early puberty at ages 10 to 14 years[1]; polycystic ovary syndrome (PCOS), by far the most common endocrine condition among adult women, present in 6% to 10% of adult women, and typically with an onset of symptoms and signs during adolescence[2-4]; type 2 diabetes mellitus (T2DM), a condition that is increasing in frequency among adolescents given the national and international epidemics of obesity[5]; hypothyroidism, most commonly caused by chronic autoimmune thyroiditis, with an elevated thyroid-stimulating hormone (TSH) level, found in 2% of adolescents[6]; and a variety of other conditions that are less frequently diagnosed during adolescence than in adulthood, such as pituitary prolactinomas. Transition of care from pediatric to adult subspecialists may be challenging for adolescents and young adults with these conditions, and care should be taken that adolescents and their parents understand and are aware of the implications of endocrine conditions on future reproductive function so that they do not "fall between the cracks" in the health care system.[7]

When considering these preexisting conditions and pregnancy, it is important to note that among women of all ages, approximately 50% of pregnancies are unplanned or unintended.[8] The percentage of unintended pregnancies is even higher among adolescents; approximately 90% of pregnancies in 15- to 17-year olds and 77% in 18- to 19-year olds are unplanned.[8] Among young adults aged 20 to 24 years, nearly two-thirds are unplanned.[8] Thus, even among young adults, it still is uncommon for an individual to have planned her pregnancy. This is of particular and critical concern among adolescents with medical conditions that affect pregnancy and in whom pregnancy affects the condition itself, such as T1DM. Any physician who provides care for adolescents must keep in mind that nearly half of all adolescents have had sexual intercourse[9] and the adolescents with chronic medical conditions are at least as sexually involved as their healthy peers[10] and thus require contraceptive counseling.[11]

Preventive guidance and the provision of appropriate advice about unintended pregnancies and the risks of sexually transmitted infections are critical for teens whose medical conditions "may make unintended pregnancy an unacceptable health risk," a phrase used by the Centers for Disease Control and Prevention (CDC).[12] Included in the list of conditions from the CDC publication, *US Medical Eligibility Criteria for Contraception (USMEC)*, are diabetes: insulin-dependent; with nephropathy/retinopathy/neuropathy or other vascular disease; or of greater than 20 years' duration.[12] Also included on this list, and a condition with significant endocrine ramifications but beyond the scope of this review, is a history of bariatric surgery within the past 2 years. For young women with underlying medical conditions, long-acting, highly effective contraceptive methods may be the best choice.[13] The American College of Obstetricians and Gynecologists and the American Academy of Pediatrics both have published committee opinion statements noting that long-acting reversible contraceptive (LARC) methods should be considered to be top-tier contraceptives for adolescents.[14,15] Per the USMEC, women with conditions that "may make unintended pregnancy an unacceptable health risk" should be advised that sole use of barrier methods for contraception and behavior-based methods of contraception (variations of natural family planning and fertility awareness methods) may *not* be the most appropriate choice for women in this group because of their relatively higher typical-use rates of failure (eg, approximately 18% for typical use of condoms).[12,16]

Physicians who care for adolescents with diabetes, PCOS, and other endocrine conditions should offer preventive guidance about contraception and pregnancy planning to all of their patients, or they should refer them to an appropriate physician who can sensitively provide this information to adolescents. Data from the National Survey of Family Growth (NSFG) found that women with diabetes or obesity are more likely to be nonusers of contraception compared to women without these conditions.[17]

The failure rates of oral contraceptive pills, the transdermal patch, and the vaginal ring were found in a recent study, the *Contraceptive CHOICE Project,* to be more than 20 times that of the failure rate of LARC methods of contraception.[18] For women with medical conditions, evidence-based recommendations for contraception for all contraceptive methods as they apply to specific medical conditions, such as diabetes, have been summarized in the USMEC.[12] For endocrine conditions, the USMEC finds the use of the progestin-only subdermal implant (Nexplanon) and levonorgestrel-containing intrauterine devices (IUDs) (Mirena and Skyla) for women with diabetes to be a category 2 option, meaning a condition for which the advantages of using the method generally outweigh the theoretical or proven risks.[12] The copper IUD (ParaGard) is rated category 1, meaning there is no restriction on the use of the method for women with diabetes. For women with thyroid disorders, all of the LARC methods are rated category 1.[12]

For those having diabetes with nonvascular disease, the USMEC rates the use of combined hormone methods (the pill, patch, ring) as category 2, with the evidence showing that for both insulin-dependent and noninsulin-dependent diabetes, use of combined hormonal methods has limited effect on daily insulin requirement and no effect on long-term diabetes control or progression to retinopathy, with limited changes in lipid profile and hemostatic markers.[12]

PREPREGNANCY PLANNING

Ideally, a pregnancy would be planned and would fit within the framework of a reproductive life plan. The CDC offers resources for health professionals to use with patients in the form of a reproductive life plan/preconception planning tool giving suggested wording for discussions with patients.[19] The CDC also offers a worksheet for individual women/patients to help them better plan for their reproductive futures.[20] For a teen with an endocrine problem, appropriate prepregnancy planning would entail postponing pregnancy by using a long-acting contraceptive method until her life situation is optimal, ideally within a stable relationship with an intimate partner who can be a part of the planning. It also would involve consultation and coordination of care with a primary physician who is familiar with all aspects of the individual's health, including an awareness of psychosocial issues, an endocrinologist who can optimize the care of the endocrine condition, and prepregnancy consultation with a specialist in maternal-fetal medicine (high-risk obstetrics) who can provide information and counseling about the potential health risks during pregnancy, information about the effect of the underlying disease on the fetus, and information about the recommended monitoring during pregnancy that would be optimal for both mother and fetus.

The CDC has urged the intake of sufficient folic acid (0.4 mg/day) for all women of reproductive age because, given the high rates of unplanned pregnancy in the United States and given that neural tube defects develop early in pregnancy (3-4 weeks after conception), before most women know that they are pregnant, the evidence finds that this will reduce the risks.[21] Folic acid supplementation is particularly important for women with diabetes, and it more strongly attenuates the risk of spina bifida for those with diabetes than does supplementation for obese women, who also have an increased risk for neural tube defects.[22]

Diabetes Mellitus

For women with T1DM, prepregnancy planning with tight glycemic control and near normoglycemia is particularly important to reduce the risks of malformations and pregnancy-related complications.[23] The American College of Obstetricians and Gynecologists recommends achieving and maintaining a hemoglobin A_{1c} (HbA_{1c}) level no greater than 6%.[24] One study found the risks of adverse outcomes to be halved with each percentage reduction in HbA_{1c} level achieved before pregnancy.[25] Preconception counseling on diabetes mellitus care and adverse pregnancy outcomes for women with T1DM led to 3-fold lower rates of congenital malformations compared to a control group.[26] In 1 study, only about one-third of women with established DM received preconception counseling.[27] It is probable that adolescents are less likely to receive such counseling, given that a higher percentage of adolescent pregnancies are unplanned. Few data have assessed the outcomes of adolescent pregnancies compared to adult pregnancies in patients with diabetes; 1 study found later presentation for prenatal care, as well as worse glycemic control throughout pregnancy, in adolescents.[28]

Screening for diabetic retinopathy, diabetic nephropathy, and thyroid dysfunction are also important, and indications for antihypertensive treatment and treatment of thyroid dysfunction need to be addressed before and during pregnancy.[29] Concurrent medications should be reviewed; in 1 study, 41% of adults with diabetes were taking 1 or more teratogenic drugs.[30] Appropriate diet and exercise should be encouraged and may be helpful in reducing the rate of preeclampsia and preterm delivery.[31] Patients should be aware that with both T1DM and T2DM, there is a greater risk of pregnancy loss/spontaneous abortion than in the general population.[32]

For adolescents with type 2 diabetes, prepregnancy planning should focus on weight reduction through an appropriate diet and exercise plan. Risks of congenital malformations and miscarriage have been associated with glycemic control in both individuals with type 1 and type 2 diabetes,[25] although women with type 2 diabetes are less likely to have diabetes-related complications than women with type 1 diabetes.[33] Perinatal deaths and rates of small-for-gestational-age (SGA) infants are increased in women with T2DM.[33]

Polycystic Ovary Syndrome

Women with PCOS are oligo-ovulatory. Although this means that they may experience a delay in conception, it does not mean that infertility is inevitable. This is a particularly important point to emphasize with adolescents, because they may consciously or subconsciously test their fertility, and an unintended pregnancy can result. The message "Do not assume that you will have difficulty getting pregnant" should be coupled with the recommendation for contraception in adolescents with PCOS. A study in Finland found that menstrual irregularity or elevated androgen levels at 16 years of age were associated with symptoms of PCOS at 26 years of age as well as infertility problems at age 26 but not with decreased pregnancy or delivery rates at age 26.[34] The benefits of combination oral contraceptives outweigh the risks for young women with PCOS who do not desire pregnancy; they very effectively regulate menses, minimize excess hair growth, and improve acne.[4] Combined oral contraceptives have several mechanisms by which they benefit PCOS: they suppress secretion of luteinizing hormone, resulting in a decrease in ovarian androgen production; the estrogen component increases sex hormone binding globulin, which results in lower levels of free testosterone; and the progestin component can compete for 5α-reductase at the level of the androgen receptor.[4] A large study in Germany found that in a population of women with subfertility, having ever used hormonal contraception was associated with increased pregnancy rates.[35]

Metformin is being used increasingly for the management of PCOS, although more evidence is needed to determine the role of this drug in either improving the hyperandrogenic symptoms of PCOS or preventing the long-term health risks associated with PCOS, such as diabetes, cardiovascular disease, or endometrial cancer, particularly for adolescents.[36] However, use of metformin as a sole agent for treating PCOS in adolescents is limited by its potential to improve ovulatory function and potentially increase the risks of unintended pregnancy. Clomiphene citrate is also generally not used in the United States for primary management of PCOS for adolescents because improving ovulation and fertility is generally not the primary issue for this age group.

Infertility in obese women is primarily the result of ovulatory dysfunction. Ovulatory function and pregnancy rates frequently improve significantly after weight loss in obese anovulatory women.[37] Adolescents with obesity and PCOS should be encouraged to manage their condition with attention to a healthy diet and regular exercise. Adolescents with obesity and PCOS are at increased risk for the development of T2DM. Although only a few studies have reported the prevalence of impaired glucose tolerance or T2DM in adolescents with PCOS, the risks seem to be increased, and adult women with PCOS have clearly been shown to have an increased risk of T2DM.[38] Behavioral contributions to the pathogenesis of impaired glucose tolerance and T2DM include dietary intake, exercise, being sedentary, sleep dysfunction, and stress.[39] Adolescents may respond to the information that a healthy diet and regular physical exercise will likely improve their future fertility if weight loss is maintained. Counseling and encouraging an adolescent to make lifestyle changes is not easy, although it is the author's experience that lifestyle changes may be easier for adolescents to make than for adults, who may have long-entrenched patterns of behavior. Motivational interviewing and a sensitive awareness of the potential effect of the diagnosis on the individual's self-esteem can be helpful.[40] New wearable technologies (pedometers and smartphone accelerometers) that monitor and track physical activity may prove to be a motivating factor, although few studies of these technologies have yet demonstrated a lasting benefit among adolescents.[40]

Preconception overweight and obesity are associated with increased risks for pregnancy complications, including preeclampsia, gestational diabetes, neural tube defects, and congenital heart defects, as well as the risks of undergoing a cesarean delivery.[41] Although a recent Cochrane review concluded that studies of lifestyle modification showed no significant effect on pregnancy rate, adolescents who are overweight or obese can be informed that lifestyle management with weight loss or use of metformin will each improve their current health (blood glucose and insulin levels).[42] Long-term follow-up of the effects of adolescent lifestyle changes on fertility are not available, but preconception assessment and nutritional intervention may improve the chances for a healthy pregnancy in the future.[41]

Adolescents with PCOS can be encouraged by the information that if and when fertility is desired, and if infertility is an issue, fertility treatment measures typically are successful. Among a large German population of "subfertile" women aged 18 to 30 years, 74.8% became pregnant within the first year after consultation.[35] Although clomiphene citrate has traditionally been used to improve ovulation in women with PCOS, metformin and clomiphene citrate have been found to be more effective in inducing ovulation than clomiphene alone.[43,44]

Some studies have found improved success with the use of the aromatase inhibitor letrozole over clomiphene.[45]

Thyroid Dysfunction

Children with conditions in which autoimmune thyroiditis and, to a lesser extent, hypothyroidism are more prevalent, including T1DM and celiac disease, should be screened. Approximately 7.3% of all US females aged 12 to 19 years had antithyroid antibodies according to the NHANES data.[6] However, a study of the natural history of euthyroid autoimmune thyroiditis demonstrated that most of those with elevated antibodies remained euthyroid, whereas 26% developed serum TSH levels 2-fold above the upper limit of normal and 10% developed only a mild elevation in serum TSH levels.[46]

ENDOCRINE CONDITIONS *DURING* PREGNANCY

Diabetes Mellitus During Pregnancy

Although maintaining tight glycemic control is extremely important before and during pregnancy for women and their fetuses, this is balanced by the need to prevent severe hypoglycemia during pregnancy in adolescents and adult women with T1DM.[23,29] Use of rapid-acting insulin analogs is regarded as safe during pregnancy, and longer-acting insulins are used as well, along with frequent self-monitoring of blood glucose, including fasting levels, before and 1 to 2 hours after each meal, and at bedtime.[24] Management of the diabetic pregnancy is ideally a collaborative effort among obstetricians, endocrinologists, dietitians, and nurse educators before and during pregnancy. Attention to diet and exercise should be strongly encouraged. Women with T1DM are at risk for gestational hypertension and preeclampsia. Pregnancy does not result in worsening of renal function for women with diabetic nephropathy and normal serum creatinine, although pregnancy-related complications, including preeclampsia and preterm delivery, occur more frequently than if kidney function were normal.[23] Pregnancy can induce worsening of diabetic retinopathy for women with T1DM, so ophthalmologic care is important. Close obstetric surveillance of fetal growth and well-being is necessary, along with careful planning for the timing and mode of delivery. Type 1 diabetes mellitus requires tight glycemic control during labor, with attention to blood pressure monitoring.[23,29]

Polycystic Ovary Syndrome During Pregnancy

Women with PCOS have an increased risk of spontaneous abortion (miscarriage) and need to be aware of this risk. In total, the risk of spontaneous abortion in women with PCOS is 3 times higher than the risk in healthy women.[47] Unfortunately, the risk of most pregnancy pathologies is also higher for patients with PCOS, including gestational diabetes, pregnancy-induced hypertension, preeclampsia, and SGA babies.[47] Use of metformin in the treatment of PCOS and gestational diabetes has led to questions about the potential risks to offspring because metformin crosses the placenta, and, although the potential risks are not well established, first trimester use has not been associated with an increased risk of major birth defects.[48-51] A Cochrane review found no conclusive evidence that metformin treatment before or during assisted reproductive technology cycles improved live birth rates in women with PCOS, but its use did increase clinical pregnancy rates and decrease the risks of ovarian hyperstimulation syndrome.[52]

Thyroid Dysfunction in Pregnancy

Overt maternal hypothyroidism is known to have adverse fetal effects, and subclinical hypothyroidism may be associated with adverse maternal and fetal effects; thus, antibody-positive women may be at increased risk for pregnancy complications.[53] It is important, therefore, that this group of women be monitored in pregnancy. There is also an association between the presence of thyroid antibodies and pregnancy loss that should be discussed in adolescents with known antibodies, but universal screening for antithyroid antibodies or possible treatment has not been recommended.[53]

Guidelines from the American Thyroid Association for the Diagnosis and Management of Thyroid Disease During Pregnancy and Postpartum, as well as from the Endocrine Society, note that pregnancy is a stress test for the thyroid, resulting in hypothyroidism for women with limited reserve or postpartum thyroiditis in women with underlying Hashimoto disease who were previously euthyroid.[53,54] The changes in thyroid physiology during a normal pregnancy should be kept in mind when interpreting thyroid function tests, and pregnancy or trimester-specific norms should be noted. The major changes in thyroid function during pregnancy include an increase in thyroid-binding globulin and stimulation of the TSH receptor by human chorionic gonadotropin, leading to an increase in both serum total thyroxine (T4) and triiodothyronine (T3) and a decrease in serum TSH. The Endocrine Society Clinical Practice Guidelines, using the US Preventive Services Task Force recommendation terminology and levels of evidence, noted level B/fair evidence for T4 replacement in women with subclinical hypothyroidism who are thyroid peroxidase antibody positive (TPO Ab+) for improving obstetric outcome and poor for fetal neurologic development but noted recommendation level C/fair evidence for thyroid peroxidase antibody negative (TPO Ab-) women for obstetric outcome.[53] Overt hypothyroidism should be treated and thyroid function test levels normalized as rapidly as possible.[53] Guidelines for the management of overt *hyper*thyroidism as a result of Graves disease or thyroid nodules recommend that antithyroid drug therapy be initiated before pregnancy if possible or adjusted to maintain the maternal thyroid levels for free T4 at or just above the upper limit of the nonpregnant reference range.[53]

SUMMARY

Because 83% of adolescent pregnancies among teens 15 to 19 years old are unintended[8] and because adolescents with chronic medical conditions are as likely to be sexually involved as are healthy teens,[10] preventing unintended pregnancies among teens with chronic endocrine conditions, including diabetes mellitus (both types 1 and 2), PCOS, and thyroid dysfunction, is critically important. Evidence-based guidelines are available to assist with assessment of the risks versus the benefits of specific options for contraception in teens with these and other medical conditions.[12] In many teens, including those with chronic medical conditions, the top-tier contraceptive methods—implants and intrauterine devices—represent the most effective, safest, and most successful contraceptive options for adolescents.[14,15]

Prepregnancy counseling can be an important tool for managing chronic endocrine conditions and lowering the risks for both mother and fetus, but it is underutilized among all women, particularly adolescents. The management of pregnancies complicated by DM, PCOS, and thyroid conditions is facilitated by a coordinated effort among obstetricians, endocrinologists, dietitians, and nurse educators. Primary physicians should be aware of their potential role in preventing unplanned pregnancies among all adolescents, but particularly among those with chronic medical conditions.

References

1. Felner EI, Klitz W, Ham M, et al. Genetic interaction among three genomic regions creates distinct contributions to early- and late-onset type 1 diabetes mellitus. *Pediatr Diabetes.* 2005;6:213-220
2. Welt CK, Carmina E. Clinical review: lifecycle of polycystic ovary syndrome (PCOS): from in utero to menopause. *J Clin Endocrinol Metab.* 2013;98:4629-4638
3. Legro RS, Arslanian SA, Ehrmann DA, et al. Diagnosis and treatment of polycystic ovary syndrome: an Endocrine Society clinical practice guideline. *J Clin Endocrinol Metab.* 2013;98: 4565-4592
4. Fauser BC, Tarlatzis BC, Rebar RW, et al. Consensus on women's health aspects of polycystic ovary syndrome (PCOS): the Amsterdam ESHRE/ASRM-Sponsored 3rd PCOS Consensus Workshop Group. *Fertil Steril.* 2012;97:28-38, e25
5. Zeitler P, Fu J, Tandon N, et al. Type 2 diabetes in the child and adolescent. *Pediatr Diabetes.* 2014;15(Suppl 20):26-46
6. Hollowell JG, Staehling NW, Flanders WD, et al. Serum TSH, T(4), and thyroid antibodies in the United States population (1988 to 1994): National Health and Nutrition Examination Survey (NHANES III). *J Clin Endocrinol Metab.* 2002;87:489-499
7. Dokras A, Witchel SF. Are young adult women with polycystic ovary syndrome slipping through the healthcare cracks? *J Clin Endocrinol Metab.* 2014;99:1583-1585
8. Finer LB, Zolna MR. Shifts in intended and unintended pregnancies in the United States, 2001-2008. *Am J Public Health.* 2014;104(Suppl 1):S43-S48
9. Kann L, Kinchen S, Shanklin SL, et al. Youth risk behavior surveillance—United States, 2013. *MMWR Surveill Summ.* 2014;63(Suppl 4):1-168
10. Suris JC, Resnick MD, Cassuto N, Blum RW. Sexual behavior of adolescents with chronic disease and disability. *J Adolesc Health.* 1996;19(2):124-131

11. Greydanus DE, Pratt HD, Patel DR. Concepts of contraception for adolescent and young adult women with chronic illness and disability. *Dis Mon.* 2012;58(5):258-320
12. Centers for Disease Control and Prevention. U.S. medical eligibility criteria for contraceptive use, 2010. *MMWR Recomm Rep.* 2010;59(RR-4):1-86
13. Lathrop E, Jatlaoui T. Contraception for women with chronic medical conditions: an evidence-based approach. *Clin Obstet Gynecol.* 2014;57:674-681
14. American College of Obstetricians and Gynecologists Committee on Gynecological Practice: Long-Acting Reversible Contraception Working Group. Committee Opinion no. 450: increasing use of contraceptive implants and intrauterine devices to reduce unintended pregnancy. *Obstet Gynecol.* 2009;114(6):1434-1438
15. American Academy of Pediatrics Committee on Adolescence. Contraception for adolescents. *Pediatrics.* 2014;134(4):e1244-e1256
16. Trussell J. Percentage of women experiencing an unintended pregnancy during the first year of typical use and the first year of perfect use of contraception, and the percentage continuing use at the end of the first year, United States. In: Hatcher R, Trussell J, Nelson AL, et al, eds. *Contraceptive Technology.* 20th ed. New York: Bridging the Gap Communications; 2011:50
17. Chuang CH, Chase GA, Bensyl DM, Weisman CS. Contraceptive use by diabetic and obese women. *Womens Health Issues.* 2005;15(4):167-173
18. Winner B, Peipert JF, Zhao Q, et al. Effectiveness of long-acting reversible contraception. *N Engl J Med.* 2012;366(21):1998-2007
19. Centers for Disease Control and Prevention; Moos M-K. Preconception health and health care: reproductive life plan tool for health professionals. Available at: www.cdc.gov/preconception/documents/rlphealthproviders.pdf. Accessed December 8, 2014
20. Moos M-K. My reproductive life plan. In: Preconception health and health care 2010. Available at: www.cdc.gov/preconception/documents/reproductivelifeplan-worksheet.pdf. Accessed November 21, 2014
21. Recommendations for the use of folic acid to reduce the number of cases of spina bifida and other neural tube defects. *MMWR Recomm Rep.* 1992;41(RR-14):1-7
22. Parker SE, Yazdy MM, Tinker SC, Mitchell AA, Werler MM. The impact of folic acid intake on the association among diabetes mellitus, obesity, and spina bifida. *Am J Obstet Gynecol.* 2013;209(3):239.e231-e238
23. Ringholm L, Mathiesen ER, Kelstrup L, Damm P. Managing type 1 diabetes mellitus in pregnancy—from planning to breastfeeding. *Nat Rev Endocrinol.* 2012;8(11):659-667
24. ACOG Practice Bulletin. Clinical management guidelines for obstetrician-gynecologists. Number 60, March 2005. Pregestational diabetes mellitus (reaffirmed 2012). *Obstet Gynecol.* 2005;105(3):675-685
25. Inkster ME, Fahey TP, Donnan PT, et al. Poor glycated haemoglobin control and adverse pregnancy outcomes in type 1 and type 2 diabetes mellitus: systematic review of observational studies. *BMC Pregnancy Childbirth.* 2006;6:30
26. Temple RC, Aldridge VJ, Murphy HR. Prepregnancy care and pregnancy outcomes in women with type 1 diabetes. *Diabetes Care.* 2006;29(8):1744-1749
27. Janz NK, Herman WH, Becker MP, et al. Diabetes and pregnancy. Factors associated with seeking pre-conception care. *Diabetes Care.* 1995;18(2):157-165
28. Carmody D, Doyle A, Firth RG, et al. Teenage pregnancy in type 1 diabetes mellitus. *Pediatr Diabetes.* 2010;11(2):111-115
29. Mathiesen ER, Ringholm L, Damm P. Therapeutic management of type 1 diabetes before and during pregnancy. *Expert Opin Pharmacother.* 2011;12(5):779-786
30. Varughese GI, Chowdhury SR, Warner DP, Barton DM. Preconception care of women attending adult general diabetes clinics—are we doing enough? *Diabetes Res Clin Pract.* 2007;76(1):142-145
31. Wolf HT, Owe KM, Juhl M, Hegaard HK. Leisure time physical activity and the risk of pre-eclampsia: a systematic review. *Matern Child Health J.* 2014;18(4):899-910
32. McGrogan A, Snowball J, de Vries CS. Pregnancy losses in women with Type 1 or Type 2 diabetes in the UK: an investigation using primary care records. *Diabet Med.* 2014;31(3):357-365

33. Gizzo S, Patrelli TS, Rossanese M, et al. An update on diabetic women obstetrical outcomes linked to preconception and pregnancy glycemic profile: a systematic literature review. *Sci World J.* 2013;2013:254901
34. West S, Lashen H, Bloigu A, et al. Irregular menstruation and hyperandrogenaemia in adolescence are associated with polycystic ovary syndrome and infertility in later life: Northern Finland Birth Cohort 1986 study. *Hum Reprod.* 2014;29:2339-2351
35. Ziller V, Heilmaier C, Kostev K. Time to pregnancy in subfertile women in German gynecological practices: analysis of a representative cohort of more than 60,000 patients. *Arch Gynecol Obstet.* 2015;291(3):657-662
36. Johnson NP. Metformin use in women with polycystic ovary syndrome. *Ann Transl Med.* 2014;2(6):56
37. Obesity and reproduction: an educational bulletin. *Fertil Steril.* 2008;90(5 Suppl):S21-S29
38. Carreau AM, Baillargeon JP. PCOS in adolescence and type 2 diabetes. *Curr Diab Rep.* 2015;15:564
39. Spruijt-Metz D, O'Reilly GA, Cook L, Page KA, Quinn C. Behavioral contributions to the pathogenesis of type 2 diabetes. *Curr Diab Rep.* 2014;14:475
40. Mani H, Potdar N, Gleeson H. How to manage an adolescent girl presenting with features of polycystic ovary syndrome (PCOS); an exemplar for adolescent health care in endocrinology. *Clin Endocrinol (Oxf).* 2014;81:652-656
41. Dean SV, Lassi ZS, Imam AM, Bhutta ZA. Preconception care: nutritional risks and interventions. *Reprod Health.* 2014;11(Suppl 3):S3
42. Domecq JP, Prutsky G, Mullan RJ, et al. Lifestyle modification programs in polycystic ovary syndrome: systematic review and meta-analysis. *J Clin Endocrinol Metab.* 2013;98(12):4655-4663
43. Tang T, Lord JM, Norman RJ, Yasmin E, Balen AH. Insulin-sensitising drugs (metformin, rosiglitazone, pioglitazone, D-chiro-inositol) for women with polycystic ovary syndrome, oligo amenorrhoea and subfertility. *Cochrane Database Syst Rev.* 2012;5:Cd003053
44. Practice Committee of the American Society for Reproductive Medicine. Use of clomiphene citrate in infertile women: a committee opinion. *Fertil Steril.* 2013;100(2):341-348
45. Franik S, Kremer JA, Nelen WL, Farquhar C. Aromatase inhibitors for subfertile women with polycystic ovary syndrome. *Cochrane Database Syst Rev.* 2014;2:Cd010287
46. Radetti G, Gottardi E, Bona G, et al. The natural history of euthyroid Hashimoto's thyroiditis in children. *J Pediatr.* 2006;149(6):827-832
47. Katulski K, Czyzyk A, Podfigurna-Stopa A, Genazzani AR, Meczekalski B. Pregnancy complications in polycystic ovary syndrome patients. *Gynecol Endocrinol.* 2015;31:87-91
48. Bertoldo MJ, Faure M, Dupont J, Froment P. Impact of metformin on reproductive tissues: an overview from gametogenesis to gestation. *Ann Transl Med.* 2014;2(6):55
49. Simmons D. Safety considerations with pharmacological treatment of gestational diabetes mellitus. *Drug Saf.* 2015;38(1):65-78
50. Cassina M, Dona M, Di Gianantonio E, Litta P, Clementi M. First-trimester exposure to metformin and risk of birth defects: a systematic review and meta-analysis. *Hum Reprod Update.* 2014;20(5):656-669
51. Holt RI, Lambert KD. The use of oral hypoglycaemic agents in pregnancy. *Diabet Med.* 2014;31(3):282-291
52. Tso LO, Costello MF, Albuquerque LE, Andriolo RB, Macedo CR. Metformin treatment before and during IVF or ICSI in women with polycystic ovary syndrome. *Cochrane Database Syst Rev.* 2014;11:Cd006105
53. De Groot L, Abalovich M, Alexander EK, et al. Management of thyroid dysfunction during pregnancy and postpartum: an Endocrine Society clinical practice guideline. *J Clin Endocrinol Metab.* 2012;97(8):2543-2565
54. Stagnaro-Green A, Abalovich M, Alexander E, et al. Guidelines of the American Thyroid Association for the diagnosis and management of thyroid disease during pregnancy and postpartum. *Thyroid.* 2011;21(10):1081-1125

Endocrine Abnormalities in Patients with Eating Disorders

Nadia Saldanha, MD*; Linda Carmine, MD

Division of Adolescent Medicine, Cohen Children's Medical Center, North Shore–Long Island Jewish Health System, Hofstra–North Shore LIJ School of Medicine, Hempstead, New York

INTRODUCTION

The endocrine consequences of eating disorders are among the most severe and potentially longest lasting of any of the medical complications associated with anorexia nervosa (AN), bulimia nervosa (BN), and binge eating disorder (BED). Endocrine complications include alterations in levels of cortisol, growth hormone (GH), insulinlike growth factor-1 (IGF-1), estradiol, testosterone, gut neuropeptides (leptin, ghrelin, peptide YY), and thyroid hormone, which lead to delayed puberty and amenorrhea and have an effect on both bone density and bone growth. Depending on the duration and degree of illness, most of the endocrine consequences can be reversed, with the exception of decreased bone density. Most of the endocrine changes are due primarily to the energy deficit created by malnutrition and thus are seen most commonly in AN. However, some neuroendocrine manifestations are seen in both BN and BED as well. This review will highlight what has been well established in the literature with regard to endocrine abnormalities in the eating disorders as well as discuss more recent findings.

EATING DISORDERS: ANOREXIA NERVOSA, BULIMIA NERVOSA, AND BINGE EATING DISORDER

The condition of self-starvation was first described in the 13th and 14th centuries when many religious young women restricted their intake to demonstrate their religious devotion. One notable example is St. Catherine of Siena, whose described restriction was central to her piety and ultimately part of her saint-

---

*Corresponding author
E-mail address: Nsaldanh12@nshs.edu

hood. In this context, the self-starvation has been referred to as *anorexia mirabilis*. In the late 1600s, the British doctor Richard Morton first described 2 cases of a syndrome of loss of appetite and extreme fasting, which is the first reference to AN in the medical literature. Of course, much has happened since then with regard to the study of the etiology of the disorder and the changing epidemiology of those affected, but currently in the United States a prevalence of 0.2% to 0.4% is reported, which makes AN the third most common chronic disease of adolescent girls.[1-3] The *Diagnostic and Statistical Manual of Mental Disorders* (Fifth Edition) (*DSM-5*) currently defines AN as a disorder in which restriction of energy intake relative to a person's requirements leads to a significantly low weight or, specifically in adolescents, a weight that is less than what is minimally expected. Other features include an intense fear of gaining weight despite being at a low weight and a lack of recognition of the severity of the illness. Notable is the absence of amenorrhea and a specific weight threshold of being less than 85% of ideal body weight, which were present in the previous *DSM-IV* criteria.[4]

Bulimia nervosa is defined by recurrent binge eating episodes that include a lack of control over eating during the binge episode. Binge eating occurs in a discrete amount of time and involves consuming a larger amount of food than what most people would eat. In addition to the binge episode there is a compensatory mechanism to prevent weight gain, which may include vomiting, laxative or diuretic use, or excessive exercising. The binge episodes and compensatory mechanisms should occur on average about once per week for 3 months to meet diagnostic criteria and should not occur during an episode of AN. Patients with BN may be normal weight, underweight, or overweight, and the degree to which they are underweight likely affects the amount of endocrine complications seen. The prevalence of BN is 1% to 1.5% among young females, and the disorder peaks in older adolescence and young adulthood.[4]

Binge eating disorder involves recurrent episodes of binge eating, as described for BN, but without the compensatory mechanism. The episodes are associated with eating more rapidly than normal, eating until feeling uncomfortably full, eating large amounts of food when not feeling hungry, eating alone because of feeling embarrassed by how much one is eating, and feeling disgusted with oneself or guilty afterward. Although most of the endocrine complications of eating disorders are seen in AN, because of the energy-deficient state some conditions specific to BN and BED will also be discussed in this review.

Although the diagnostic criteria for eating disorders are primarily psychiatric, the medical complications affect almost all organ systems and can complicate treatment. These include electrolyte abnormalities such as hypokalemia, seen especially in patients with purging, and hyponatremia, which can be seen in patients who water load in an attempt to increase their weight. Gastrointestinal complications range from less severe manifestations, such as transient elevations in amylase and liver enzymes or delayed gastric emptying and decreased intestinal motility, often causing abdominal pain and constipation, to less common but more severe findings such as gastric dilation and rupture or the superior mesenteric artery syndrome. Cardiac complications include bradycardia and orthostatic hypotension, electrocardiographic changes such as prolonged QT intervals and decreased left ventricular forces, as well as an increased risk of pericardial effusion and congestive heart failure. Patients with AN often report a decreased ability to concentrate or feeling in a "fog." Magnetic resonance imaging of the brain can show pseudocortical atrophy and enlarged ventricles. Hematologic changes include anemia, thrombocytopenia, and most commonly leukopenia.[5,6]

The endocrine complications of eating disorders are the most pervasive and potentially the longest lasting. The other medical complications tend to resolve with treatment and weight gain, but endocrine abnormalities can take longer or may have effects on the body even after the eating disorder has resolved. Endocrine complications of eating disorders include delayed puberty, hypothalamic amenorrhea, and impaired bone metabolism. The hypothalamic-pituitary-ovarian (HPO) axis is directly affected in both hypothalamic amenorrhea and bone metabolism, and the alterations seen in the hypothalamic-pituitary-adrenal (HPA) axis, the hypothalamic-pituitary-thyroid (HPT) axis, and the gut neuropeptides indirectly contribute to the effects of malnutrition on bone metabolism.

HYPOTHALAMIC AMENORRHEA

The age at which girls achieve menarche had reportedly decreased in developed countries from the mid-1800s to the 1960s. Presumably because of improved nutrition and eradication of infections, studies evaluating the changes in menarcheal age over the past 50 years, during which the age of menarche has continued to fall (although more slowly), have postulated that race, genetics, environmental chemicals, and overnutrition all are contributing factors.[7-11] According to the American Academy of Pediatrics, an absence of puberty at age 13 years or absence of menarche at 15 years now should be considered the time at which a medical evaluation would be initiated, because 98% of girls will have achieved menarche by age 15 years. Additional criteria for evaluation include an adolescent who has not had thelarche by age 13 years, an adolescent having menarche with more than 3 years since thelarche, and an adolescent who has not had menarche by age 14 years in whom there is suspicion of an eating disorder or excessive exercise, hirsutism, or genital outflow tract obstruction.[12] The menstrual cycle should be consistent and remain between 20 to 45 days, with approximately 30 mL of blood flow, not to exceed 80 mL. Menstrual irregularity in adolescent girls is a frequent occurrence with a myriad of etiologies, but because of concerns of osteopenia, prolonged amenorrhea requires evaluation and management.

The hypothalamic neuroendocrine systems controlling pituitary gonadotropin secretion are integral to the development and functioning of the reproductive system. Neurotransmitters and neuropeptides control the pulsatile release of gonadotropin-releasing hormone (GnRH), presumably from the median eminence of the hypothalamus, the GnRH pulse generator. Norepinephrine, dopamine, and gamma-aminobutyric acid neurons affect GnRH release at the arcuate nucleus and the median eminence of the hypothalamus, both directly and indirectly. In addition, dopamine interacts with endogenous opioids, such as beta-endorphins, in their inhibition of GnRH secretion, as demonstrated in studies using naloxone to stimulate GnRH and luteinizing hormone (LH) release. Corticotropin-releasing hormone (CRH) also exerts a suppressive effect on GnRH, likely through its stimulation of endogenous opioid receptors.[13]

Hypothalamic suppression and functional hyperandrogenism are the 2 most frequent causes of amenorrhea in nonpregnant adolescents. A Swedish study that evaluated menstrual disorders in more than 200 adolescent girls found amenorrhea in 58% and oligomenorrhea in 42%, and determined that 68% of the girls with amenorrhea and 38% of those with oligomenorrhea had an eating disorder. For girls with reported weight loss, the study also found an eating disorder in 83% of the amenorrheic girls and 61% of the oligomenorrheic girls.[14] Although the girls with amenorrhea were more likely to present with laboratory findings consistent with hypothalamic suppression, the girls with oligomenorrhea were more likely to have a higher LH to follicle-stimulating hormone (FSH) ratio, to have a higher testosterone to steroid hormone-binding globulin ratio, and to meet criteria for polycystic ovarian syndrome (55% vs 38%). This hyperandrogenic state is characterized by estrogen sufficiency and high LH, which is associated with high GnRH pulsatility.

The amenorrhea of hypothalamic suppression is a direct manifestation of decreased pulsatility of GnRH secretion, resulting in an altered gonadotropin cycle and a subsequent estrogen-deficient state. The gonadotropin pattern is represented by decreased frequency and intensity of LH pulses and a decreased LH to FSH ratio. The follicular phase becomes prolonged, and, without adequate stimulation, ovulation and the luteal phase may not occur. An energy deficit based on inadequate nutrition, excessive exercise, or chronic illness may result in suppression of the HPO axis, leading to reduced menstrual frequency or amenorrhea. The mechanism of this suppression is complex and not fully understood, but neurotransmitters, including leptin, CRH, norepinephrine, beta-endorphins, and dopamine, are each involved in the regulation of GnRH. Whereas the energy depletion of weight loss and exercise are thought to exert their effects on the HPO axis through *leptin*, stress and exercise may exert their effects through the HPA axis, norepinephrine, beta-endorphins, and CRH.[15,16]

Leptin may directly affect GnRH pulsation frequency and amplitude such that low leptin levels associated with energy deficiency will result in low GnRH pulsations. The determination of which women will develop hypothalamic amenorrhea is still not clear. The evidence for a differential in percentage of body fat between adolescents with and those without menses does not exist, and up to 20% of women with restrictive eating patterns will become amenorrheic before weight loss. Early studies of AN and GnRH pulsatility indicated that the degree of pulsatile immaturity was not directly correlated with the duration of illness, degree of "fatness," or deviation from ideal weight. Furthermore, resumption of menses also was not directly correlated with weight restoration.[17] Although leptin has a clear role in GnRH pulse frequency and levels of leptin have been found to be lower in amenorrheic women with lower body fat mass, there is significant overlap in leptin levels between those who recover menses and those who do not.

The type of eating disorder also may not be the determining factor in altering menstrual function based on hypothalamic suppression such that the energy deficit associated with any eating disorder type may lead to this dysfunction. In a study of high school girls taking a National Eating Disorders survey, those reporting vomiting as a weight control behavior 1 to 3 times per month were one and a half times more likely than those without vomiting to have irregular menses, and girls vomiting more than once per week were 3 times more likely after adjustment for body mass index (BMI), age, and race, including only those with a healthy BMI.[18] These authors and others have postulated that stimulation of the emesis center in the area postrema of the medulla causes a release of dopaminergic and opioid activity that may result in these alterations of menstrual function.[19] Alternatively, 1 small research study demonstrated that severe restriction of dietary fat while maintaining overall calories, in a sample matched for BMI with a control group, was associated with functional hypothalamic amenorrhea previously thought to be solely on a psychogenic basis. In addition to the HPO axis suppression related to lower GnRH and LH pulses, the group with amenorrhea showed alterations in GH, IGF-1, cortisol, and insulin similar to those of amenorrheic athletes.[20]

With regard to stress, the role of the HPA axis has been studied in athletes as well as in amenorrheic women with stress and weight loss. Preservation of energy is the evolutionary justification for suppression of the reproductive system under stress. Stress results in the release of norepinephrine and activation of the HPA axis and its primary regulatory neuropeptide CRH, which leads to increased levels of glucocorticoids, which in turn suppress pituitary release of LH and ovarian release of estrogen and progesterone. Corticotropin-releasing hormone is also found in ovarian tissue and other reproductive organs, having a direct effect on all aspects of reproductive function. Increased CRH directly inhibits GnRH pulsatility and indirectly inhibits GnRH through the activation of endorphins, which further inhibit GnRH. Corticotropin-releasing hormone has been found to inhibit appetite and enhance thermogenesis as well as to inhibit the release of GH, thyrotropin-releasing hormone (TRH), and thyroid-stimulating hormone (TSH) via somatostatin. Glucocorticoids have multiple and diverse effects, with both negative feedback on CRH and further suppression of GH and TSH.[21] In addition to stimulation of the HPA axis, stress and energy deficit both result in suppression of the HPT axis, further contributing to suppression of the HPO axis and amenorrhea.

The female athlete triad, first described in the 1990s, refers to women who have an energy deficit as a result of inadequate nutrition for their level of exercise, menstrual irregularity, and osteoporosis. The energy deficit may be intentional, in association with a restrictive eating disorder, or may be a result of excessive exercise, with an inability to accomplish adequate intake. The etiology of the menstrual irregularity or amenorrhea is hypothalamic suppression, with the concern for an increased risk of fractures as a result of the hypoestrogenic state leading to reduced bone mineralization. Sports that depend on lean body mass likely affect the HPO axis through the energy-deficit mechanism, which may rely on leptin or neurotransmitter effects. Ballet, figure skating, and gymnastics are classic sports in which athletes maintain a low body weight in order to optimize performance. Without a balance to help maintain healthy endocrine and musculoskeletal systems, young athletes are at risk for serious injuries. For example, collegiate runners frequently do not know the required caloric intake to keep up with their energy expenditures while running as many as 40 to 65 miles per week, which may result in stress fractures.[22]

Alternatively, swimmers, who have a different somatotype, have been shown to have menstrual irregularity but have normal to elevated LH and estradiol levels, as well as elevated dehydroepiandrosterone sulfate (DHEAS) and androstenedione. It is likely that hyperandrogenism, possibly through stimulation of the HPA axis, rather than hypothalamic amenorrhea is the mechanism of amenorrhea in these athletes.[23]

To be differentiated from functional hypothalamic amenorrhea, hypothalamic suppression may also be caused by the effects of medication or chronic illness. Medications, particularly psychotropic medications, may suppress the HPO axis through dopamine and its effect on prolactin secretion by the pituitary. Dopamine, which normally inhibits prolactin secretion, is decreased with use of these medications resulting in significantly elevated prolactin levels, which lead to suppression of the HPO axis through suppression of GnRH pulsations and inhibition of the GnRH effect on the pituitary. In 1 study of 50 patients on antipsychotic medication, 54% had menstrual irregularities and 12% had amenorrhea.[24] Chronic illness in adolescence has many potential avenues that lead to an energy-deficit state and thus result in hypothalamic suppression with menstrual irregularities and amenorrhea in a similar pattern to those with stress or eating disorders. Chronic illness may result in malabsorption, poor appetite, delayed growth and development, metabolic abnormalities, or hormonal dysfunction.

Furthermore, certain disorders, such as autism, may be associated with disordered eating, which leads to the same metabolic effects as AN with hypothalamic suppression and amenorrhea.

Whereas some authors have determined that return of menstrual function for some adolescents is likely dependent on factors such as weight restoration (either returning to the prepubertal growth trajectory or 2 kg more than the weight noted at the time of the onset of amenorrhea),[25,26] others have found that fat mass is an independent predictor of recovery of menses. In a longitudinal prospective study evaluating predictors of recovery of menses in girls with AN, a final percentage of body fat greater than 24.4% predicted menses recovery, whereas less than 18.1% predicted failure of menses recovery in all girls studied. In addition, those with higher baseline cortisol levels, after adjusting for baseline fat and leptin levels, had greater gains in fat mass with weight restoration, which independently predicted recovery of menses. Higher baseline cortisol levels were not associated with an increase in disease severity.[27]

BONE METABOLISM

More than any other organ system, the endocrine consequences of eating disorders can be especially devastating to long-term bone health. Depending on the timing and duration of illness, unlike in some of the other organ systems affected acutely, there may be lasting effects on the skeletal system even with appropriate recovery of the eating disorder. Bone density changes are primarily seen in AN. Bone density changes in patients with BN have been reported, but only in patients in whom there was a prior history of AN.[28] Bone mass may not fully return to normal levels with weight gain, calcium supplementation, and hormonal therapy, and, in younger patients who may not achieve their optimal peak bone mass, there is a risk for osteoporosis later in life.[29] Girls who develop AN during adolescence tend to have lower bone density than those who develop the disorder as adults.[30] Long-term studies have shown that there is an increase in fracture risk that persists for at least 10 years after the diagnosis is made.[31] The effects on bone may be more pronounced than other organ systems, as many of the hormonal axes affected by malnutrition work in concert on bone metabolism. Bone is also a highly metabolically active tissue, and the formation of new bone is suppressed in an energy-deficient state as an adaptive response.[32]

Low bone mineral density is seen at the spine and hip in patients in an energy-deficient state, indicating that both trabecular and cortical sites are affected. The hypogonadal state seen when adolescents are nutritionally depleted plays a role in the pathogenesis of bone loss. Both low estrogen and low testosterone are predictive of low bone mineral density in patients with eating disorders.[33] However, multiple studies have shown that estrogen replacement and use of oral contraceptive pills do not correct the estrogen deficit and positively affect bone metabolism. This is believed to result from the lowering of IGF-1 caused by the estrogen in oral contraceptive pills. Insulinlike growth factor-1 enhances bone formation through its action on mature osteoblasts, and circulating levels of IGF-1 are necessary for the preservation of cortical bone mass. However, physiologic estrogen replacement does increase bone accrual rates in girls with AN. This results in maintenance of bone mineral density as measured by Z-scores, but no increase is seen, so catch-up for existing losses does not occur, likely because of the effect of other hormones.[32,33] Estrogen decreases osteoclastic bone resorption and may affect bone by reducing sclerostin levels, as seen in adult women. Sclerostin, a protein secreted by osteocytes that negatively regulates bone formation, has been found to be higher in patients with AN.[34,35] The relationship between sclerostin and bone turnover markers seems to be disrupted in adolescent girls with AN compared to healthy weight controls; however, a larger study showed no difference in sclerostin levels between these groups and no increase in the setting of estrogen administration.[36] Studies of testosterone replacement in adult women have similarly not shown an improvement in bone mineral density.[33] These findings suggest that other endocrinopathies are also playing a role in bone metabolism in patients with eating disorders.

Despite the significant decrease in bone mineral density in patients with AN, studies have shown that levels of both vitamin D and parathyroid hormone are normal in these patients.[37,38] As previously mentioned, IGF-1 levels are lowered in patients with AN. Low IGF-1 has been shown to be associated with lower levels of bone formation and lower bone mineral density. Insulinlike growth factor-1 has anabolic effects on bone, so the lowered levels lead to lower bone mass.[35] Growth hormone resistance has also been shown in bone in these patients, and this combination may contribute to the poor bone mineralization that is seen.[39] The elevated cortisol levels seen in AN also contribute to decreased bone mass. Cortisol decreases calcium absorption in the intestine, decreases osteoblast proliferation, and inhibits GH secretion, adding an additional mechanism by which IGF-1 is decreased. Cortisol may also act indirectly by decreasing gonadotropin secretion.[35]

Bone mineral density has also been shown to be negatively associated with peptide YY, a neuropeptide known to be increased in energy-deficient states and inversely associated with adiponectin, which has been found to be elevated when controlling for fat mass in patients with AN. Adiponectin may contribute to decreased bone mass by increasing levels of an osteoclast activator and decreasing levels of a receptor that inhibits osteoclast-activating effects.[32,35] Leptin, another adipokine, is associated with both lower fat mass and lower bone density in this population.[39] In a study of patients with hypothalamic amenorrhea, administration of leptin was associated with an increase in osteocalcin, a marker of bone formation.[32,40] However, another study found that leptin decreased osteoblast proliferation and bone formation, contradicting the idea that lower leptin has a negative effect on bone.[32,41] Thus, the complex interactions of multiple hormonal systems on bone density in patients with eating disorders is still to be fully understood.

GROWTH HORMONE AND INSULINLIKE GROWTH FACTOR-1

Growth hormone is released from the anterior pituitary in a pulsatile manner in response to both growth hormone-releasing hormone, which has a stimulatory effect, and somatostatin, which has an inhibitory effect. Ghrelin, together with growth hormone-releasing hormone, also affects GH secretion. Insulinlike growth factor-1 is secreted in response to GH primarily from the liver, but also from other cells, including chondrocytes in bones. Growth hormone has direct and indirect effects on the growth plate, leading to increased proliferation of prechondrocytes and an increase in chondrocyte differentiation with the aid of IGF-1.[42]

In adolescents with AN, the endocrine changes that occur are an adaptive mechanism in response to the energy-deficient state, with the goal of conserving energy and maintaining euglycemia. Growth hormone levels in these patients are higher than in controls, with those who are the most malnourished having the highest levels. However, insulinlike growth factor-1 levels in these patients are much lower. It has been suggested that there is an acquired resistance to GH in the malnourished state as a result of downregulation of GH receptor expression.[32] Studies have shown that both basal and pulsatile release of GH are increased in women with AN and are higher specifically in adolescent girls with AN than in controls, even at the time of the physiologic peak of GH.[17] Other studies have shown that when patients with AN are given supraphysiologic doses of recombinant human GH, there is no increase in IGF-1, further supporting the idea that there is an acquired resistance to GH in this disorder. These higher doses of GH lead to a reduction in fat mass and leptin, believed to be the result of IGF-1 independent effects of GH, as there are no benefits to lean body mass or bone growth.[17,39] In a starvation state, IGF-1 secretion is blocked by the liver, which, through negative feedback, also affects GH secretion.[32] One of the roles of GH is to maintain euglycemia in a low-energy state via gluconeogenesis, which further explains its elevated levels in patients with AN. Weight gain does reverse the GH resistance seen in patients with AN via an increase in IGF-1, which reduces the levels of GH.

Because AN most commonly occurs during adolescence, it would be expected to have an effect on linear growth and attainment of predicted growth potential. In other disorders with low levels of IGF-1, delayed growth is seen; however, in those other disorders, GH is also usually lowered as well. An older study showed that patients who developed AN before menarche and exhibited growth retardation at the time of diagnosis did show catch-up growth after treatment, although these patients did not attain their full genetic height potential.[43] Other larger studies, however, have shown that growth is ultimately unaffected in females with AN. One large study showed that even with a loss of up to 45% of body weight, adolescents with AN were able to reach their predicted height.[44] The same study found a decline in height percentile in males with AN, which was postulated to occur because malnutrition would have a greater effect on males as a result of the longer duration of bone growth. In a more recent, larger case control study, height potential was preserved. This was believed to be the result of a delay in skeletal maturation, caused by the hypogonadal state, which allows for a longer period of bone growth. They also found that although IGF-1 levels were lower than in controls, they may not be low enough to affect bone growth. Growth hormone levels were elevated and not a predictor of bone growth, supporting the idea that there is a resistance to GH at the growth plate.[42] The differing results may be due to a smaller study population or a longer duration of illness in the patients who did not achieve their predicted growth.

HYPOTHALAMIC-PITUITARY-ADRENAL AXIS

Cortisol is a glucocorticoid secreted from the adrenal gland that stimulates gluconeogenesis and decreases glucose utilization in muscle. It also breaks down protein and fat into amino acids and glycerol, which are used as gluconeogenic substrates. In an energy-deficient state, this allows for increased production and conservation of glucose for use by essential organs.

In patients with AN, cortisol levels are elevated when measured from blood, urine, and saliva. This increase in cortisol may help in conjunction with GH to maintain euglycemia.[34] Corticotropin-releasing hormone levels are elevated when measured in cerebrospinal fluid, which acts on the release of cortisol. Corticotropin-releasing hormone levels may be elevated because of elevated levels of ghrelin, which is seen in AN. Evidence from many studies has shown that dexamethasone does not fully suppress cortisol in patients with AN, suggesting that there is a higher set-point for cortisol in this condition. Diurnal variation, however, is maintained.[32,34,39] The adrenocorticotropic hormone (ACTH) response in AN is inappropriately low, which suggests feedback at the pituitary level. Despite the chronic elevation of cortisol, patients with AN do not exhibit Cushing-like features. However, these patients do tend to accumulate more truncal than extremity fat during recovery. Higher cortisol levels have also been shown to predict weight gain and resumption of menses.[17,32] Another study, however, showed that the increase in CRH contributed to weight loss because it has anorexigenic features.[39] Hypercortisolemia is also associated with depression, anxiety, and reduced bone mineral density in patients with AN.[17] It has been proposed, as well, that the effect of both GH and cortisol on proinflammatory cytokines and lipid status may increase the cardiovascular risk of patients with AN despite their being underweight.[3] Upon weight restoration, cortisol levels return to normal, and there is no indication for pharmacologic treatment during illness.

The HPA axis is also affected in patients with BN. Normal and increased secretion have been reported, and some of the variability may be due, in part, to whether levels were measured when the patient was more actively bingeing. Increased visceral fat and adrenal gland volume have also been shown in patients with BN.[32]

GUT NEUROPEPTIDES: GHRELIN AND PEPTIDE YY

Ghrelin is a peptide secreted by the stomach with orexigenic (increases appetite) properties that inhibits gonadotropin secretion and promotes GH and ACTH secretion. It is secreted in a pulsatile manner, with peak levels at 8 pm and rising levels before meals in healthy patients. It stimulates GH secretion through receptors in the hypothalamus and pituitary.[39] Ghrelin and other gut neuropeptides travel to the brain to control metabolism and food intake by providing signals to measure nutritional status and energy demands.[32] Ghrelin is inversely associated with BMI, fat mass, and insulin levels. It has also been proposed that the normal ghrelin suppressive secretory response to food is heightened in patients with AN, which would cause an increased sensation of satiety in patients with AN as demonstrated in a study that showed a reduction in ghrelin in patients in a hyperinsulemic state.[17] This difference has also been shown when looking at different types of eating disorders, with ghrelin being increased in restrictive AN, unchanged in binge-purge type AN, and reduced in BN.

Ghrelin has been studied as a therapeutic agent in AN because of its effect on increasing appetite, but several small studies have reported conflicting results. In patients with AN, ghrelin levels are elevated compared to normal-weight controls, partially explained by chronic self-induced starvation. In a study of adolescents, ghrelin was significantly higher in patients with AN compared both to those who were partially recovered and to constitutionally thin controls. When patients were given ghrelin infusions, the rise in ghrelin was the same among all groups, but there was a significantly greater increase in GH response in both the thin and partially recovered patients than in those with active AN. The same study also found that patients with AN or partially recovered from AN felt less hungry when given ghrelin, which goes against the assumption that as an orexigenic hormone it would increase appetite. This decreased effect on GH may be explained by prolonged exposure to an elevated ghrelin level, causing a desensitization to its actions.[45] In a study of 5 patients with AN who were motivated to gain weight but restricted their intake because of abdominal discomfort, intravenous (IV) administration of ghrelin did increase appetite and reduce postprandial bloating.[46] Given the small size of the study, further studies are needed to confirm this effect. Weight gain is associated with a reduction in ghrelin levels, which supports the idea that ghrelin is increased in patients with AN as an adaptive response because in a starvation state it increases both GH and ACTH, which together work to maintain euglycemia.[39]

Peptide YY is another peptide secreted by the distal gut. It has anorexigenic (decreases appetite) properties, and its levels rise 15 to 30 minutes after food intake, which induces satiety. Levels have been reported to be higher, lower, and unchanged in patients with AN[47-49] but have been consistently shown to be inversely related to both BMI and fat mass. Even in the studies that showed higher levels in patients with AN, the levels remained high even with weight gain, suggesting that the levels do not rise as an adaptive response to a starvation state. Mechanisms for a role of peptide YY in AN have been proposed, but a definitive effect has not yet been proven.[50]

ADIPOKINES: LEPTIN AND ADIPONECTIN

Leptin has been well studied in eating disorders and has been found to be low in both AN and BN and elevated in BED. It is a polypeptide made primarily in fat cells that is believed to be a signal of nutritional status to the central nervous system; it acts on other hormones directly in a food deprivation state. It is secreted in proportion to the amount of adipose tissue and is a peripheral signal of the amount of energy reserves the body has.[50] It has been found to correlate positively with percent body fat in normal and overweight subjects and negatively with those experiencing weight loss.[32,51,52] Multiple studies have shown that leptin has an effect on the HPO axis, HPA axis, FH, and thyroid function. Leptin has a diurnal pattern of secretion with levels rising throughout the day and then falling at night. In patients with AN, both low basal and pulsatile levels of leptin have been reported, which is reversed with weight gain. These lowered levels of leptin are believed to be an adaptive response to an energy-deficient state as leptin decreases appetite, so in a malnourished state leptin levels are lowered in order to prevent the body from being susceptible to its appetite suppressant effects. However, an interesting finding of smaller studies of males with AN was that their leptin levels were not lower than in healthy controls, suggesting a further area of research.[53]

Leptin also stimulates GnRH, so these lowered levels may play a role in the hypogonadism seen in energy-deficit disorders. Studies have looked at a therapeutic effect of leptin on these patients and have found that administration of recombinant leptin led to LH pulsatility and ovulation in patients with hypothalamic amenorrhea.[32,34] Other effects of leptin include stimulating the HPT axis and inhibiting the HPA axis, which may also explain the depressed function of the thyroid and increased activity of the adrenal gland seen in AN.[54] More recent data have shown that leptin may regulate the ability of GH to stimulate IGF-1. In a sample of patients in an energy-deficient state, administration of leptin increased circulating levels of IGF-1.[50] This same effect was not seen when leptin was given to patients with normal levels of leptin, so there may be a threshold below which leptin levels need to be in order for this effect on IGF-1 to be seen.

In patients with BN, leptin levels tend to be lower than in healthy controls but not as low as in patients with AN. This is likely because body weight is more stable in these patients. However in those who are normal weight, levels have been reported to be either normal or increased. Levels are affected by the severity of disease and correlate positively with BMI. In patients with a higher number of binge/purge episodes per day, leptin tends to be hyposecreted despite no significant change in body weight or BMI.[54] Leptin has not been as well studied in BED, but levels tend to be elevated compared to healthy controls. Studies have shown that levels are similar in obese binge eating and non-binge eating women, suggesting more research is needed.[52]

Adiponectin is a protein hormone produced in adipose tissue that is circulated in lower levels in patients with obesity and modulates insulin sensitivity. It has been shown to be high, normal, or low in those who are underweight, but more recent data suggest that levels are higher in energy-deficient patients.[34,54-56] The variability in the measurements may be the result of the degree of fat mass in the patients being studied. The role of adiponectin in patients with eating disorders remains unclear. It has been hypothesized that elevated adiponectin could contribute to the etiology of AN or that the elevated levels are the result of a compensatory mechanism for the increased insulin sensitivity seen in these patients. In a study of 9 women with AN, adiponectin levels were decreased, but not significantly, compared to age-matched controls. The authors suggested that perhaps, despite having fewer fat cells, those cells may have produced more adiponectin.[55] In a study of patients with BN, levels of adiponectin were found to positively correlate with the severity of binge/purge episodes but were normal or even decreased in other studies.[57]

Other hormones that may play a role in patients with eating disorders that are related directly to body weight include irisin and resistin. Irisin is secreted from skeletal muscle and is part of an energy expenditure cascade that is involved with the browning of white fat, a process that increases thermogenesis. In a study investigating the relationship between irisin and BMI, irisin levels were shown to be lower in subjects with AN. There was no relationship with ghrelin, but there was a positive correlation with insulin. The lower levels of irisin may be an adaptive mechanism of the body to conserve energy by reducing the browning of white fat.[34,58] Resistin is a hormone made in adipose tissue that affects energy homeostasis and insulin. It has been shown to be lower in patients with AN, but its role is unclear.[32,59]

HYPOTHALAMIC-PITUITARY-THYROID AXIS

The same deprivations and stressors that affect the HPO and HPA axes may cause alterations in the function of the HPT axis, resulting in alterations of thyroid hormones. In addition, as with other stressors, energy deprivation may lead to reversal of the usual peripheral conversion of T4 (thyroxine) to T3 (triiodothyronine) such that a greater amount of T4 is converted to rT3 (reverse triiodothyronine), creating a sick euthyroid syndrome condition. Although there is evidence of suppression of TRH, there also is evidence of inadequate response of thyrotropin (TSH) to the TRH that is available.[60] Thus, both central and peripheral forces are affecting thyroid hormone function in patients with malnutrition. Symptoms of hypothyroidism, such as bradycardia, hypothermia, and hypotension, are frequently seen with malnutrition, but restoration of nutrition reverses the hormonal dysfunction. Weight restoration is associated with an increase in T3 and the metabolic rate. Treatment with thyroid hormone is not recommended because it leads to further weight loss and loss of muscle mass.[32]

Just as with the HPO axis, hypoleptinemia signals to the hypothalamus an energy-deficient state, resulting in conservation through suppression of activity in the HPT axis, with a decreased release of TRH. Results of research evaluating the importance of leptin in the etiology of the thyroid dysfunction and the benefit of leptin therapy in restoration of thyroid function have varied. A review of research related to the relationship of leptin to neuroendocrine function determined that leptin has a significant regulatory effect on TSH, but its role with regard to circulating levels of T3 and T4 may be more complex.[50] Furthermore, the effect of leptin administration may be related to the extent of leptin deficiency.

TREATMENT AND ENDOCRINE COMPLICATIONS OF RECOVERY

Treatment of eating disorders is multifaceted, with a need initially for medical stabilization, nutritional rehabilitation, and psychological therapy. Medical stabilization may require inpatient treatment to correct electrolyte abnormalities or to treat a patient who has significant bradycardia and malnutrition. Therapy is a key part of treatment of eating disorders, and various types have been shown to be effective. Family-based therapy (FBT) is often better with younger patients, and dialectical behavior therapy (DBT) has shown benefit, especially with BN. Cognitive behavior therapy (CBT) is another treatment modality of benefit to these patients. Selective serotonin reuptake inhibitors (SSRIs), antipsychotics, and mood stabilizers may also be used, depending on the presence of any premorbid psychiatric disorders. If the patient is depressed as a consequence of an eating disorder, SSRIs may be used, or weight gain and treatment of the eating disorder may be enough to help the depressed mood.

One particular feature of nutritional rehabilitation that has possible endocrine complications is refeeding syndrome. During starvation, insulin decreases and glucagon increases, which results in increased breakdown of glycogen and gluconeogenesis. Adipose tissue releases large quantities of fatty acids and glycerol, and muscle releases amino acids leading to ketone bodies and free fatty acids as the main source of energy instead of glucose. Overall in a starvation state there is catabolism of adipose tissue and muscle, resulting in loss of lean body mass.[61] During refeeding, there is a shift from fat to carbohydrate metabolism. This increase in glucose causes increased cellular uptake of glucose, phosphate, potassium, magnesium, and water, as well as protein synthesis. As a result, hypophosphatemia, hypomagnesemia, and hypokalemia can develop, all of which can cause severe cardiac side effects. For this reason, patients at increased risk for refeeding syndrome because of the degree of their weight loss may begin their nutritional rehabilitation in an inpatient setting where they can be closely monitored.

CLINICAL IMPLICATIONS

Much of what is discussed in this article is the focus of current research, and many of the hormones being measured are done so only in an investigative setting. Routinely, when evaluating a patient with an eating disorder one should check a complete blood count, complete metabolic panel, magnesium and phosphorus levels, TSH, T4, free T4, and T3 levels, and, if the patient is presenting with amenorrhea, prolactin, estradiol, LH, and FSH levels. Both T3 and estradiol are most often depressed, and serial measurements can be used as a marker of treatment success or failure. Current recommendations do not include routine measurement of other hormones such as leptin.

With regard to treatment, weight gain is ultimately the most effective treatment of the medical consequences. Oral contraceptives are not indicated, as previously mentioned, because they do not provide a benefit with regard to improved bone mineralization, and the return of menses is an important marker of therapeutic success and helps identify the appropriate goal weight for the patient. Vitamin D and calcium should be supplemented, but it is important to note that supplementation alone will not improve bone mineral density. Some guidelines suggest performing a DEXA after 6 months of amenorrhea. Although many women with AN recover normal reproductive function with weight restoration, approximately 15% remain amenorrheic, which is an issue that is still not fully understood.[62]

CONCLUSION

Eating disorders are psychiatric conditions with significant medical complications, largely related to the degree of energy deficiency. The endocrine consequences are among the most pervasive and potentially longest lasting, with hypothalamic amenorrhea and disordered bone metabolism of primary concern. With appropriate medical, nutritional, and psychological treatment, the prognosis for adolescents is good, and most of the medical complications are reversed.

References

1. Pearce JM. Richard Morton: origins of anorexia nervosa. *Eur Neurol.* 2004;52:191-192
2. Meczekalski B, Podfigurna-Stopa A, Katulski K. Long-term consequences of anorexia nervosa. *Maturitas.* 2013;75:215-220
3. Misra M, Aggarwal A, Miller KK, et al. Effects of anorexia nervosa on clinical, hematologic, biochemical, and bone density parameters in community-dwelling adolescent girls. *Pediatrics.* 2004;114:1574-1583
4. American Psychiatric Association. *Diagnostic and Statistical Manual of Mental Disorders.* 5th ed. Arlington, VA: American Psychiatric Publishing; 2013
5. Fisher M. Treatment of eating disorders in children, adolescents, and young adults. *Pediatr Rev.* 2006;27:5-16
6. Goldstein MA, Dechant EJ, Beresin EV. Eating disorders. *Pediatr Rev.* 2011;32:508-521
7. Adams Hillard PJ. Menstruation in adolescents: what's normal, what's not. *Ann N Y Acad Sci.* 2008;1135:29-35
8. Denham M, Schell LM, Deane G, et al. Relationship of lead, mercury, mirex, dichlorodiphenyldichloroethylene, hexachlorobenzene, and polychlorinated biphenyls to timing of menarche among Akwesasne Mohawk girls. *Pediatrics.* 2005;115:e127-e134
9. Biro F. Secular trends in menarche. *J Pediatr.* 2005;147:725-726
10. Herman-Giddens ME. The decline in the age of menarche in the United States: should we be concerned? *J Adolesc Health.* 2007;40:201-203
11. Anderson SE, Must A. Interpreting the continued decline in the average age at menarche: results from two nationally representative surveys of U.S. girls studied 10 years apart. *J Pediatr.* 2005;147:753-760
12. American Academy of Pediatrics Committee on Adolescence; American College of Obstetricians and Gynecologists Committee on Adolescent Health Care; Diaz A, Laufer MR, Breech LL. Menstruation in girls and adolescents: using the menstrual cycle as a vital sign. *Pediatrics.* 2006;118:2245-2250
13. Genazzani AR, Petraglia F, Gamba O, et al. Neuroendocrinology of the menstrual cycle. *Ann N Y Acad Sci.* 1997;816:143-150
14. Wiksten-Almstromer M, Hirschberg AL, Hagenfeldt K. Menstrual disorders and associated factors among adolescent girls visiting a youth clinic. *Acta Obstet Gynecol Scand.* 2007;86:65-72
15. Usdan L, Khaodhiar L, Apovian CM. The endocrinopathies of anorexia nervosa. *Endocr Pract.* 2008;14:1055-1063
16. Golden NH, Carlson JL. The pathophysiology of amenorrhea in the adolescent. *Ann N Y Acad Sci.* 2008;1135:163-178
17. Miller KK. Endocrine effects of anorexia nervosa. *Endocrinol Metab Clin North Am.* 2013;42:515-528
18. Austin SB, Ziyadeh NJ, Vohra S, et al. Irregular menses linked to vomiting in a nonclinical sample: findings from the National Eating Disorders Screening Program in high schools. *J Adolesc Health.* 2008;42:450-457
19. Gendall KA, Bulik CM, Joyce PR, McIntosh VV, Carter FA. Menstrual cycle irregularity in bulimia nervosa. Associated factors and changes with treatment. *J Psychosom Res.* 2000;49:409-415
20. Laughlin G, Dominguez CE, Yen SS. Nutritional and endocrine-metabolic aberrations in women with functional hypothalamic amenorrhea. *J Clin Endocrinol Metab.* 1998;83:25-32

21. Tsigos C, Chrousos GP. Hypothalamic-pituitary-adrenal axis, neuroendocrine factors and stress. *J Psychosom Res.* 2002;53:865-871
22. Kazis K, Iglesias E. The female athlete triad. *Adolesc Med.* 2003;14:87-95
23. Constantini NW, Warren MP. Menstrual dysfunction in swimmers: a distinct entity. *J Clin Endocrinol Metab.* 1995;80:2740-2744
24. Thangavelu K, Geetanjali S. Menstrual disturbance and galactorrhea in people taking conventional antipsychotic medications. *Exp Clin Psychopharmacol.* 2006;14:459-460
25. Golden N, Jacobson MS, Schebendach J, et al. Resumption of menses in anorexia nervosa. *Arch Pediatr Adolesc Med.* 1997;151:16-21
26. Swenne I. Weight requirements for return of menstruations in teenage girls with eating disorders, weight loss and secondary amenorrhoea. *Acta Paediatr.* 2004;93:1449-1455
27. Misra M, Prabhakaran R, Miller KK, et al. Role of cortisol in menstrual recovery in adolescent girls with anorexia nervosa. *Pediatr Res.* 2006;59:598-603
28. Naessén S, Carlström K, Glant R, Jacobsson H, Hirschberg AL. Bone mineral density in bulimic women—influence of endocrine factors and previous anorexia. *Eur J Endocrinol.* 2006;155:245-251
29. Soyka L, Misra M, Frenchman A, et al. Abnormal bone mineral accrual in adolescent girls with anorexia nervosa. *J Clin Endocrinol Metab.* 2002;87:4177-4185
30. Biller BM, Saxe V, Herzog DB, et al. Mechanisms of osteoporosis and in adult and adolescent women with anorexia nervosa. *J Clin Endocrinol Metab.* 1989;68:548-554
31. Vestergaard P, Emborg C, Støving RK, et al. Fractures in patients with anorexia nervosa, bulimia nervosa, and other eating disorders—a nationwide register study. *Int J Eat Disord.* 2002;32:301-308
32. Warren MP. Endocrine manifestations of eating disorders. *J Clin Endocrinol Metab.* 2011;96:333-343
33. Misra M, Kilbanski A. Anorexia nervosa and bone. *J Endocrinol.* 2014;221:R163-R176
34. Singhal V, Misra M, Kilbanski A. Endocrinology of anorexia nervosa in young people: recent insights. *Curr Opin Endocrinol Diabetes Obes.* 2014;21:64-70
35. Fazeli P, Kilbanski A. Anorexia nervosa and bone metabolism. *Bone.* 2014;66:39-45
36. Faje AT, Fazeli PK, Katzman DK, et al. Sclerostin levels and bone turnover markers in adolescents with anorexia nervosa and healthy adolescent girls. *Bone.* 2012;5:474-479
37. Haagensen AL, Feldman HA, Ringelheim J, Gordon CM. Low prevalence of vitamin D deficiency among adolescents with anorexia nervosa. *Osteoporos Int.* 2008;19:289-294
38. Carmichael K, Carmichael D. Bone metabolism and osteopenia in eating disorders. *Medicine (Baltimore).* 1995;74:254-267
39. Misra M, Kilbanski A. Endocrine consequences of anorexia nervosa. *Lancet Diabetes Endocrinol.* 2014;2:581-592
40. Welt C, Chan JL, Bullen J, et al. Recombinant human leptin in women with hypothalamic amenorrhea. *N Engl J Med.* 2004;351:987-997
41. Wolf G. Energy regulation by the skeleton. *Nutr Rev.* 2008;66:229-233
42. Prabhakaran R, Misra M, Miller KK, et al. Determinants of height in adolescent girls with anorexia nervosa. *Pediatrics.* 2008;121:e1517-e1523
43. Lantzouni E, Frank GR, Golden NH, Shenker RI. Reversibility of growth stunting in early onset anorexia nervosa: a prospective study. *J Adolesc Health.* 2002;31:162-165
44. Pfeiffer RJ, et al. Effect of anorexia nervosa on linear growth. *Clin Pediatr (Phila).* 1986;25:7-12
45. Miljic D, Pekic S, Djurovic M, et al. Ghrelin has partial or no effect on appetite, growth hormone, prolactin, and cortisol release in patients with anorexia nervosa. *J Clin Endocrinol Metab.* 2006;91:1491-1495
46. Hotta M, Ohwada R, Akamizu T, Shibasaki T, Kangawa K. Therapeutic potential of ghrelin in restricting-type anorexia nervosa. *Methods Enzymol.* 2012;514:381-398
47. Lawson, EA, Eddy KT, Donoho D, et al. Appetite-regulating hormones cortisol and peptide YY are associated with disordered eating psychopathology, independent of body mass index. *Eur J Endocrinol.* 2011;164:253-261

48. Misra M. Effects of hypogonadism on bone metabolism in female adolescents and young adults. *Nat Rev Endocrinol.* 2012;8:395-404
49. Misra M, Miller KK, Tsai P, et al. Elevated peptide YY levels in adolescent girls with anorexia and nervosa. *J Clin Endocrinol Metab.* 2006;91:1027-1033
50. Khan S, Hamnvik OP, Brinkoetter M, Mantzoros CS. Leptin as a modulator of neuroendocrine function in humans. *Yonsei Med J.* 2012;53:671-679
51. Eckert E, Pomeroy C, Raymond N, et al. Leptin in anorexia nervosa. *J Clin Endocrinol Metab.* 1998;83:791-795
52. Bluher S, Mantzoros C. Role of leptin in regulating neuroendocrine function in humans. *J Nutr.* 2004;134:2469S-2474S
53. Misra M, Klibanski A. Neuroendocrine consequences of anorexia nervosa in adolescents. *Endocr Dev.* 2010;17:197-214
54. Monteleone P, Castaldo E, Maj M. Neuroendocrine dysregulation of food intake in eating disorders. *Regul Pept.* 2008;149:39-50
55. Amitani H, Askawa A, Ogiso K, et al. The role of adiponectin multimers in anorexia nervosa. *Nutrition.* 2013;29:203-206
56. Misra M, Miller KK, Cord J, et al. Relationships between serum adipokines, insulin levels, and bone density in girls with anorexia nervosa. *J Clin Endocrinol Metab.* 2007;92:2046-2052
57. Nogueira J, Maraninchi M, Lorec AM, et al. Specific adipocytokines profiles in patients with hyperactive and/or binge/purge form of anorexia nervosa. *Eur J Clin Nutr.* 2010;64:840-844
58. Stengel A, Hofmann T, Goebel-Stengel M, et al. Circulating levels of irisin in patients with anorexia nervosa and different stages of obesity—correlation with body mass index. *Peptides.* 2013;39:125-130
59. Housova J, Anderlova K, Krizová J, et al. Serum adiponectin and resistin concentration in patients with restrictive and binge/purge form of anorexia nervosa and bulimia nervosa. *J Clin Endocrinol Metab.* 2005;90:1366-1370
60. Usdan L, Khaodhiar L, Apovian CM. The endocrinopathies of anorexia nervosa. *Endocr Pract.* 2008;14:1055-1063
61. Crook MA, Hally V, Panteli JV. The importance of the refeeding syndrome. *Nutrition.* 2001;17:632-637
62. Jocoangeli F, Masala S, Staar Messasalma F, et al. Amenorrhea after weight recovery in anorexia nervosa: role of body composition and endocrine abnormalities. *Eat Weight Disord.* 2006;11:e20-e26

Turner Syndrome and Klinefelter Syndrome

Suzanne E. Kingery, MD; Kupper A. Wintergerst, MD*

Division of Pediatric Endocrinology, Department of Pediatrics, University of Louisville School of Medicine, Louisville, Kentucky

TURNER SYNDROME

Turner syndrome (TS) is one of the most common chromosomal disorders in females, affecting 1 of every 2000 live births.[1] It is characterized by the complete or partial absence of the second X chromosome plus a constellation of physical features. The most common karyotype, 45,X, affects approximately 50% of females with TS, although other variants include mosaicism 45,X/46,XX; X isochromosome 46,X,i(Xq); deletions 46,XXp- or 46,XXq-; and Y chromosomal material 45,X/46XY.[2] Particular phenotypic features of TS include short stature, ovarian failure, and lymphatic, cardiac, renal, endocrine, and skeletal anomalies.[3]

The classic karyotype 45,X is diagnosed at a younger age, on average, than other chromosomal variants, since the signs for classic TS are more easily identified.[4] Despite the classic phenotype features of TS, the mean age at diagnosis is still rather late, 15.1 years.[4] This is because many of these features are absent in nonclassic variants, requiring a higher index of suspicion. Indications for prenatal karyotyping include increased nuchal translucency or the presence of a cystic hygroma. Postnatal indications for karyotype include growth failure and pubertal delay or pubertal arrest. The most common reason to screen in childhood and adolescence is short stature.[5] Other indications for screening are lymphedema in phenotypic females or in girls with left-sided cardiac anomalies.[5]

Short stature is almost universal in girls with TS. It is the result of mild intrauterine growth restriction, slow growth in infancy, deceleration in height velocity in childhood, and then the absence of a pubertal height spurt.[6] On average, girls with TS are 20 cm (8 in) shorter than their midparental height.[6] Recent studies

---

*Corresponding author
E-mail address: Kupper.wintergerst@louisville.edu

have identified that this short stature is caused at least in part by the absence of the short-stature-homeobox (*SHOX*) gene, which is located on the distal end of the short arm of the X chromosome.[7] This gene is likely a dose-dependent gene: one copy results in short stature, and multiple copies, as seen in Klinefelter syndrome, result in tall stature. The *SHOX* gene is expressed in the cells of the limbs and pharyngeal arches and is likely also responsible for some of the skeletal abnormalities seen in TS, such as mesomelia, micrognathia, cubitus valgus, high arched palate, short metacarpals, and Madelung deformity.[7] Table 1 outlines these and other associated physical, autoimmune, and developmental characteristics of TS.

Although *SHOX* gene haploinsufficiency has not been associated with defects in the growth hormone insulinlike growth factor-1 (IGF-1) axis, females with TS

Table 1
Summary of clinical features of Turner syndrome

- Short stature
- Primary ovarian failure
  - Delayed puberty/pubertal arrest
  - Infertility
- Lymphedema
- Webbed neck
- Cardiac anomalies
  - Congenital heart disease
    - Bicuspid aortic valve
    - Aortic coarctation
    - Dilated aorta
  - Hypertension
- Skeletal anomalies
  - Cubitus valgus
  - Nail hypoplasia/hyperconvex
  - High arched palate
  - Madelung deformity
  - Short fourth metacarpal/metatarsal
- Autoimmunity
  - Thyroid disorders
  - Celiac disease
- Renal anomalies
  - Duplicated collecting duct
  - Horseshoe kidney
- Auditory anomalies
  - Hearing loss (both conductive and sensorineural)
  - Low set/malrotated ears
- Psychoeducational impairments
  - Selective impairment in nonverbal skills
  - Attention-deficit/hyperactivity disorder

Note: There is variation in the clinical features of patients with Turner syndrome: some patients may experience almost all of the characteristics whereas others may experience only a few of these features.

respond well to treatment with growth hormone therapy. Growth hormone was first approved in 1996 by the US Food and Drug Administration (FDA) for treatment of girls with TS, based only on historical and prospective studies. Nearly 9 years after growth hormone was approved for girls with TS, the first randomized controlled trial was published in 2005. In that study, patients with TS either were treated with growth hormone 0.3 mg/kg/week or received no growth hormone therapy.[8] All study participants received sex steroid replacement at 13 years of age.[8] An average height gain of 7.2 cm was seen in girls treated with growth hormone therapy from a starting age of about 10 years and treated for an average of 5.7 years.[8]

Girls with TS often experience growth failure shortly after birth. In a toddler growth hormone study published in 2007, 88 girls with TS between the ages of 9 months and 4 years (median age 1.98 years) received either growth hormone 0.35 mg/kg/week or no growth hormone therapy.[9] After 2 years of growth hormone treatment, treated girls gained 1.6 ± 0.6 standard deviations (SD) in height versus nontreated growth hormone TS controls. Because treatment with growth hormone therapy can significantly improve height potential, current guidelines recommend treatment with growth hormone as soon as growth failure is observed.[10]

Oxandrolone, which is a nonaromatizable anabolic steroid, has also historically been used in girls with TS. However, it must be used with caution because it is an anabolic steroid and can cause virilization. In a study of 92 girls treated with growth hormone and randomized to also receive either oxandrolone or placebo starting around age 9 years (age range 7-13 years), oxandrolone increased final height by 4.6 cm.[11] In contrast, delaying pubertal induction until age 14 increased height by only 3.8 cm. Thus, for girls older than 9 years or with extreme short stature, adding a nonaromatizable anabolic steroid should be considered.

Although up to one-third of girls with TS can undergo spontaneous puberty and less than 5% can have a spontaneous pregnancy, almost all women with TS ultimately have gonadal failure.[12] Ovarian failure in TS can begin as early as 18 weeks' gestation, with continued degeneration of the ovarian follicles to fibrous tissue thereafter. Biochemical evidence of primary ovarian failure can be seen with the rise of luteinizing hormone (LH) and follicle-stimulating hormone (FSH) in infancy and early childhood. Luteinizing hormone and FSH then slowly decline until age 6, but increase again at the time of normal puberty.[13] Because of the importance of estrogen therapy on growth, bone mineralization, physical development, psychological development, and improvement in motor speed and verbal and nonverbal memory and processing, delaying estrogen therapy is unwarranted.[10] Estrogen form, dosing, and timing should ideally reflect those of normal puberty.

The use of estrogen in girls with TS has historically been delayed because of potential reduction of height caused by the premature closure of growth plates with estrogen. In a large study of 232 subjects, girls received 0.27 or 0.36 mg/kg/week of growth hormone therapy with either low-dose estrogen (starting at age 8 or older) or oral placebo.[14] The average age at the start of the study was 9.7 ± 2.8 years. Mean near-final heights of subjects who received the lower growth hormone dose, with or without estrogen, were 145.1 ± 5.4 cm and 149.9 ± 6.0 cm, respectively. Those who received the higher growth hormone dose, with or without estrogen, achieved mean near-final heights of 149.1 ± 6.0 cm and 150.4 ± 6.0 cm, respectively. Higher doses of growth hormone resulted in taller final heights, and this effect seemed to be only slightly mitigated by the addition of estrogen therapy.

The form of estrogen therapy administered might also play a role in height preservation. The StaTur Study followed 704 girls with TS treated with growth hormone at 0.26 ± 0.06 mg/kg/week.[15] Puberty was induced at age 15 years using 1 of 4 types of estrogen therapy: oral ethinyl estradiol, oral estradiol, percutaneous estradiol, or estrogen-progestin combinations. The use of percutaneous versus oral estrogens was associated with greater height by a gain of +2.1 cm.[15] However, there were far fewer patients in the percutaneous or estrogen-progestin group than in the oral ethinyl estradiol or oral estradiol group.

More recent literature suggests that estrogen therapy may not be detrimental to height preservation and that it actually may improve final height. In a study of 149 girls with TS aged 5 to 12.5 years, girls were randomized to receive 1 of 4 treatment groups: (1) double placebo; (2) estrogen alone, with low-dose oral estradiol started at age 5 followed by an escalating pubertal dose starting at 12 years; (3) growth hormone alone at 0.1 mg/kg 3 times per week; or (4) growth hormone and estrogen.[16] The study found that the average height gain for growth hormone therapy alone versus placebo was 0.78 ± 0.13 SD (5.0 cm). For growth hormone plus estrogen versus growth hormone alone, the average height gain was 0.32 ± 0.17 SD (2.1 cm). These new data suggest that using a percutaneous form of estrogen with small escalating doses of estrogen therapy may actually increase final height in TS.

Congenital cardiac defects affect one-third to one-half of all women with TS. The most common cardiac abnormalities are bicuspid aortic valve and aortic coarctation. Cardiac defects are 4-fold more common in girls with lymphatic issues (ie, webbed neck).[17] Hypertension also is common.[18] Ho et al[19] found that structural anomalies were present even in patients who were asymptomatic from a cardiovascular standpoint, namely, 50% of these patients had angulation and elongation of the aortic arch and 13% had a partial anomalous pulmonary connection.[19] Although these abnormalities are not associated with any particular condition or increased risk, there is concern that these abnormalities represent an abnormal aortic wall that may be prone to dilation and dissection.

Indeed, compared with healthy female controls, women with TS not treated with growth hormone are an average 20 cm shorter than their female counterparts, yet they have been shown to have the same aortic size diameter.[20] Normalized for body surface area (BSA), women with TS had significantly greater ascending aorta and descending aortic diameters (aortic size index), resulting in a 100-fold higher rate of aortic dissection. In a publication by Carlson and Silberbach[21] in 2007, 85 cases of aortic dissections were reported among women with TS between 1961 and 2006. Even more striking was that the average age of dissection in these women was 30.7 years (age range 4-67 years).[21] In this review of the risk factors for aortic dissection, nearly 15% of women with TS had hypertension alone, 30% had congenital heart disease alone, and 34% had both hypertension and congenital heart disease.[21] However, 11% of the women with aortic dissection had neither known hypertension nor known congenital heart disease.

Of equal concern was the finding that among women with TS, the risk of maternal death from aortic dissection or rupture is 2% or higher.[22] In 2012, the Practice Committee of the American Society for Reproductive Medicine published guidelines in which they asserted that TS is a relative contraindication for pregnancy because of the increased risk of morbidity and mortality associated with pregnancy.[23] In women with TS who do achieve pregnancy, up to 60% face complications, including pregnancy-induced hypertension, aortic rupture, gestational diabetes mellitus, eclampsia, and liver failure.[22] Unfortunately, women with TS rate infertility as one of their most prominent issues in adulthood.[24] Because of the high cardiac risk, even in asymptomatic females, all girls with TS should be evaluated by a cardiologist at diagnosis.[10] Patients should be reevaluated when they transition to adult care, before they attempt pregnancy, or when they develop of hypertension. Girls who have undergone only echocardiography should be reevaluated using magnetic resonance imaging when they are old enough to cooperate with the procedure, because magnetic resonance imaging is thought to provide more detailed imaging of the heart vessels. Otherwise, cardiac imaging should be obtained every 5 to 10 years.[10]

Girls and women with TS also have lower bone mineral density, likely related to prolonged estrogen deficiency. Because they have been shown to have an increased fracture rate across all age groups, evaluation of bone mineral density is also recommended when they are transitioning to adult care.[25]

Autoimmune disease is more prevalent in females with TS. Thyroid disorders are among the most frequently seen, in more than one-fourth of women with TS. In a study by Livadas et al[26] in 2005, hypothyroidism was detected in 24% of patients and hyperthyroidism in 2.5% of patients. Strikingly, greater than 60% of women with TS have positive thyroid antibodies. In addition, more than 5% of women with TS also have celiac disease (CD).[27] Recent studies have found that patients with TS with CD exhibit more atypical symptoms, including anemia, anorexia, and delayed growth.[27] Less than half of the patients with TS and CD showed classic symptoms, such as loose stools, abdominal pain, or bloating. Because of this increased risk of autoimmunity, girls with TS older than 4 years of age should be screened yearly for thyroid disorders and every 3 to 5 years for CD.[10]

Congenital malformations in the urinary system are common, occurring in up to 40% of girls with TS.[28] Collecting system malformations are seen most often and occur in approximately 20% of patients; horseshoe kidney occurs in about 10% of patients.[28] Given the high incidence of renal anomalies, renal ultrasound should be performed at diagnosis. Because these urinary malformations predispose patients to infections, frequent monitoring for urinary tract infections is recommended in patients identified with a congenital urinary anomaly.[10]

Hearing problems are frequent in females with TS. Congenital ear malformations, including the presence of small, tortuous eustachian tube canals, have been reported, accompanied by a high prevalence of otitis media.[29] Girls who experience recurrent ear infections then are at an increased risk for conductive hearing loss over time.[29] Furthermore, women with TS are at high risk for developing sensorineural hearing loss, even in the absence of ear malformations.[10] Given the high risk of hearing problems, audiologic evaluation at diagnosis is recommended. If the patient has a history of otitis media or hearing problems, then annual evaluation is also recommended. Because of the risk of sensorineural hearing loss, even in the absence of any ear problems, audiologic surveillance is recommended every 2 to 3 years.[10]

Cognitive development and function seem to be factors. Although girls with TS have normal intelligence, they have a particular cognitive profile with selective impairment in nonverbal skills. Girls with TS have difficulties in visuospatial organization, social cognition, problem-solving, and motor skills.[30] In addition, almost one-fourth of girls with TS have been diagnosed with attention-deficit/hyperactivity disorder.[31] In psychological development, these girls are at higher risk for social isolation, immaturity, anxiety, and decreased self-esteem, and they are less likely to marry.[32] Current guidelines recommend comprehensive psychoeducational evaluation before school entry (or at diagnosis) and stress the importance of age-appropriate pubertal induction and addressing the ramifications of TS, especially infertility.[10]

Women with TS have an overall increased risk of mortality. In a study of more than 3000 women with TS diagnosed between 1959 and 2002, 296 deaths occurred.[33] This death rate represents a 3-fold higher mortality rate than in the general population. Cardiac disease accounted for 41% of excess mortality, and the greatest risk for cardiac mortality was aortic aneurysm.[33] Respiratory and endocrine abnormalities, specifically diabetes mellitus, accounted for the second and third most common causes of death in patients with TS.[33]

Table 2

Medical management and monitoring in Turner syndrome

All patients	Genetic counseling and education regarding Turner syndrome to parents
	Cardiovascular evaluation as indicated
	Audiologic evaluation as indicated
	Monitoring for growth and puberty
	Renal evaluation as indicated
Infants and toddlers	Consideration for growth hormone therapy when growth failure demonstrated
Childhood	Thyroid function test annually
	Celiac screen every 2-5 years
	Orthodontic evaluation as indicated
	Psychoeducational evaluation annually
Adolescents and adults	Thyroid function test annually
	Celiac screen every 2-5 years
	Hepatic and renal function testing annually
	Fasting glucose and lipid profile assessment annually
	Monitoring ovarian function both clinically and with biochemical markers
	Age-appropriate pubertal induction and estrogen replacement when hypogonadism demonstrated
	Bone mineral density evaluation as indicated

Guidelines adapted from Bondy CA; Turner Syndrome Study Group. Care of girls and women with Turner syndrome: a guideline of the Turner Syndrome Study Group. *J Clin Endocrinol Metab.* 2007;92:10-25.

Overall, girls and women with TS face a number of challenges that evolve from early childhood, through adolescence, and on through adulthood. It is important for their physicians to provide the necessary supportive care during development and to monitor these individuals closely throughout their lives (Table 2). Ongoing support, particularly during childhood and adolescence, provides those with TS the best opportunity to grow into healthy adults.

KLINEFELTER SYNDROME

Klinefelter syndrome (KS) is one of the most common chromosomal abnormalities in males. Although no firm guidelines exist for clinical diagnosis, KS is most often characterized by an array of clinical and developmental characteristics (Table 3), including small testes, hypogonadism, infertility, gynecomastia, and learning difficulties.[34] Klinefelter syndrome occurs when at least 1 extra X chromosome is added to a normal male karyotype, 46,XY. The classic and most commonly identified form is that in which there is 1 extra X chromosome resulting in the karyotype of 47,XXY.[35] However, other karyotypes have been observed, such as 48,XXYY; 48,XXXY; and 49,XXXXY.

Table 3
Summary of clinical features of Klinefelter syndrome

- Tall stature
- Hypogonadism
  - Small testes
  - Infertility
  - Microphallus
  - Cryptorchidism
  - Delayed puberty/pubertal arrest
- Gynecomastia
- Endocrinopathies
  - Metabolic syndrome
  - Type 2 diabetes
- Autoimmunity
  - Systemic lupus erythematosus
- Psychoeducational impairments
  - Selective impairment in verbal skills
  - Delayed expressive language development
  - Attention-deficit/hyperactivity disorder
  - Psychiatric conditions (anxiety, depression, autism spectrum disorders)

Note: There is variation in the clinical features of patients with Klinefelter syndrome: some patients may experience almost all of the characteristics, whereas others may experience only a few of these features.

Approximately 80% of males with KS carry 1 additional X chromosome, 47,XXY, whereas the other 20% of cases have the higher grade aneuploidies or demonstrate mosaicism.[35] Studies suggest that the incidence of KS ranges from 1 per 630-660 newborn males.[1,36] Given such a high prevalence, it is noteworthy that these studies suggest that only about 25% of the expected numbers of males with KS are ever diagnosed, and less than 10% are diagnosed before puberty.[37] The study from Denmark also notes that most patients with KS are diagnosed later in life.[1] Although the reasons for such delays in diagnosis are unknown, many speculate it could be related to the variable or mild phenotypes.

The diagnosis of KS is made by cytogenetic analysis, either on lymphocytes from peripheral blood or on amniocytes or chorionic villi from prenatal specimens. Indications to request a karyotype to assess for KS are based on age. The most common reasons for chromosomal analysis in infancy include hypospadias, small phallus, and cryptorchidism.[38] Developmental delay in expressive language skills or behavioral and social problems in toddlers or school-age children may also prompt karyotype analysis.[39] Evaluation for KS is indicated in adolescents with delayed or incomplete pubertal development, gynecomastia, or small testes.[40] Because KS is one of the most common causes of male infertility, adults with infertility should also prompt karyotype analysis.[41]

One of the classic features of KS is tall stature with a eunuchoid body habitus. Growth in infants with KS usually is normal. By the age of 3 years, growth velocity typically has accelerated, which results in taller than average males from age 5 years and onward.[42] Males with KS have a mean final height of 179.2 ± 6.2 cm.[43] The increase in height primarily results from increased leg length, which can be noted on physical examination before the onset of puberty.[44] The exact mechanism for the increase in height and the abnormal proportions is still unknown. In 1976, Tanner et al[45] noted that males with hypogonadism have increased leg length. However, the increased leg length seen in KS is present before puberty, making androgen deficiency an unlikely cause of this growth pattern. In a study published in 2008, Aksglaede et al[44] demonstrated that males with KS also have normal IGF-1 and insulinlike growth factor binding protein-3 levels from infancy to adulthood. Thus, it also is unlikely that aberrations in the growth hormone–IGF-1 axis are the cause of this abnormal growth.

More recent research in genomics has revealed the *SHOX* gene is involved in regulating growth.[46] This *SHOX* gene is located on the short arm of the X chromosome in a region known as the pseudoautosomal region 1 (PAR1).[46] The PAR1 is known to escape X inactivation and thereby can exert a gene dosage effect on sex chromosomal disorders.[47] For instance, the haploinsufficiency of *SHOX* seen in TS, 45,X, results in short stature.[48] In a study of males with KS, the number of sex chromosomes was associated with increased height, except in cases of 5 sex chromosomes (4 Xs and 1 Y).[48] More than 10% of the genes located on the X chromosome are expressed in the testis and very likely could play a role in the clinical features seen in KS.[49]

KS is associated with hypergonadotropic hypogonadism. The testicular volume typically is reduced in infants and prepubertal males with KS because of degeneration of germ cells starting in fetal life.[49] This degeneration continues through childhood and accelerates during puberty, resulting in extensive fibrosis and hyalinization of the seminiferous tubules.[50] Puberty typically is associated with an increase in testicular volume but is followed by testicular volume reduction, likely induced by the deterioration of testicular function.[51] This results in a severely reduced testes volume of 3 mL in adults.[51]

Early studies demonstrated that males with KS had a blunted "minipuberty" during the first 3 months of life, with low testosterone but normal anti-müllerian hormone and inhibin B hormone levels.[52] However, more recent data suggest that there is no difference between males with or without KS in "minipuberty" with regard to these hormone levels.[53] However, this subsequent study did note a small difference in the ratio of testosterone to LH and between FSH and inhibin B, which may represent an abnormality in hormone release even though the testosterone level is within normal limits.

Males with KS have an increased frequency of underdeveloped male genitalia, particularly cryptorchidism and microphallus. Frequency of cryptorchidism in published studies range from 4.5% to as high as 68%.[49,54] Frequency of microphallus in KS ranges similarly from 4.5% of referrals to as high as 56%.[49,55] In 1 study, although only 1 male infant met the criteria for true microphallus, 22 other infants had a penile length of -0.9 SD.[49] Another study reported a normal size of phallus at birth but poor growth of the phallus during the subsequent years.[56] Although males with microphallus benefit from testosterone therapy with a gain in penile length, data regarding the use of testosterone during the "minipuberty" during infancy in all patients with KS still are limited.

At the start of puberty, males with KS typically have normal levels of LH, FSH, anti-müllerian hormone, inhibin B, insulin-like factor 3, and testosterone. However, as puberty progresses FSH and LH rise and the levels of testosterone and insulinlike factor 3 decline in comparison to other males.[57] Thus, by midpuberty, patients with KS have a relative testosterone deficiency manifested by increases in LH and FSH while the testosterone level plateaus. Inhibin B levels decrease significantly during puberty and become almost undetectable by the end of puberty.[58] These decreased inhibin B levels signify the impairment in spermatogenesis that is seen in most male with KS.[44] By adulthood, most males with KS have significantly elevated LH and FSH levels and a low or low-normal testosterone level. Adults with KS are characterized by hypergonadotropic hypogonadism. Estradiol levels typically are high by early puberty and generally remain elevated, even in males without gynecomastia.[57]

Testosterone therapy usually is indicated in late adolescence into early adulthood when there is evidence of androgen deficiency. The question of the timing of testosterone therapy initiation remains a challenge. Specifically, there is a lack of placebo-controlled trials showing the effectiveness of early testosterone replacement as LH and FSH begin to rise while the testosterone level remains in the normal or low-normal range.

As previously noted, Sertoli cells are also affected by hyalinization and fibrosis, and, as a result, most males with KS are infertile. Because of the lack of spermatogenesis, semen analysis typically reveals azoospermia. In a study of 131 males with KS, only 8.4% had spermatozoa in their semen.[35] The few subjects capable of spermatogenesis had an increased risk for chromosomal abnormalities.[59] However, recent reproductive technology has allowed for biologic paternity in male KS couples. Techniques such as testicular sperm extraction (TESE) followed by intracytoplasmic sperm injection have resulted in relatively good success. One study reported a sperm recovery rate of nearly 66%, with a live birth of a child in 45%.[60] Another technique, called microdissection TESE, has resulted in sperm recovery rates as high as 70%.[61] Although testicular histopathology is predictive of successful sperm retrieval, TESE has been successful even when no sperm were seen on histologic sections.[61] Cryopreservation of semen samples containing a low number of sperm in early puberty is possible, and many experts recommend that this should be offered to appropriate patients before testosterone therapy. However, it can be difficult for young boys in early puberty to provide a semen sample, and puberty marks the start of a rapid depletion of Sertoli cells, which can lead to a low success rate. Although studies for fertility preservation before the onset of puberty are ongoing, these options are still considered experimental.

Males with KS are at increased risk for learning impairments, although the neuropsychological phenotype is quite variable. Boys with KS most commonly have difficulties in language development, with more specific learning disabilities in the areas of spelling and reading.[62] Because of these learning issues, boys with KS are more likely to require extra educational help in school, specifically speech and language therapy.[63] Delays in speech milestones can be seen in younger boys, whereas difficulties in expressive language are more common in older boys and adolescents. Interestingly, males with KS have greater difficulties in both identifying and verbalizing emotions.[64] Visual and spatial abilities, as well as math skills, typically are normal.[65] Overall, though, the cognitive ability of males with KS is near normal. In a registry study that also assessed social outcomes, patients with KS had fewer partnerships and fatherhoods, as well as lower educational levels and lower incomes, than age-matched controls.[66] Males with KS also seem to have higher psychiatric morbidity. One study noted a frequency of KS in inpatient psychiatric wards of 0.8% among patients with schizophrenia.[67] Another study noted that up to 54% of boys with KS in adolescence had mild to moderate psychiatric disorders.[68] Other psychiatric conditions seen more frequently in males with KS include schizotypal traits, depression, anxiety, autism spectrum disorder, and attention-deficit/hyperactivity disorder.[69] Monitoring for learning disabilities, providing psychoeducational testing in school-aged boys, and providing ongoing psychological support all are recommended for males with KS.

Patients with KS are at a higher risk for breast cancer than their peers. Although the exact cause of this risk is still unknown, gynecomastia, elevated estrogen-to-testosterone ratios, obesity, and a lack of physical activity, as well as the exposure to exogenous androgens, all have been proposed as potential contributing factors.[70] Swerdlow et al[71] studied breast cancer rates in males with KS in the United Kingdom and found that the standardized mortality rate was 61.7 (confidence interval 7.5-222.7).

Endocrinopathies are seen more prominently in males with KS, especially diabetes mellitus. Studies have shown that adults with KS have an almost 5-fold increased risk for developing metabolic syndrome than age-matched peers.[72] In a study of 89 children aged 4 to 12 years, insulin resistance was found in 24%, metabolic syndrome in 7%, and elevated low-density lipoprotein cholesterol in 37%.[73] Many of the studies also indicated that males with KS have increased truncal obesity and total fat, which is also known to be associated with an increased risk of metabolic derangements.[72] Of note, the greater body fat mass can already be seen before puberty.[74] However, other studies have observed an inverse relationship between insulin resistance and testosterone levels in the serum.[75] Indeed, type 2 diabetes is frequently seen in hypogonadotropic patients.[72] The mechanism by which how hypogonadism leads to increased truncal obesity or increased truncal obesity leads to lower testosterone levels, called the hypogonadal-obesity circle, has not been fully elucidated.[76] More studies are needed to clarify whether early androgen deficiency is the cause of the insulin resistance and metabolic syndrome or other factors are playing a role.

Patients with KS are at higher risk for having autoimmune disorders, including systemic lupus erythematosus. One study noted that males with KS had a 14-fold increased risk for systemic lupus erythematosus in comparison to the general male population.[77] This risk is similar to that seen in the female population, which could suggest a gene dosage effect of the X chromosome on autoimmune disorders.[78]

Osteopenia and osteoporosis can been seen frequently in males with KS. This increased risk of bone demineralization has been linked to the androgen deficiency.[79] Not surprisingly, adult males with KS often have decreased bone mineral density, which typically improves with testosterone treatment.[80] In a study of 24 children and adolescents (aged 4.3-18.6 years) with KS, lumbar bone mineral density and whole body bone mineral content were found to be normal, which suggests that the decreased bone mineral density may not be present until after puberty.[74] However, data on the effect of exogenous testosterone on fracture rate and the development of osteoporosis are limited.

Males with KS have a reduced life expectancy. One study noted a lower median survival of 2.1 years in comparison to age-matched peers, or an increased mortality risk of 1.40 (confidence interval 1.13-1.74).[81] This increased mortality was the result of diabetes mellitus, pulmonary diseases, neurologic problems, cerebrovascular diseases, or infectious causes. More specific causes of death were identified as epilepsy, pulmonary embolism, peripheral vascular disease, vascular insufficiency of the intestine, and cardiovascular congenital anomalies.[82] In another study from the United Kingdom, cancer mortality was increased for breast cancer, non-Hodgkin lymphoma, and lung cancer.[83] Increased morbidity and mortality could be related to hypogonadism, the non-inactivated gene on the extra X chromosome, the learning impairments, or the lower socioeconomic status commonly seen in patients with KS.[66]

In general, the diagnosis of KS requires physicians to maintain a high index of suspicion in males demonstrating associated physical, medical, social, or developmental characteristics. Medical management for issues particular to KS from infancy to adulthood can potentially improve overall health and quality of life (Table 4). Early intervention, at least in adolescence, can potentially influence

Table 4

Medical management and monitoring in Klinefelter syndrome

All patients	Genetic counseling and education regarding Klinefelter syndrome support to parents
	Monitoring for growth and puberty
	Ongoing psychological support with consideration for psychological referral
Infants and toddlers	Treatment of cryptorchidism if needed
	Testosterone therapy for micropenis if needed
Childhood	Psychoeducational evaluation annually
	Speech therapy or social skills training if needed
Adolescents and adults	Monitoring for hypogonadism both clinically and with biochemical markers
	Age-appropriate pubertal induction and androgen replacement when hypogonadism demonstrated
	Fertility counseling with consideration for cryopreservation or testicular sperm extraction
	Fasting glucose and lipid profile annually
	Thyroid function, hemoglobin, and hematocrit testing annually
	Exercise and nutritional assessment
	Bone mineral density evaluation as indicated
	Counseling regarding increased risk for autoimmune diseases, metabolic syndrome, and breast cancer

Guidelines adapted from Aksglaede L, Link K, Giwercman A, et al. 47,XXY Klinefelter syndrome: clinical characteristics and age-specific recommendations for medical management. *Am J Med Genet C Semin Med Genet.* 2013;163c:55-63.

social and physical development and may also affect future fertility and critical monitoring of disorders associated with adults diagnosed with KS.

References

1. Nielsen J, Wohlert M. Sex chromosome abnormalities found among 34,910 newborn children: results from a 13-year incidence study in Arhus, Denmark. *Birth Defects Orig Art Ser.* 1990;26: 209-223
2. Gravholt CH. Epidemiological, endocrine and metabolic features in Turner syndrome. *Eur J Endocrinol.* 2004;151:657-687
3. Batch J. Turner syndrome in childhood and adolescence. *Best Pract Res Clin Endocrinol Metab.* 2002;16:465-482
4. Stochholm K, Juul S, Juel K, Naeraa RW, Gravholt CH. Prevalence, incidence, diagnostic delay, and mortality in Turner syndrome. *J Clin Endocrinol Metab.* 2006;91:3897-3902
5. Gravholt CH. Clinical practice in Turner syndrome. *Nat Clin Pract Endocrinol Metab.* 2005;1: 41-52
6. Brook CG, Murset G, Zachmann M, Prader A. Growth in children with 45,XO Turner's syndrome. *Arch Dis Child.* 1974;49:789-795
7. Zinn A, Ross J. Critical regions for Turner syndrome phenotypes on the X chromosome. In: Saenger P, Pasquino A, eds. *Optimizing Health Care for Turner Patients in the 21st Century. Proceedings from the 5th International Symposium on Turner Syndrome. Naples, Italy.* Amsterdam: Elsevier Science; 2000:19-28

8. Stephure DKl; Canadian Growth Hormone Advisory Committee. Impact of growth hormone supplementation on adult height in turner syndrome: results of the Canadian randomized controlled trial. *J Clin Endocrinol Metab.* 2005;90:3360-3366
9. Davenport ML, Crowe BJ, Travers SH, et al. Growth hormone treatment of early growth failure in toddlers with Turner syndrome: a randomized, controlled, multicenter trial. *J Clin Endocrinol Metab.* 2007;92:3406-3416
10. Bondy CA; Turner Syndrome Study Group. Care of girls and women with Turner syndrome: a guideline of the Turner Syndrome Study Group. *J Clin Endocrinol Metab.* 2007;92:10-25
11. Gault EJ, Perry RJ, Cole TJ, et al. Effect of oxandrolone and timing of pubertal induction on final height in Turner's syndrome: randomised, double blind, placebo controlled trial. *BMJ.* 2011;342:d1980
12. Pasquino AM, Passeri F, Pucarelli I, Segni M, Municchi G. Spontaneous pubertal development in Turner's syndrome. Italian Study Group for Turner's Syndrome. *J Clin Endocrinol Metab.* 1997;82:1810-1813
13. Fechner PY, Davenport ML, Qualy RL, et al. Differences in follicle-stimulating hormone secretion between 45,X monosomy Turner syndrome and 45,X/46,XX mosaicism are evident at an early age. *J Clin Endocrinol Metab.* 2006;91:4896-4902
14. Quigley CA, Crowe BJ, Anglin DG, Chipman JJ. Growth hormone and low dose estrogen in Turner syndrome: results of a United States multi-center trial to near-final height. *J Clin Endocrinol Metab.* 2002;87:2033-2041
15. Soriano-Guillen L, Coste J, Ecosse E, et al. Adult height and pubertal growth in Turner syndrome after treatment with recombinant growth hormone. *J Clin Endocrinol Metab.* 2005;90:5197-5204
16. Ross JL, Quigley CA, Cao D, et al. Growth hormone plus childhood low-dose estrogen in Turner's syndrome. *N Engl J Med.* 2011;364:1230-1242
17. Loscalzo ML, Van PL, Ho VB, et al. Association between fetal lymphedema and congenital cardiovascular defects in Turner syndrome. *Pediatrics.* 2005;115:732-735
18. Sybert VP. Cardiovascular malformations and complications in Turner syndrome. *Pediatrics.* 1998;101:E11
19. Ho VB, Bakalov VK, Cooley M, et al. Major vascular anomalies in Turner syndrome: prevalence and magnetic resonance angiographic features. *Circulation.* 2004;110:1694-1700
20. Matura LA, Ho VB, Rosing DR, Bondy CA. Aortic dilatation and dissection in Turner syndrome. *Circulation.* 2007;116:1663-1670
21. Carlson M, Silberbach M. Dissection of the aorta in Turner syndrome: two cases and review of 85 cases in the literature. *J Med Genet.* 2007;44:745-749
22. Chevalier N, Letur H, Lelannou D, et al. Materno-fetal cardiovascular complications in Turner syndrome after oocyte donation: insufficient prepregnancy screening and pregnancy follow-up are associated with poor outcome. *J Clin Endocrinol Metab.* 2011;96:E260-E267
23. Practice Committee of American Society For Reproductive Medicine. Increased maternal cardiovascular mortality associated with pregnancy in women with Turner syndrome. *Fertil Steril.* 2012;97:282-284
24. Sutton EJ, McInerney-Leo A, Bondy CA, et al. Turner syndrome: four challenges across the lifespan. *Am J Med Genet A.* 2005;139a:57-66
25. Marshall D, Johnell O, Wedel H. Meta-analysis of how well measures of bone mineral density predict occurrence of osteoporotic fractures. *BMJ.* 1996;312:1254-1259
26. Livadas S, Xekouki P, Fouka F, et al. Prevalence of thyroid dysfunction in Turner's syndrome: a long-term follow-up study and brief literature review. *Thyroid.* 2005;15:1061-1066
27. Bonamico M, Pasquino AM, Mariani P, et al. Prevalence and clinical picture of celiac disease in Turner syndrome. *J Clin Endocrinol Metab.* 2002;87:5495-5498
28. Bilge I, Kayserili H, Emre S, et al. Frequency of renal malformations in Turner syndrome: analysis of 82 Turkish children. *Pediatr Nephrol.* 2000;14:1111-1114
29. Stenberg AE, Nylen O, Windh M, Hultcrantz M. Otological problems in children with Turner's syndrome. *Hear Res.* 1998;124:85-90

30. Rovet JF. The psychoeducational characteristics of children with Turner syndrome. *J Learn Disabil.* 1993;26:333-341
31. Russell HF, Wallis D, Mazzocco MM, et al. Increased prevalence of ADHD in Turner syndrome with no evidence of imprinting effects. *J Pediatr Psychol.* 2006;31:945-955
32. Carel JC, Elie C, Ecosse E, et al. Self-esteem and social adjustment in young women with Turner syndrome—influence of pubertal management and sexuality: population-based cohort study. *J Clin Endocrinol Metab.* 2006;91:2972-2979
33. Schoemaker MJ, Swerdlow AJ, Higgins CD, Wright AF, Jacobs PA; United Kingdom Clinical Cytogenetics Group. Mortality in women with turner syndrome in Great Britain: a national cohort study. *J Clin Endocrinol Metab.* 2008;93:4735-4742
34. Visootsak J, Graham JM Jr. Klinefelter syndrome and other sex chromosomal aneuploidies. *Orphanet J Rare Dis.* 2006;1:42
35. Lanfranco F, Kamischke A, Zitzmann M, Nieschlag E. Klinefelter's syndrome. *Lancet.* 2004;364:273-283
36. Coffee B, Keith K, Albizua I, et al. Incidence of fragile X syndrome by newborn screening for methylated FMR1 DNA. *Am J Med Genet.* 2009;85:503-514
37. Bojesen A, Juul S, Gravholt CH. Prenatal and postnatal prevalence of Klinefelter syndrome: a national registry study. *J Clin Endocrinol Metab.* 2003;88:622-626
38. Caldwell PD, Smith DW. The XXY (Klinefelter's) syndrome in childhood: detection and treatment. *J Pediatr.* 1972;80:250-258
39. Walzer S, Wolff PH, Bowen D, et al. A method for the longitudinal study of behavioral development in infants and children: the early development of XXY children. *J Child Psychol Psychiatry.* 1978;19:213-229
40. Robinson A, Bender BG, Linden MG. Summary of clinical findings in children and young adults with sex chromosome anomalies. *Birth Defects Orig Art Ser.* 1990;26:225-228
41. Okada H, Fujioka H, Tatsumi N, et al. Klinefelter's syndrome in the male infertility clinic. *Hum Reprod.* 1999;14:946-952
42. Ratcliffe SG, Butler GE, Jones M. Edinburgh study of growth and development of children with sex chromosome abnormalities. IV. *Birth Defects Orig Art Ser.* 1990;26:1-44
43. Schibler D, Brook CG, Kind HP, Zachmann M, Prader A. Growth and body proportions in 54 boys and men with Klinefelter's syndrome. *Helv Paediatr Acta.* 1974;29:325-333
44. Aksglaede L, Skakkebaek NE, Juul A. Abnormal sex chromosome constitution and longitudinal growth: serum levels of insulin-like growth factor (IGF)-I, IGF binding protein-3, luteinizing hormone, and testosterone in 109 males with 47,XXY, 47,XYY, or sex-determining region of the Y chromosome (SRY)-positive 46,XX karyotypes. *J Clin Endocrinol Metab.* 2008;93:169-176
45. Tanner JM, Whitehouse RH, Hughs PC, Carter BS. Relative importance of growth hormone and sex steroids for the growth at puberty of trunk length, limb length, and muscle width in growth hormone-deficient children. *J Pediatr.* 1976;89:1000-1008
46. Rappold GA, Durand C, Decker E, Marchini A, Schneider KU. New roles of SHOX as regulator of target genes. *Pediatr Endocrinol Rev.* 2012;9(Suppl 2):733-738
47. Rao E, Weiss B, Fukami M, et al. Pseudoautosomal deletions encompassing a novel homeobox gene cause growth failure in idiopathic short stature and Turner syndrome. *Nat Genet.* 1997;16:54-63
48. Ottesen AM, Aksglaede L, Garn I, et al. Increased number of sex chromosomes affects height in a nonlinear fashion: a study of 305 patients with sex chromosome aneuploidy. *Am J Med Genet A.* 2010;152a:1206-1212
49. Ross JL, Samango-Sprouse C, Lahlou N, et al. Early androgen deficiency in infants and young boys with 47,XXY Klinefelter syndrome. *Horm Res.* 2005;64:39-45
50. Aksglaede L, Wikstrom AM, Rajpert-De Meyts E, et al. Natural history of seminiferous tubule degeneration in Klinefelter syndrome. *Hum Reprod Update.* 2006;12:39-48
51. Aksglaede L, Skakkebaek NE, Almstrup K, Juul A. Clinical and biological parameters in 166 boys, adolescents and adults with nonmosaic Klinefelter syndrome: a Copenhagen experience. *Acta Paediatr.* 2011;100:793-806

52. Lahlou N, Fennoy I, Carel JC, Roger M. Inhibin B and anti-Mullerian hormone, but not testosterone levels, are normal in infants with nonmosaic Klinefelter syndrome. *J Clin Endocrinol Metab.* 2004;89:1864-1868
53. Aksglaede L, Petersen JH, Main KM, Skakkebaek NE, Juul A. High normal testosterone levels in infants with non-mosaic Klinefelter's syndrome. *Eur J Endocrinol.* 2007;157:345-350
54. Bastida MG, Rey RA, Bergada I, et al. Establishment of testicular endocrine function impairment during childhood and puberty in boys with Klinefelter syndrome. *Clin Endocrinol.* 2007;67:863-870
55. Battin J, Malpuech G, Nivelon JL, et al. [Klinefelter syndrome in 1993. Results of a multicenter study on 58 cases and review of the literature]. *Ann Pediatr (Paris).* 1993;40:432-437
56. Ratcliffe SG. The sexual development of boys with the chromosome constitution 47,XXY (Klinefelter's syndrome). *Clin Endocrinol Metab.* 1982;11:703-716
57. Salbenblatt JA, Bender BG, Puck MH, et al. Pituitary-gonadal function in Klinefelter syndrome before and during puberty. *Pediatr Res.* 1985;19:82-86
58. Christiansen P, Andersson AM, Skakkebaek NE. Longitudinal studies of inhibin B levels in boys and young adults with Klinefelter syndrome. *J Clin Endocrinol Metab.* 2003;88:888-891
59. Staessen C, Tournaye H, Van Assche E, et al. PGD in 47,XXY Klinefelter's syndrome patients. *Hum Reprod Update.* 2003;9:319-330
60. Ramasamy R, Ricci JA, Palermo GD, et al. Successful fertility treatment for Klinefelter's syndrome. *J Urol.* 2009;182:1108-1113
61. Schiff JD, Palermo GD, Veeck LL, et al. Success of testicular sperm extraction [corrected] and intracytoplasmic sperm injection in men with Klinefelter syndrome. *J Clin Endocrinol Metab.* 2005;90:6263-6267
62. Bender BG, Linden MG, Robinson A. Neuropsychological impairment in 42 adolescents with sex chromosome abnormalities. *AM J Med Genet.* 1993;48:169-173
63. Rovet J, Netley C, Keenan M, Bailey J, Stewart D. The psychoeducational profile of boys with Klinefelter syndrome. *J Learn Disabil.* 1996;29:180-196
64. van Rijn S, Aleman A, Swaab H, et al. What it is said versus how it is said: comprehension of affective prosody in men with Klinefelter (47,XXY) syndrome. *J Int Neuropsychol Soc.* 2007;13:1065-1070
65. Itti E, Gaw Gonzalo IT, Pawlikowska-Haddal A, et al. The structural brain correlates of cognitive deficits in adults with Klinefelter's syndrome. *J Clin Endocrinol Metab.* 2006;91:1423-1427
66. Bojesen A, Stochholm K, Juul S, Gravholt CH. Socioeconomic trajectories affect mortality in Klinefelter syndrome. *J Clin Endocrinol Metab.* 2011;96:2098-2104
67. DeLisi LE, Friedrich U, Wahlstrom J, et al. Schizophrenia and sex chromosome anomalies. *Schizophr Bull.* 1994;20:495-505
68. Bender BG, Harmon RJ, Linden MG, Robinson A. Psychosocial adaptation of 39 adolescents with sex chromosome abnormalities. *Pediatrics.* 1995;96(2 Pt 1):302-308
69. Bruining H, Swaab H, Kas M, van Engeland H. Psychiatric characteristics in a self-selected sample of boys with Klinefelter syndrome. *Pediatrics.* 2009;123:e865-870
70. Aksglaede L, Link K, Giwercman A, Jorgensen N, Skakkebaek NE, Juul A. 47,XXY Klinefelter syndrome: clinical characteristics and age-specific recommendations for medical management. *Am J Med Genet C Semin Med Genet.* 2013;163c:55-63
71. Swerdlow AJ, Hermon C, Jacobs PA, et al. Mortality and cancer incidence in persons with numerical sex chromosome abnormalities: a cohort study. *Ann Hum Genet.* 2001;65(Pt 2):177-188
72. Bojesen A, Kristensen K, Birkebaek NH, et al. The metabolic syndrome is frequent in Klinefelter's syndrome and is associated with abdominal obesity and hypogonadism. *Diabetes Care.* 2006;29:1591-1598
73. Bardsley MZ, Falkner B, Kowal K, Ross JL. Insulin resistance and metabolic syndrome in prepubertal boys with Klinefelter syndrome. *Acta Paediatr.* 2011;100:866-870
74. Aksglaede L, Molgaard C, Skakkebaek NE, Juul A. Normal bone mineral content but unfavourable muscle/fat ratio in Klinefelter syndrome. *Arch Dis Child.* 2008;93:30-34

75. Grossmann M, Thomas MC, Panagiotopoulos S, et al. Low testosterone levels are common and associated with insulin resistance in men with diabetes. *J Clin Endocrinol Metab.* 2008;93:1834-1840
76. Wang C, Jackson G, Jones TH, et al. Low testosterone associated with obesity and the metabolic syndrome contributes to sexual dysfunction and cardiovascular disease risk in men with type 2 diabetes. *Diabetes Care.* 2011;34:1669-1675
77. Rovensky J. Rheumatic diseases and Klinefelter's syndrome. *Autoimmun Rev.* 2006;6:33-36
78. Sawalha AH, Harley JB, Scofield RH. Autoimmunity and Klinefelter's syndrome: when men have two X chromosomes. *J Autoimmun.* 2009;33:31-34
79. Finkelstein JS, Klibanski A, Neer RM, et al. Osteoporosis in men with idiopathic hypogonadotropic hypogonadism. *Ann Intern Med.* 1987;106:354-361
80. Behre HM, Kliesch S, Leifke E, Link TM, Nieschlag E. Long-term effect of testosterone therapy on bone mineral density in hypogonadal men. *J Clin Endocrinol Metab.* 1997;82:2386-2390
81. Bojesen A, Juul S, Birkebaek N, Gravholt CH. Increased mortality in Klinefelter syndrome. *J Clin Endocrinol Metab.* 2004;89:3830-3834
82. Swerdlow AJ, Higgins CD, Schoemaker MJ, Wright AF, Jacobs PA. Mortality in patients with Klinefelter syndrome in Britain: a cohort study. *J Clin Endocrinol Metab.* 2005;90:6516-6522
83. Swerdlow AJ, Schoemaker MJ, Higgins CD, Wright AF, Jacobs PA. Cancer incidence and mortality in men with Klinefelter syndrome: a cohort study. *J Nat Cancer Inst.* 2005;97:1204-1210

Disorders of Sex Development: Why Adolescent Medicine Specialists Should Care

David E. Sandberg, PhD

University of Michigan, Pediatrics & Communicable Diseases and Child Health Evaluation & Research (CHEAR) Unit, Ann Arbor, Michigan

INTRODUCTION

Disorders of sex development (DSD) is an umbrella term covering congenital conditions in which development of chromosomal, gonadal, or anatomic sex is atypical.[1] Until 2005, *intersex* was adopted as the preferred umbrella term for variations in somatic sex characteristics that prevent easy classification of the person as male or female. The term was used by both physicians and patients in preference to the gonadal-based terminology of male or female pseudohermaphroditism and true hermaphroditism, which, nevertheless, continue to be used as diagnostic labels in the *International Statistical Classification of Diseases and Related Health Problems-10* (ICD-10).[2]

The clinical management of patients with DSD generates many controversies and questions regarding best practices. This review is written from the perspective that adolescent medicine specialists are well equipped to deliver primary and transition care to these patients and their families by virtue of their scope of practice and expertise. The goal of this review is to familiarize the reader with recent developments in this area of clinical care and to make the case that the adolescent medicine specialist's knowledge of cognitive, emotional, and psychosexual development during the adolescent years, emerging sexuality, and issues related to transition from pediatric to adult care are particularly well suited to the needs of this population.

E-mail address: dsandber@med.umich.edu

Copyright © 2015 American Academy of Pediatrics. All rights reserved. ISSN 1934-4287

WHAT ARE DISORDERS OF SEX DEVELOPMENT?*

Definitions and Categories

Disorders of sex development are the consequence of errors in the process of *sex determination* (ie, process in which the bipotential gonad develops into a testis or an ovary) or *sex differentiation* (ie, process of differentiation of the internal genital ducts and external genitalia).[3] In response to advances in molecular diagnosis, changes in surgical techniques, and growing controversy regarding the model of patient care, the Lawson Wilkins Pediatric Endocrine Society (renamed the Pediatric Endocrine Society in 2010) and the European Society for Paediatric Endocrinology, in 2005, convened a consensus conference on the clinical management of intersex conditions.[1] Conference participants included international experts from various specialties, including mental health, as well as patient advocate representatives. The *Consensus Statement on Management of Intersex Disorders* (hereafter referred to as the "Consensus") was published the following year (2006) and is an endorsed policy statement of the American Academy of Pediatrics.[4]

One of the consensus conference working groups focused on nomenclature. Among the salient recommendations was removal of terms perceived as offensive, such as "hermaphrodite," "pseudo-hermaphrodite," "sex reversal," and "intersex." In their place, all variations in somatic sex development were incorporated under a new umbrella term, "disorders of sex development" (DSD), defined as "congenital conditions in which development of chromosomal, gonadal, or anatomic sex is atypical."[1] This definition underscores the fact that both sex chromosomes and gonads are key etiologic parameters responsible for variations in biologic sex development. In the new scheme, karyotype serves as the basis for categorizing DSD: *sex chromosome DSD*; *46,XY DSD*; and *46,XX DSD* (Table 1). Depending on which specific conditions are subsumed under the superordinate category, DSD in the aggregate, have an estimated incidence ranging from 0.018% to 1.7% of live births.[5]

There is some confusion as to whether hypospadias (in which the urethral meatus terminates on the undersurface of the penis) is a DSD. This can be inferred from the Consensus, which asserts that "apparent male genitalia with bilateral undescended testes, micropenis, isolated perineal hypospadias, or mild hypospadias with undescended testis" only "suggest DSD"[1(p.e490)] rather than the phenotype meeting the definitional requirements of DSD.

---

* The acronym DSD is used in this chapter to refer exclusively to a category of medical conditions sharing common features. In this context, DSD carries no implications for the identity of the person, some of whom prefer the term *intersex*. In general, we adopt the principle of "people-first" language, which refers to the person first, and the potentially associated disability second.

Table 1

Disorders of sex development (DSD) nomenclature

Sex Chromosome DSD	46,XY DSD	46,XX DSD
45,X (Turner syndrome and variants)	Disorders of gonadal (testicular) development: (1) complete gonadal dysgenesis (Swyer syndrome); (2) partial gonadal dysgenesis; (3) gonadal regression; and (4) ovotesticular DSD	Disorder of gonadal (ovarian) development: (1) ovotesticular DSD; (2) testicular DSD (eg, SRY+, duplicate SOX9); and (3) gonadal dysgenesis
47,XXY (Klinefelter syndrome and variants)	Disorders in androgen synthesis or action: (1) androgen biosynthesis defect (eg, 17-hydroxysteroid dehydrogenase deficiency, 5αRD2 deficiency, StAR mutations); (2) defect in androgen action (eg, CAIS, PAIS); (3) luteinizing hormone receptor defects (eg, Leydig cell hypoplasia, aplasia); and (4) disorders of anti-Müllerian hormone and anti-Müllerian hormone receptor (persistent Müllerian duct syndrome)	Androgen excess: (1) fetal (eg, 21-hydroxylase deficiency, 11-hydroxylase deficiency); (2) fetoplacental (aromatase deficiency, POR [P450 oxidoreductase]); and (3) maternal (luteoma, exogenous, etc)
45,X/46,XY (MGD, ovotesticular DSD)		Other (eg, cloacal exstrophy, vaginal atresia, MURCS [Müllerian, renal, cervicothoracic somite abnormalities], other syndromes)
46,XX/46,XY (chimeric, ovotesticular DSD)		

Although consideration of karyotype is useful for classification, unnecessary reference to karyotype should be avoided; ideally, a system based on descriptive terms (eg, androgen insensitivity syndrome) should be used wherever possible. StAR indicates steroidogenic acute regulatory protein.

From Lee PA, Houk CP, Ahmed SF, Hughes IA, in collaboration with the participants in the International Consensus Conference on Intersex. Consensus statement on management of intersex disorders. *Pediatrics*. 2006;118:e488-e500.

In the DSD framework, neither atypical genital appearance nor uncertainties about assignment to an "optimal" gender of rearing are necessary features of classified conditions. For instance, Klinefelter and Turner syndromes, and their variants, are categorized as *sex chromosome DSD*. Both conditions are associated with gonadal dysgenesis, yet the external genitalia appear typical and the sex announcement at birth is never in question. Additional examples that reflect the dissociation of DSD from the feature of "ambiguous genitalia" (or uncertainty regarding gender assignment) include 46,XY women with pure gonadal dysgenesis (Swyer syndrome), 46,XX men with a translocation of the SRY gene, and complete androgen insensitivity syndrome (CAIS). All of these conditions are associated with a typical female genital phenotype, and all the individuals reared as girls from birth.

It would be misleading to give the impression that the DSD terminology, or its definition, has been universally accepted. Although the new terminology has enjoyed broad acceptance by medical and research communities, some people born with "intersex traits" are strongly opposed to what they perceive as the unnecessary pathologization of their intersex identity and damaging consequences associated with current clinical management strategies.[6-8]

Timing of Diagnosis

Disorders of sex development are most commonly discovered at birth. Triggers for an evaluation include atypical genital appearance or discordance between results of prenatal diagnostic testing (eg, ultrasound, amniocentesis) and genital appearance at the time of delivery. The presence at birth of a congenital anomaly affecting a child's genital appearance or future reproductive function can engender a "psychosocial emergency" for parents and physicians.[9,10] Atypical genital anatomy may represent, for both the physician and the family, the most challenging aspect of otherwise complex and even life-threatening conditions (most notably classic 21-hydroxylase congenital adrenal hyperplasia).[11]

Clinical presentations identified beyond the newborn period include a phenotypically typical female with inguinal hernia(s) found to contain testes, primary amenorrhea in girls and lack of adrenarche during adolescence, absent müllerian structures on ultrasound examination in an otherwise phenotypically typical female exhibiting normal breast development and pubertal growth occurring at the appropriate age (eg, CAIS),[12] or a contrasexual (ie, masculinizing) puberty in girls (eg, 5α-reductase-2 deficiency [5α-RD-2] or 17β-hydroxysteroid dehydrogenase-3 deficiency [17β-HSD-3]).[3]

Distinctions Between Transgender and Disorders of Sex Development

The DSM-5[13] diagnostic category of "Gender Dysphoria" (previously *Gender Identity Disorder in Children* or *Gender Identity Disorder in Adolescents or Adults*[14]) is applied to persons experiencing a conflict between their gender identity (ie, self-identification as either girl/woman or boy/man) versus their sex and gender of rearing that were announced at birth. Atypical gender-role behavior (ie, behaviors that differ in frequency or level between boys/men and girls/women in this culture and time, such as toy play or maternal interest) is a well-recognized behavioral feature of particular DSD syndromes (eg, tomboyish behavior in girls with congenital adrenal hyperplasia).[15] Furthermore, substantial evidence suggests that this shift in gender-typed behavior is the consequence of the organizational effects of androgens on steroid-sensitive brain regions during sensitive (prenatal) periods of brain development.[16] Far less evidence suggests a prenatal action of androgens on development of gender identity. Accordingly, the Consensus warns against viewing gender-atypical behavior as an indicator of gender dysphoria.[1(p.e492)]

The frequencies of gender dysphoria and gender change in persons with DSD vary dramatically according to DSD syndrome and gender assignment.[17,18] For example, with very limited exceptions, people with CAIS who were reared as girls identify as girls/women across the lifespan.[19] Similarly, there are no reported cases of people with a 46,XY karyotype and micropenis, reared as either a boy or girl, who self-reassigned their gender later in life.[19] At the other end of the continuum of gender identity stability are the syndromes associated with errors in testosterone biosynthesis, such as 5α-RD-2 or 17β-HSD-3.[3] In these 2 syndromes, between 56% and 63% and 39% and 64%, respectively, of affected persons assigned as girls at birth changed their gender, usually during adolescence or adulthood.[20] It is commonly assumed that gender self-reassignment is the consequence of a combination of prenatal and pubertal exposure to endogenous testosterone; however, other equally plausible alternative explanations have yet to be systematically assessed.[20-22]

Although there are some overlapping features in the putative etiology of gender dysphoria in persons with or without DSD, the presence of factors unique to those with DSD suggests the possibility that the pathway to gender dysphoria differs between groups.[23,24] Although more complete explanations for gender dysphoria in persons with DSD and those without require further research, it is indisputable that those affected with DSD have experienced very different life events than individuals without DSD. From the moment of detection, DSD can trigger a series of events that dramatically distinguish those born with atypical sex anatomies from those born physically typical. These events can consign the affected person and their parents to monitoring by physicians, much like anyone with a chronic illness. For the individual born with atypical genitalia or with discordance between karyotype and genital phenotype, the question that immediately faces physicians and parents is to which gender the infant should be assigned. The individual's history may include a change of the gender announcement at birth, with parents having to re-announce the gender of their child to siblings, grandparents, and friends. There may also be the necessity for lifesaving medication, as in the case of infants with congenital adrenal hyperplasia. There are also salient issues surrounding surgical reconstruction of the genitals and the possibility of contrasexual pubertal development or hormone treatment to induce puberty and maintain a general state of good health. As a consequence, the context within which a child with DSD grows and develops is much different from that of a child without a DSD. The extent to which these experiences contribute to gender dysphoria in a subset of patients with DSD remains unclear and understudied.

CLINICAL MANAGEMENT

Key to appreciating the complexity and challenge of clinical management in DSD is recognition that a diagnosis frequently does not imply a clear treatment recommendation. There are multiple choice points, and quality care requires that parents of infants and children (and, later, mature minors) understand that each decision carries the potential for serious risks, that outcomes (functional and psychological) are uncertain, that only very rarely does an emergency require immediate treatment (ie, although treatments may be considered therapeutic, they are elective), and that treatment approaches continue to be controversial.

Gender Assignment

The Consensus states that all newborns should receive a gender assignment, with the decision being informed by expert evaluation delivered by a multidisciplinary team working closely with the parents. Gender assignment decisions typically are guided by a combination of diagnosis and long-term adult follow-up studies that focus on gender identity stability and other psychosexual outcomes.[19,20,25,26] As noted earlier, gender identity refers to a person's inner sense of being a boy/man or girl/woman.[27] Unfortunately, for some conditions classified as DSD, adult gender identity cannot confidently be predicted, and atypical gender-role behavior in childhood is a poor predictor.[18,28-30] This is because little is known about the relative contribution of biologic (eg, genes, prenatal sex hormone exposure) and nonbiologic influences (eg, parental beliefs, attitude and preferences, peer influences, cultural context) on gender identity development and stability. Critical stages in the development or potential interactions of the various factors also are unclear.

Gender assignment does not pose insurmountable problems in most DSD conditions. However, in some conditions (eg, partial androgen insensitivity syndrome, 5α-RD-2, or 17β-HSD-3), the choice may be difficult because so little is known about postnatal events in the social environment that potentially intervene between early biologic events to modulate gender identity outcomes. For instance, should a child with 5α-RD-2 who is born with female-appearing external genitalia be gonadectomized to prevent a masculinizing puberty and reared as a girl? This choice is associated with lost capacity for spontaneous puberty, loss of potential fertility,[31] and the need for lifelong sex hormone replacement therapy. Alternatively, if reared as a boy, what would be the person's experience living with markedly atypical external genitalia? In such cases, dihydrotestosterone ointment (unavailable in the United States) applied directly to the genital tissue has been shown to result in increased phallic length, although it remains substantially below norms.[32] In such decisions, nonmedical factors such as the ability of parents to cope with uncertainties, personal and cultural values in the particular societal context, and medical factors such as surgical possibilities (5α-RD-2 is frequently associated with proximal hypospadias), potential for fertility, and need for hormone replacement need to be included. Even considering all these factors, one cannot be certain that the chosen gender assignment will result in a good quality of life. Unfortunately, the evidence on quality-of-life outcome of adults with DSD that could be used to inform such decisions is sparse and biased toward reports of patients from consanguineous pedigrees in developing countries. Under circumstances of limited medical care, these children, commonly reared as girls from birth, experience a masculinizing puberty that is associated with a gender change in later adolescence and young adulthood. The salient advantages of living as men in these patriarchal societies (eg, Dominican Republic, Brazil, Papua New Guinea, and the Middle East) has repeatedly been suggested as an alternative to a biologic explanation for postpubertal gender change.[20,21]

It is clear that atypical gender-role behavior (which refers to behaviors that differ in frequency or level between males and females in a particular culture and time, such as toy play or maternal interest) is not a proxy for gender dysphoria in DSD. Yet, awareness of the child's DSD may lead parents and physicians to erroneously regard gender behavior that is inconsistent with the gender of rearing as an indication of an error in the gender assignment. Gender reassignment should not occur without an assessment by an experienced mental health practitioner, ideally the designated mental health member of the multidisciplinary DSD team.[1]

To the extent that the aforementioned DSD-specific medical and associated experiences potentially contribute to developing gender dysphoria and influence the quality of life of those affected, it is incumbent on physicians, particularly those knowledgeable of mental health factors, to consider these in conceptualizing the etiology of the dysphoria and in designing the intervention. For suggestions regarding such an assessment and treatment strategies, see Mazur et al[23] and Meyer-Bahlburg.[33] The *Standards of Care* of the World Professional Association of Transgender Health (WPATH), a professional organization in the field of gender dysphoria, are potentially useful in guiding the assessment and treatment process.[34,35]

Genital Surgery

Questions about surgery to "normalize" genital appearance and function can arise shortly after birth. Surgeons, and other members of the DSD health care team described in the Consensus, have the responsibility to provide families with surgical options (including abstaining from performing any procedure for reasons other than medical necessity in the immediate term).[1] As in the case of birth defects, in general, parents of children with DSD commonly experience distress over the atypical appearance of their child's genitals. The desire to surgically "correct" or "fix" the difference is observed across countries and cultures.[36-38] Long-term follow-up studies of the results of genital surgery performed in early life suggest that complications are common and that the procedures can compromise sexual function and satisfaction.[39-41] It is clear that a motivating factor in the decision for early surgery is the belief among pediatric surgeons and parents that withholding surgery in early life would lead to negative psychosocial outcomes for both patients and their families. Because so little information is available regarding the outcomes of those who had not undergone early genital surgery, predictions of negative outcomes if surgery is not performed remains untested.

Hormone Replacement

Sex hormone replacement therapy is required in many individuals with DSD because the gonad never developed (ie, streak gonads as in Turner syndrome), failed,[42] or were removed because of risk of gonadal tumors.[43] Children require preparation before the time that puberty is pharmacologically induced and need to know that their puberty may be associated with some, but not all, typical somatic changes (eg, absence of menses in girls with CAIS or Mayer-Rokitansky-Küster-Hauser syndrome). Optimizing preparation and subsequent involvement of the patient in this aspect of care are essential in increasing the likelihood that adherence to the hormone replacement regimen remains high during the transition from pediatric to adult care and beyond. Again, the training and experience of pediatric and adolescent medicine specialists make them suited to be participants in the DSD health care team.

Sexuality

Although adolescents with physical disabilities may experience delays in puberty and a degree of social isolation, investigations in a nationally representative sample have shown that these youth, on the whole, are as likely to be sexually active as their nondisabled peers, yet there is evidence that they may not be considered equal to their nondisabled peers as targets for sexual education and counseling.[44] Youth with DSD can experience negative genital self-appraisal and sexual inhibition,[45-47] and exhibit delays and arrests in acquisition of psychosexual milestones.[48] The Consensus underscores that "quality of life encompasses falling in love, dating, attraction, ability to develop intimate relationships, sexual functioning, and the opportunity to marry and raise children, regardless of biological indicators of sex."[1(p.e493)] Accordingly, members of the health care team are encouraged to provide adolescents with opportunities to speak confidentially about possible concerns, including fear of stigmatization and rejection. To avert negative sexual experiences, youth will benefit from advice and counseling on building relationships. Consideration should be given to incorporating a sex therapist as a member of the DSD team to normalize sexuality as a component of comprehensive care.

There is evidence that early (ie, prenatal) atypical sex hormone exposure is associated with higher rates of nonheterosexual orientation.[49] However, data necessary to support a causative link between prenatal sex hormone exposure and sexual orientation are lacking.[16] Regardless of explanations for this relationship, parents may struggle contemplating this possibility already when the child is very young. They may not openly express their thoughts and feelings on the subject and will benefit from having misunderstandings and misinformation directly addressed.

Fertility

Infertility in DSD can be the direct consequence of errors in the process of sex determination or sex differentiation.[3] Failure to contribute to a pregnancy can also be the result of suboptimal hormone replacement therapy,[11] reduced interest in parenting,[50] reduced heterosexual activity[49] or sexual arousability,[51-53] atypical genital anatomy (eg, inadequate introitus[54]), or pain or reduced genital sensitivity during intercourse.[55,56] To the extent that DSD can be associated with lack of arousability or avoidance of sexual relations, it is important that these features not be confused with low libido.

Advances in reproductive medicine, and particularly in assisted reproductive technology (ART), have revolutionized management of infertility. These advances deliver hope for fertility in patient groups unable to achieve biologic parenthood. Nevertheless, new opportunities demand that there be judicious application of ART coupled with expert genetic counseling. Major gaps in evidence regarding the application of ART in DSD serve as obstacles to informed decision-making.

Psychosocial Adaptation

Advances in therapeutics for specific pediatric conditions have strongly contributed to a disease-specific ("categorical") approach to chronic pediatric conditions.[57] In the case of DSD, this approach led to enhanced understanding of the genetic origins of DSD[58,59] along with advances in genital surgical techniques.[60] Much of what is known about the psychological development of persons affected with DSD stems from research elucidating the influence of atypical sex hormone exposure during steroid-sensitive periods of brain development.[15] Prenatal androgens masculinize the genitalia, and experimental research has shown that androgens organize the development of regions of the brain responsible for sex differences in behavior across a wide range of mammalian species.[61] Because of inherent restrictions on experimental research in humans, investigators have relied on DSD as a model for testing hormonal hypotheses related to the influence of early androgen exposure on behaviors exhibiting sex-related variability, particularly psychosexual differentiation (ie, gender identity, gender role, and sexual orientation).[61,62]

In comparison to knowledge about psychosexual differentiation stemming from this type of research, we face major gaps in our understanding of other factors that likely contribute to specific and global adaptation in people with DSD. Consider the psychosocial research literature on congenital adrenal hyperplasia because of 21-hydroxylase deficiency: psychosexual differentiation has received the most attention in research on psychological outcomes.[62] In addition, there has been little reliance on theory or research strategies derived from developmental psychology (typical and atypical) or pediatric psychology that considers the interaction of biologic and environmental factors.[63,64] Such approaches routinely consider risk and protective factors, cognitive appraisal, and coping processes that are critical for testing competing theories about developmental pathways. The focus of the extant research literature stands in apparent contrast with calls from patient stakeholders to attend to more global indicators of adaptation. Disorders of sex development and related consensus statements and clinical care guidelines recognize the stress on patients and family associated with chronic medical conditions presenting at birth.[1,11,65]

A broadened clinical and research agenda in DSD is warranted, in part, to respond to justifiable criticism by former patients and advocates that poor psychosocial or psychosexual outcomes may be less a function of atypical sex hormone exposure or surgical procedures than the consequence of a complex interaction among experiences (eg, medical/surgical decision-making, experience of DSD as stigmatizing and associated with feelings of secrecy and shame, financial hardships attendant with a chronic medical condition, mental health, or marital problems that predate the child's birth) that modulate outcomes within and across developmental stages.

SHIFTING APPROACHES IN DISORDERS OF SEX DEVELOPMENT MANAGEMENT

The Consensus notes that cultural and social factors modulate outcomes in affected persons and therefore recommends that these influences be taken into account in both medical care and clinical research design. The statement encourages physicians and researchers to examine a wide range of psychological endpoints, including "sexual function, and social and psychosexual adjustment, mental health, quality of life, and social participation."[1(p.e493)]

In addition to the recommended broadening of psychological domains that should be tracked as measures of quality care, the concept of "patient centeredness" has increasingly become a focus of clinical management strategies in DSD. Defined as respect for patients' values, preferences, and expressed needs; coordination and integration of care; information, communication, and education; and emotional support—relieving fear and anxiety, the Institute of Medicine identifies patient-centeredness as a core feature of quality health care.[66]

Earlier (ie, from the mid-1950s to the early 1990s), decisions regarding gender assignment and genital surgery in DSD were guided by the *optimal gender policy*, which is concerned with the stability of gender identity, positive psychosocial adjustment, and the potential for complete sexual function.[21] This approach assumes the following: (1) gender identity is not firmly established at birth but rather is the outcome of how a child is reared; (2) stable gender identity and positive psychological adaptation require that genital appearance match assigned gender from an early age; and (3) a stable gender identity and the capacity for full sexual function are prerequisites for a positive quality of life. The optimal gender policy called for "uncompromising adherence to the (gender assignment) decision,"[67(p.334)] which has frequently, but erroneously, been interpreted as implying that select details of the condition needed to be kept from the parents and patient to avoid uncertainty about the gender assignment decision.[68] These assumptions have contributed to the prevalent practice of early genital surgery[69] but have been questioned in recent years.[70,71] The optimal gender policy may also be viewed as reflecting a kind of paternalism that is largely discouraged in modern health care delivery and constitutes an ethically dubious practice. Challenges to this approach have come from former patients claiming to have been physically and psychologically injured by this model of care.[72-74]

Specific complaints from patient stakeholders center on the lack of information, or worse, the misinformation, they were given about their condition as they grew older.[74-76] They have also reported feeling stigmatized and shamed by the secrecy surrounding their condition and its management. Many also attribute poor sexual function to damaging genital surgery[56,77] or repeated, insensitive genital examinations,[78,79] which were performed without their consent. The issue of consent centers on timing: should these momentous decisions, most particularly irreversible decisions such as genital surgery, be made early by parental surrogates, or should they wait until the child can provide input? Such grievances by former patients and their advocates have had a substantial influence on the medical community, culminating in representatives of the advocacy community participating in the DSD consensus conference and helping to shape the published statement.[1]

Shared Decision-Making in Disorders of Sex Development

Whereas the axis of decision-making in the newborn rests with the parents and the child's physicians, ascertainment of a DSD in adolescence requires that the affected youth be fully informed and involved in the decision-making process.[80] Adolescent medicine specialists, by virtue of their training in male and female reproductive health care and transitional health issues, are well positioned to facilitate such challenging discussions.

The years since publication of the Consensus have seen a burgeoning of DSD health care teams in both North America and Europe.[81,82] However, as yet there are no examples of a shared decision-making process being operationalized for DSD. Agreement among physicians has been elusive for many DSD-related decisions, and some of these interventions, although considered therapeutic, nonetheless are elective. It is just these circumstances that call for shared decision-making and specialized support tools that can facilitate this difficult process.

Parents making proxy decisions for their child can have diminished ability to understand and arrive at decisions because of the fear, anxiety, and denial that can accompany this complicated and unfamiliar set of diagnoses (Figure 1). With identification of a DSD, the parents may find all of their usual sources of social support (including extended family and friends) less accessible because of the expectation that gossip and stigma will surround their child and, by implication, their family. This set of circumstances can contribute to parents becoming secretive about the child's condition and avoidant of social contacts that may have previously been experienced as supportive. Adding to the challenges of informed decision-making are multiple physicians from different specialties offering decision recommendations, making it difficult for parents who are in crisis to clearly sift through the information. Physicians do not always communicate clearly and may offer too much (or too little) information or provide information in a confusing manner. Finally, assimilating parents' values and preferences is important if optimal decisions are to be reached.[83] Decision support tools encourage values clarification and can be used to educate parents about the complexities of DSD and assist them in understanding the decisions and options that are possible for their child. This approach will hopefully result in longer-term decisional satisfaction and decreased likelihood of regret.[84]

A significant barrier to shared decision-making for parents is the lack of readily accessible information. In 1 retrospective, semistructured interview study, par-

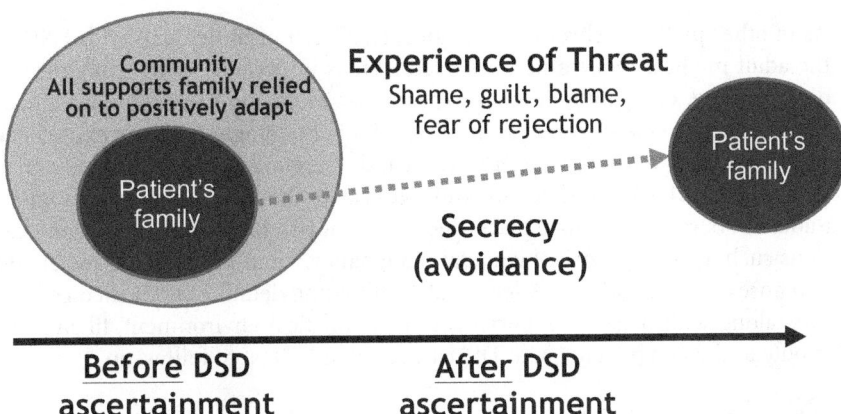

Fig 1. Schematic of the emotional and behavioral reaction of parents to identification of their child's disorder of sex development (DSD).

ents of children with DSD expressed their desire for a "survival guide or playbook" that would explain their child's condition to them in understandable terms with practical information.[85] Another small, semistructured interview study showed that parents felt they received inadequate information regarding their child's condition and were unclear about the expected appearance of their child's genitals after surgery.[86] The lack of clear information has been noted as one of the most stressful and frustrating aspects of parenting a child with a DSD.[9]

Parental emotional distress, fueled by confusion and lack of comprehension, may interfere with the decision-making process. A medicalized approach, which defines the condition solely or predominately as a medical problem requiring treatment, is more likely to lead to early surgery than an approach emphasizing the importance of the social context and both child and family resilience when provided with coping strategies from professionals and their community.[87] There is also a perception that a newborn with atypical genitalia requires early surgery.[10,21,72,88,89] Parents may feel stigmatized by the birth of a child affected with DSD and seek to act as quickly as possible to "normalize" their child without properly weighing the risks and benefits of surgery.[90] A decision fueled by the pressure for rapid action may not follow the family's values and preferences. Alternatively, parents may assume a diagnosis implies a certain treatment path and may not realize that a choice exists.[9] Poorly informed decisions (eg, inadequate discussion of potential complications) or decisional conflict represent risk factors for decisional regret.[91,92] To address these challenges to informed and balanced decision-making, an effort, supported by the Patient-Centered Outcomes Research Institute (PCORI), is currently underway to create a decision support tool for parents of young children with DSD and their providers.[93]

Transition

As in other pediatric chronic conditions, transition of individuals with DSD to the adult medical home and adult specialists is imperfect. Apart from adrenal disorders (eg, congenital adrenal hyperplasia) requiring life-sustaining glucocorticoid replacement, persons with DSD of other etiologies may not experience negative consequences in the short term and, therefore, may easily avoid maintaining contact with physicians knowledgeable about DSD. Although easily understood, such avoidance places the person at risk for longer-term complications such as osteoporosis,[94] gonadal malignancy,[43] and poor psychosocial and psychosexual adaptation.[95] A legacy of withholding details of their medical history, along with negative experiences in the medical environment, likely contribute to the fact patients with DSD are frequently "lost to follow-up."[9,79,96,97]

Other features of DSD that may first present as a challenge during adolescence or young adulthood are anticipatory anxiety related to the desire for romantic and sexual relations because of atypical genital anatomy, function (eg, genital pain from earlier surgery, inadequate vaginal introitus), or infertility, and fears of others learning of their condition together with self-perceptions that the DSD challenges the person's authenticity of being a man or a woman.[98,99]

Without adequate patient "education"[†] regarding all aspects of their medical history in an iterative and developmentally sensitive manner, expectations regarding strong medical and psychological follow-up should be limited.[100] A plan for educating the patient should be prepared at the time of the diagnosis.[1] Although adolescents may be reticent regarding contact with patient-support organizations, the potential benefits of speaking with others who have shared similar experiences should be reintroduced if initially rejected.[101]

The Society for Adolescent Health and Medicine (SAHM) published a 2003 position paper, "Transition to Adult Health Care for Adolescents and Young Adults With Chronic Conditions,"[102] which endorsed the 2002 national "Consensus Statement on Health Care Transitions for Young Adults with Special Health Care Needs"[103] and added 7 additional recommendations.

In total, the principles articulated regarding the transition to adult health care for adolescents and young adults with chronic conditions are complete, although their operationalization is left to others. Information specific to the health care transition process in DSD can be found in Hullmann et al[104] and Crouch and Creighton.[105]

Roles for Adolescent Medicine in Disorders of Sex Development

It is hoped that the adolescent medicine specialist reading this review will immediately recognize the multiple opportunities for their specialty in serving as extended members of the DSD health care team, especially during the patient's adolescent years and in preparing for transition to an adult medical home and associated adult specialists. Multidisciplinary health care teams, along the lines described in the Consensus,[1] are becoming more common across the United States, and they typically are located in pediatric academic medical centers where adolescent medicine is already generally well represented.

Adolescent medicine specialists can play a strategic role in helping families to understand and accept the role of the mental health specialist member of the comprehensive DSD team. Because of their training in the biopsychosocial model of care and as physician members of the team, they are skilled in com-

---

[†]The term *education* is used in preference to the more common *disclosure* because the latter can imply revealing something that was earlier hidden or kept a secret. Secrecy surrounding DSD has been identified by former patients as very damaging because of it being interpreted as a sign of shame.[8]

municating, to parents, the benefits of fully integrating the medical with psychosocial components of care from the earliest stages of the family's engagement with the health care team. The stigma commonly perceived in relationship to accessing mental health services is greatly reduced when these are integrated within the model of care.[106-108]

Finally, and key to their particular qualifications to assist patients and families affected by DSD, is the familiarity of adolescent medicine specialists with the developmental trajectories of physically healthy youth and those whose development has been perturbed by chronic illness.[109] Their training and experience in guiding patients and families through adolescent development—typical or atypical—qualifies them to assume a role in the care of these patients, which commonly occurs at tertiary care centers. Because adolescent medicine specialists are trained to manage both primary and subspecialty health care needs, they are certain to emphasize the importance of both specialty care and the medical home in planning for the transition to adult providers.[110]

In summary, the clinical management of people born with DSD is in a state of flux. The model of care promoted in the Consensus is unequivocally biopsychosocial, yet this goal remains aspirational. The involvement of adolescent medicine specialists in caring for such patients and their families likely will facilitate evolution in the model of care to one that is patient- and family-centered. Hopefully, the content of this review provides the reader with sufficient background to encourage further study and collaboration with other pediatric and adolescent specialists caring for this patient population.

ACKNOWLEDGMENTS

The author thanks Victoria Kuipers for literature review support and Melissa Gardner for comments on an earlier draft. This work was supported, in part, by a grant from the *Eunice Kennedy Shriver* National Institute of Child Health and Human Development (R01 HD068138) and a Patient-Centered Outcomes Research Institute (PCORI) Award (#1360).

References

1. Lee PA, Houk CP, Ahmed SF, Hughes IA; in collaboration with the participants in the International Consensus Conference on Intersex. Consensus statement on management of intersex disorders. *Pediatrics*. 2006;118(2):e488-e500
2. World Health Organization. *ICD-10: International Statistical Classification of Diseases and Related Health Problems/World Health Organization*. 10th ed. Geneva, Switzerland: Geneva World Health Organization; 1992
3. Achermann J, Hughes I. Disorders of sex development. In: Melmed S, Polonsky K, Larsen P, Kronenberg H, eds. *Williams Textbook of Endocrinology*. 12th ed. Philadelphia, PA: WB Saunders Co; 2011:868-934

4. Lee PA, Houk CP, Ahmed SF, Hughes IA; International Consensus Conference on Intersex organized by the Lawson Wilkins Pediatric Endocrine Society and the European Society for Paediatric Endocrinology. Consensus statement on management of intersex disorders. *Pediatrics.* 2006;118(2):e488-e500
5. Sax L. How common is intersex? A response to Anne Fausto-Sterling. *J Sex Res.* 2002;39(3):174-178
6. Davis G. The power in a name: diagnostic terminology and diverse experiences. *Psychol Sex.* 2013;5(1):15-27
7. Karkazis K. *Fixing Sex: Intersex, Medical Authority, and Lived Experience.* Durham, NC: Duke University Press; 2008
8. Feder EK. *Making Sense of Intersex: Changing Ethical Perspectives in Biomedicine.* Bloomington, IN: Indiana University Press; 2014
9. Crissman HP, Warner L, Gardner M, et al. Children with disorders of sex development: A qualitative study of early parental experience. *Int J Pediatr Endocrinol.* 2011;2011(1):10
10. Sanders C, Carter B, Goodacre L. Parents' narratives about their experiences of their child's reconstructive genital surgeries for ambiguous genitalia. *J Clin Nurs.* 2008;17(23):3187-3195
11. Speiser PW, Azziz R, Baskin LS, et al. Congenital adrenal hyperplasia due to steroid 21-hydroxylase deficiency: an Endocrine Society clinical practice guideline. *J Clin Endocrinol Metab.* 2010;95(9):4133-4160
12. Hughes IA, Davies JD, Bunch TI, et al. Androgen insensitivity syndrome. *Lancet.* 2012;380(9851):1419-1428
13. American Psychiatric Association. *Diagnostic and Statistical Manual of Mental Disorders.* 5th ed. Arlington, VA: American Psychiatric Publishing; 2013
14. American Psychiatric Association. *Diagnostic and Statistical Manual of Mental Disorders: DSM-IV-TR. Fourth Edition, Text Revision.* Washington, DC: American Psychiatric Association; 2000
15. Berenbaum SA, Beltz AM. Sexual differentiation of human behavior: Effects of prenatal and pubertal organizational hormones. *Front Neuroendocrinol.* 2011;32(2):183-200
16. Hines M. Gonadal hormone influences on human neurobehavioral development: outcomes and mechanisms. In: Pfaff DW, Christen Y, eds. *Multiple Origins of Sex Differences in Brain*: Springer Berlin Heidelberg; 2013:59-69
17. Meyer-Bahlburg HF. Introduction: gender dysphoria and gender change in persons with intersexuality. *Arch Sex Behav.* 2005;34(4):371-373
18. de Vries AL, Doreleijers TA, Cohen-Kettenis PT. Disorders of sex development and gender identity outcome in adolescence and adulthood: understanding gender identity development and its clinical implications. *Pediatr Endocrinol Rev.* 2007;4(4):343-351
19. Mazur T. Gender dysphoria and gender change in androgen insensitivity or micropenis. *Arch Sex Behav.* 2005;34(4):411-421
20. Cohen-Kettenis PT. Gender change in 46,XY persons with 5α-reductase-2 deficiency and 17β-hydroxysteroid dehydrogenase-3 deficiency. *Arch Sex Behav.* 2005;34(4):399-410
21. Zucker KJ. Intersexuality and gender identity differentiation. *Annu Rev Sex Res.* 1999;10:1-69
22. Meyer-Bahlburg HF. Gender assignment and reassignment in 46,XY pseudohermaphroditism and related conditions. *J Clin Endocrinol Metab.* 1999;84(10):3455-3458
23. Mazur T, Colsman M, Sandberg DE. Intersex: definition, examples, gender stability, and the case against merging with transsexualism. In: Ettner R, Monstrey S, Eyler AE, eds. *Principles of Transgender Medicine and Surgery.* Binghamton, NY: Haworth Press; 2007:235-259
24. Meyer-Bahlburg HF. Intersexuality and the diagnosis of gender identity disorder. *Arch Sex Behav.* 1994;23(1):21-40
25. Dessens AB, Slijper FM, Drop SL. Gender dysphoria and gender change in chromosomal females with congenital adrenal hyperplasia. *Arch Sex Behav.* 2005;34(4):389-397
26. Meyer-Bahlburg HFL. Gender identity outcome in female-raised 46,XY persons with penile agenesis, cloacal exstrophy of the bladder, or penile ablation. *Arch Sex Behav.* 2005;34(4):423-438

27. Ruble D, Martin C, Berenbaum S. Gender development. In: Damon W, Lerner R, Eisenberg N, eds. *Handbook of Child Psychology: Social, Emotional, and Personality*. 6th ed. New York John Wiley & Sons; 2006:858-932
28. Berenbaum SA. Psychological outcome in children with disorders of sex development: implications for treatment and understanding typical development. *Ann Rev Sex Res*. 2006;17:1-38
29. Cohen-Kettenis P. Psychological long-term outcome in intersex conditions. *Hormone Res*. 2005;64(Suppl. 2):27-30
30. Richter-Appelt H, Discher C, Gedrose B. Gender identity and recalled gender related childhood play-behaviour in adult individuals with different forms of intersexuality. *Anthropol Anz*. 2005;63(3):241-256
31. Matsubara K, Iwamoto H, Yoshida A, Ogata T. Semen analysis and successful paternity by intracytoplasmic sperm injection in a man with steroid 5alpha-reductase-2 deficiency. *Fertil Steril*. 2010;94(7):2770.e2777-2710
32. Mendonca BB, Inacio M, Costa EM, et al. Male pseudohermaphroditism due to steroid 5alpha-reductase 2 deficiency. Diagnosis, psychological evaluation, and management. *Medicine*. 1996;75(2):64-76
33. Meyer-Bahlburg HFL. Treatment guidelines for children with disorders of sex development. *Neuropsychiatr Enfance 'Adolesc*. 2008;56(6):345-349
34. Coleman E, Bockting W, Botzer M, et al. Standards of care for the health of transsexual, transgender, and gender-nonconforming people, version 7. *Int J Transgend*. 2012;13(4):165-232
35. Meyer-Bahlburg HFL. Variants of gender differentiation in somatic disorders of sex development: recommendations for version 7 of the World Professional Association for Transgender Health's standards of care. *Int J Transgend*. 2009;11(4):226-237
36. Nelson P, Glenny AM, Kirk S, Caress AL. Parents' experiences of caring for a child with a cleft lip and/or palate: a review of the literature. *Child Care Health Dev*. 2012;38(1):6-20
37. Rumsey N, Harcourt D. Visible difference amongst children and adolescents: issues and interventions. *Dev Neurorehabil*. 2007;10(2):113-123
38. Stone MB, Botto LD, Feldkamp ML, et al. Improving quality of life of children with oral clefts: perspectives of parents. *J Craniofacial Surg*. 2010;21(5):1358-1364
39. Diamond M, Garland J. Evidence regarding cosmetic and medically unnecessary surgery on infants. *J Pediatr Urol*. 2014;10(1):2-6
40. Tourchi A, Hoebeke P. Long-term outcome of male genital reconstruction in childhood. *J Pediatr Urol*. 2013;9(6, Pt B):980-989
41. Creighton SM, Michala L, Mushtaq I, Yaron M. Childhood surgery for ambiguous genitalia: glimpses of practice changes or more of the same? *Psychol Sex*. 2013;5(1):34-43
42. Hiort O, Birnbaum W, Marshall L, et al. Management of disorders of sex development. *Nat Rev Endocrinol*. 2014;10(9):520-529
43. Cools M, Wolffenbuttel KP, Drop SLS, Oosterhuis JW, Looijenga LHJ. Gonadal development and tumor formation at the crossroads of male and female sex determination. *Sex Devel*. 2011;5(4):167-180
44. Cheng MM, Udry JR. Sexual behaviors of physically disabled adolescents in the United States. *J Adolesc Health*. 2002;31(1):48-58
45. Schonbucher VB, Weber DM, Landolt MA. Psychosocial adjustment, health-related quality of life, and psychosexual development of boys with hypospadias: a systematic review. *J Pediatr Psychol*. 2008;33(5):520-535
46. van der Zwan YG, Callens N, van Kuppenveld J, et al. Long-term outcomes in males with disorders of sex development. *J Urol*. 2013;190(3):1038-1042
47. van der Zwan YG, Janssen EH, Callens N, et al. Severity of virilization is associated with cosmetic appearance and sexual function in women with congenital adrenal hyperplasia: a cross-sectional study. *J Sex Med*. 2013;10(3):866-875
48. Kleinemeier E, Jürgensen M, Lux A, Widenka P-M, Thyen U. Psychological adjustment and sexual development of adolescents with disorders of sex development. *J Adolesc Health*. 2010;47(5):463-471

49. Meyer-Bahlburg HF, Dolezal C, Baker SW, New MI. Sexual orientation in women with classical or non-classical congenital adrenal hyperplasia as a function of degree of prenatal androgen excess. *Arch Sex Behav.* 2008;37(1):85-99
50. Mathews GA, Fane BA, Conway GS, Brook CG, Hines M. Personality and congenital adrenal hyperplasia: possible effects of prenatal androgen exposure. *Horm Behav.* 2009;55(2):285-291
51. Nordenstrom A. Adult women with 21-hydroxylase deficient congenital adrenal hyperplasia, surgical and psychological aspects. *Curr Opin Pediatr.* 2011;23(4):436-442
52. Minto CL, Liao LM, Woodhouse CR, Ransley PG, Creighton SM. The effect of clitoral surgery on sexual outcome in individuals who have intersex conditions with ambiguous genitalia: a cross-sectional study. *Lancet.* 2003;361(9365):1252-1257
53. Fagerholm R, Santtila P, Miettinen PJ, et al. Sexual function and attitudes toward surgery after feminizing genitoplasty. *J Urol.* 2011;185(5):1900-1904
54. Jaaskelainen J, Tiitinen A, Voutilainen R. Sexual function and fertility in adult females and males with congenital adrenal hyperplasia. *Horm Res.* 2001;56(3-4):73-80
55. Nordenskjold A, Holmdahl G, Frisen L, et al. Type of mutation and surgical procedure affect long-term quality of life for women with congenital adrenal hyperplasia. *J Clin Endocrinol Metab.* 2008;93(2):380-386
56. Crouch NS, Liao LM, Woodhouse CR, Conway GS, Creighton SM. Sexual function and genital sensitivity following feminizing genitoplasty for congenital adrenal hyperplasia. *J Urol.* 2008;179(2):634-638
57. Stein RE. The 1990s: a decade of change in understanding children with ongoing conditions. *Arch Pediatr Adolesc Med.* 2011;165(10):880-883
58. Arboleda VA, Sandberg DE, Vilain E. DSDs: genetics, underlying pathologies and psychosexual differentiation. *Nat Rev Endocrinol.* 2014;10(10):603-615
59. Baxter RM, Arboleda VA, Lee H, et al. Exome sequencing for the diagnosis of 46,XY disorders of sex development. *J Clin Endocrinol Metab.* 2014;100(0):e333-e344
60. Vidal I, Gorduza DB, Haraux E, et al. Surgical options in disorders of sex development (DSD) with ambiguous genitalia. *Best Pract Res Clin Endocrinol Metab.* 2009;24(2):311-324
61. Hines M. Gonadal hormones and sexual differentiation of human brain and behavior. In: Pfaff DW, Arnold AP, Fahrbach SE, Etgen AM, Rubin RT, eds. *Hormones, Brain and Behavior.* 2nd ed. San Diego, CA: Academic Press; 2009:1869-1910
62. Stout SA, Litvak M, Robbins NM, Sandberg DE. Congenital adrenal hyperplasia: classification of studies employing psychological endpoints. *Intl J Pediatr Endocrinol.* 2010;2010(doi:10.1155/2010 /191520). Available at: www.hindawi.com/journals/ijpe/2010/191520. Accessed May 24, 2015
63. Pickles A, Hill J. Developmental pathways. In: Cicchetti D, Cohen D, eds. *Developmental Psychopathology Theory and Method.* 2nd ed. Hoboken, NJ: John Wiley & Sons, Inc; 2006:211-243
64. Rose BM, Holmbeck GN, Coakley RM, Franks EA. Mediator and moderator effects in developmental and behavioral pediatric research. *J Devel Behav Pediatr.* 2004;26:58-67
65. Auchus R, Witchel S, Leight K, et al. Guidelines for the development of comprehensive care centers for congenital adrenal hyperplasia: guidance from the CARES Foundation Initiative. *Int J Pediatr Endocrinol.* 2010;2010:275213
66. Institute of Medicine Committee on Quality of Health Care in America. *Crossing the Quality Chasm: A New Health System for the 21st Century.* Washington, DC: The National Academies Press; 2001
67. Money J, Hampson JG, Hampson JL. Imprinting and the establishment of gender role. *AMA Arch Neurol Psychiatry.* 1957;77(3):333-336
68. Creighton S, Minto C. Managing intersex. Most vaginal surgery in childhood should be deferred. *Br Med J.* 2001;323(7324):1264-1265
69. American Academy of Pediatrics Section on Urology. Timing of elective surgery on the genitalia of male children with particular reference to the risks, benefits, and psychological effects of surgery and anesthesia. *Pediatrics.* 1996;97(4):590-594
70. Creighton S, Chernausek SD, Romao R, Ransley P, Salle JP. Timing and nature of reconstructive surgery for disorders of sex development—introduction. *J Pediatr Urol.* 2012;8(6):602-610

71. Mouriquand P, Caldamone A, Malone P, Frank JD, Hoebeke P. The ESPU/SPU standpoint on the surgical management of Disorders of Sex Development (DSD). *J Pediatr Urol.* 2014;10(1):8-10
72. Stein MT, Sandberg DE, Mazur T, Eugster E, Daaboul J. A newborn infant with a disorder of sexual differentiation. *J Dev Behav Pediatr.* 2003;24(2):115-119
73. Karkazis K, Tamar-Mattis A, Kon AA. Genital surgery for disorders of sex development: implementing a shared decision-making approach. *J Pediatr Endocrinol Metab.* 2010;23(8):789-805
74. Frader J, Alderson P, Asch A, et al. Health care professionals and intersex conditions. *Arch Pediatr Adolesc Med.* 2004;158(5):426-428
75. Dreger AD. *Hermaphrodites and the Medical Invention of Sex.* Cambridge, MA: Harvard University Press; 1998
76. Chase C. What is the agenda of the intersex patient advocacy movement? *Endocrinologist.* 2003;13(3):240-242
77. Crouch NS, Minto CL, Laio LM, Woodhouse CR, Creighton SM. Genital sensation after feminizing genitoplasty for congenital adrenal hyperplasia: a pilot study. *BJU Int.* 2004;93(1):135-138
78. Money J, Lamacz M. Genital examination and exposure experienced as nosocomial sexual abuse in childhood. *J Nerv Mental Dis.* 1987;175(12):713-721
79. Creighton S, Alderson J, Brown S, Minto CL. Medical photography: ethics, consent and the intersex patient. *BJU Int.* 2002;89(1):67-71
80. American Academy of Pediatrics Committee on Bioethics. Informed consent, parental permission, and assent in pediatric practice. *Pediatrics.* 1995;95(2):314-317. Reaffirmed October 2006
81. Pasterski V, Prentice P, Hughes IA. Consequences of the Chicago consensus on disorders of sex development (DSD): current practices in Europe. *Arch Dis Child.* 2010;95(8):618-623
82. Moran ME, Karkazis K. Developing a multidisciplinary team for disorders of sex development: planning, implementation, and operation tools for care providers. *Adv Urol.* 2012;2012:604135
83. Siminoff LA, Step MM. A communication model of shared decision making: accounting for cancer treatment decisions. *Health Psychol.* 2005;24(4 Suppl):S99-S105
84. Feldman-Stewart D, Tong C, Siemens R, et al. The impact of explicit values clarification exercises in a patient decision aid emerges after the decision is actually made. *Med Dec Making.* 2012;32(4):616-626
85. Boyse KL, Gardner M, Marvicsin DJ, Sandberg DE. "It was an overwhelming thing": parents' needs after infant diagnosis with congenital adrenal hyperplasia. *J Pediatr Nurs.* 2014;29(5):436-441
86. Duguid A, Morrison S, Robertson A, et al. The psychological impact of genital anomalies on the parents of affected children. *Acta Pædiatr.* 2007;96(3):348-352
87. Streuli JC, Vayena E, Cavicchia-Balmer Y, Huber J. Shaping parents: impact of contrasting professional counseling on parents' decision making for children with disorders of sex development. *J Sex Med.* 2013;10(8):1953-1960
88. Sanders C, Carter B, Goodacre L. Searching for harmony: parents' narratives about their child's genital ambiguity and reconstructive genital surgeries in childhood. *J Adv Nurs.* 2011;67(10):2220-2230
89. Hiort O, Thyen U, Holterhus PM. The basis of gender assignment in disorders of somatosexual differentiation. *Horm Res.* 2005;64(Suppl 2):18-22
90. Sandberg DE, Mazur T. A noncategorical approach to the psychosocial care of persons with DSD and their families. In: Kreukels BPC, Steensma TD, de Vries ALC, eds. *Gender Dysphoria and Disorders of Sex Development.* New York: Springer; 2014:93-114
91. Lorenzo AJ, Pippi Salle JL, Zlateska B, et al. Decisional regret after distal hypospadias repair: single institution prospective analysis of factors associated with subsequent parental remorse or distress. *J Urol.* 2014;191(5 Suppl):1558-1563
92. Lorenzo AJ, Braga LHP, Zlateska B, et al. Analysis of decisional conflict among parents who consent to hypospadias repair: single institution prospective study of 100 couples. *J Urol.* 2012;188(2):571-575

93. Sandberg DE. Decision support for parents receiving genetic information about child's rare disease. 2012. Available at: www.pcori.org/research-results/2012/decision-support-parents-receiving-genetic-information-about-childs-rare. Accessed May 17, 2014
94. Bertelloni S, Dati E, Baroncelli GI. Disorders of sex development: hormonal management in adolescence. *Gynecol Endocrinol.* 2008;24(6):339-346
95. Liao L-M, Tacconelli E, Wood D, Conway G, Creighton SM. Adolescent girls with disorders of sex development: a needs analysis of transitional care. *J Pediatr Urol.* 2010;6(6):609-613
96. Thyen U, Lux A, Jurgensen M, Hiort O, Kohler B. Utilization of health care services and satisfaction with care in adults affected by disorders of sex development (DSD). *J Gen Intern Med.* 2014;29(Suppl 3):S752-S759
97. Roen K, Pasterski V. Psychological research and intersex/DSD: recent developments and future directions. *Psychol Sex.* 2013;5:102-116
98. Chadwick PM, Liao LM, Boyle ME. Size matters: experiences of atypical genital and sexual development in males. *J Health Psychol.* 2005;10(4):529-543
99. Alderson J, Madill A, Balen A. Fear of devaluation: Understanding the experience of intersexed women with androgen insensitivity syndrome. *Br J Health Psychol.* 2004;9(1):81-100
100. Sandberg DE, Gardner M, Cohen-Kettenis PT. Psychological aspects of the treatment of patients with disorders of sex development. *Semin Reprod Med.* 2012;30(05):443-452
101. Baratz AB, Sharp MK, Sandberg DE. Disorders of sex development peer support. In: Hiort O, Ahmed S, editors. *Understanding Differences and Disorders of Sex Development (DSD).* Basel, Switerland: Karger; 2014:99-112
102. Rosen DS, Blum RW, Britto M, Sawyer SM, Siegel DM. Transition to adult health care for adolescents and young adults with chronic conditions: position paper of the Society for Adolescent Medicine. *J Adolesc Health.* 2003;33(4):309-311
103. American Academy of Pediatrics, American Academy of Family Physicians, American College of Physicians-American Society of Internal Medicine. A consensus statement on health care transitions for young adults with special health care needs. *Pediatrics.* 2002;110(Suppl 3):1304-1306
104. Hullmann SE, Chalmers LJ, Wisniewski AB. Transition frompediatric to adult care for adolescents and young adults with a disorder of sex development. *J Pediatr Adolesc Gynecol.* 2012;25(2):155-157
105. Crouch NS, Creighton SM. Transition of care for adolescents with disorders of sex development. *Nat Rev Endocrinol.* 2014;10(7):436-442
106. Jonovich SJ, Alpert-Gillis LJ. Impact of pediatric mental health screening on clinical discussion and referral for services. *Clin Pediatr.* 2014;53(4):364-371
107. Keller D, Sarvet B. Is there a psychiatrist in the house? Integrating child psychiatry into the pediatric medical home. *J Am Acad Child Adolesc Psychiatr.* 2013;52(1):3-5
108. Johnson SB. Increasing psychology's role in health research and health care. *Am Psychol.* 2013;68(5):311-321
109. Pinquart M. Achievement of developmental milestones in emerging and young adults with and without pediatric chronic illness—a meta-analysis. *J Pediatr Psychol.* 2014;39(6):577-587
110. American Academy of Pediatrics, American Academy of Family Physicians, American College of Physicians; Transitions Clinical Report Authoring Group. Supporting the health care transition from adolescence to adulthood in the medical home. *Pediatrics.* 2011;128(1):182-200

Endocrine Consequences of Treatment for Childhood Cancer

Susan E. Stred, MD

Clinical Professor of Pediatrics, Pediatric Endocrinology Center, SUNY Upstate Medical University, Syracuse, New York

INTRODUCTION

More than 80% of children and adolescents diagnosed with cancer will become long-term survivors.[1] There are nearly 400,000 survivors in the United States alone.[1] Of these, it is generally accepted that at least 50% will develop 1 or more endocrine disorders consequent to their treatment.

It can be challenging for primary care practitioners to stay current with recommended surveillance for childhood cancer survivors.[2] Survivors may have poor knowledge of the details of their antineoplastic therapies and the attendant risks for late effects.[3] Psychological barriers, learning disabilities, and challenges to health literacy may make it more difficult for survivors to grasp the gravity of the need for lifelong surveillance for sequelae. For those with intellectual disabilities consequent to antineoplastic treatment, particularly for survivors of brain tumors diagnosed in very early childhood, knowledge of their condition and potential consequences may be limited. Therefore, primary care physicians are key in providing appropriate anticipatory guidance and surveillance for late effects.

Many oncology centers offer annual visits for comprehensive survivor surveillance into young adulthood. In the absence of this resource, it is strongly recommended that primary care physicians seek a treatment summary, and *tailored patient-specific surveillance recommendations*, from the treating cancer center.[2] The Children's Oncology Group (COG) publishes guidelines for the medical

---

E-mail address: streds@upstate.edu

care of survivors of childhood cancer, with the most recent Long-Term Follow-Up Guidelines (version 4.0) published in October 2013.[4] A comprehensive template for recording cancer treatments and determining appropriate follow-up is located in Appendix I of this online resource (www.survivorshipguidelines.org/pdf/COG_LTFU_Guidelines_AppendixI_v4.pdf).

It is important to keep in mind that antineoplastic treatment modalities are constantly being modified, and recent therapeutic options may result in reduced risk for complications compared to those being discussed in this article. Although valuable for its size and for the care taken in data collection, the largest cohort study, the Childhood Cancer Survivor Study (CCSS), includes individuals whose cancer treatment is now 45 years in the past. Thus, we can glean useful information on type and general magnitude of risk of various therapeutic modalities, but published risk ratios are likely to be imprecise for the survivor group currently in their teens. Nevertheless, certain important sequelae are common enough to represent appropriate foci for this article.

Young people who have undergone bone marrow transplant (BMT) are at increased risk for significant chronic health conditions compared to age-matched cancer survivors treated with other modalities and to unaffected siblings. Most hematopoietic allografts require conditioning with total body irradiation (TBI). Recipients of transplants from unrelated donors are at the highest risk for all adverse health conditions,[5] including endocrinopathies. Having undergone TBI and having active chronic graft-versus-host disease were critical modifiers in determining future disease risk.[5]

Recommendation: Obtain a treatment summary and patient-specific recommendations from the cancer treatment center. Charts of young people who are survivors of TBI and allogeneic BMT should be flagged for more detailed surveillance.

HYPOTHALAMIC-PITUITARY AXIS

There are no identified sequelae of chemotherapy on the hypothalamic-pituitary axis. However, anterior pituitary hormones and/or their hypothalamic releasing factors are sensitive to radiotherapy (Figure 1), and hypothalamic-pituitary dysfunction after cranial radiation therapy (CRT) or TBI is common. The degree of severity correlates with the total radiation dose delivered and the length of time since treatment (reviewed in Darzy and Shalet[6]). Growth hormone is the anterior pituitary hormone most vulnerable to radiotherapy, and growth hormone deficiency may represent the sole manifestation of neuroendocrine injury.

Recommendation: It is logical that survivors, after receiving CRT ≥40 Gray (Gy), in addition to those who had pituitary mass lesions or intracranial surgery, be under the ongoing care of a pediatric endocrinologist.

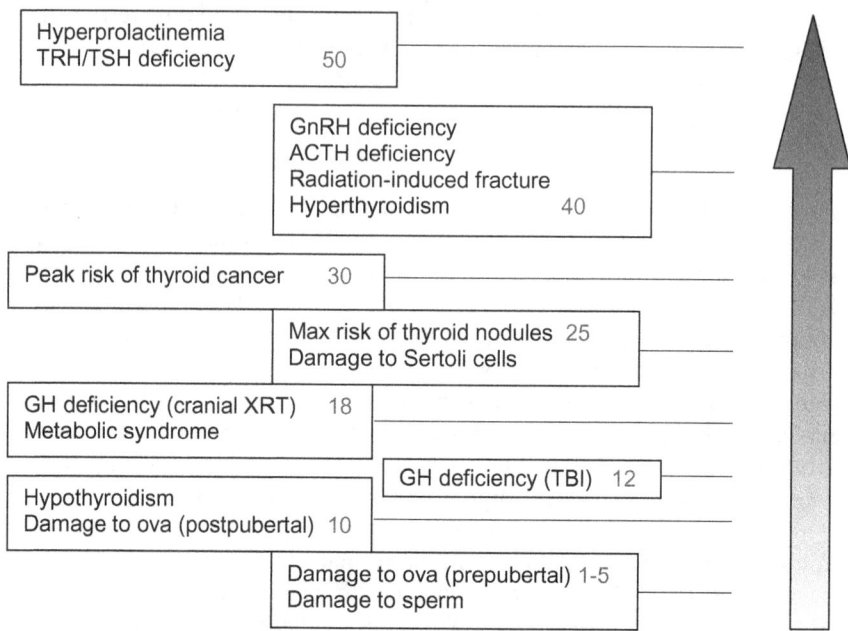

Fig 1. Hierarchy of risk of endocrine sequelae of radiation therapy, by cumulative radiation dose in Gray (Gy) units.

SHORT STATURE

Disrupted growth has been a well-recognized adverse consequence of treatment of childhood cancer for many decades. As noted earlier, growth hormone is the anterior pituitary hormone that is most sensitive to radiotherapy, with deficiencies recognized within 3 years in survivors of CRT > 18 Gy or TBI >10 Gy.[7,8] Treatment regimens have been adjusted over the years, with a dramatic reduction in radiotherapy protocols, specifically to address this issue. Nevertheless, it is estimated that 10% to 15% of current leukemia patients may still be exposed to radiation therapy (XRT) to the brain or craniospinal axis, or to TBI before BMT.[9] Radiation therapy may also be used for solid tumors of the trunk and abdominal cavity, subjecting the skeleton, particularly the spine, to radiation exposure. Radiated vertebrae have reduced growth potential, resulting in disproportionate short stature.

In an analysis of a cohort of CCSS leukemia survivors by Chow et al[9] (Table 1), the odds of adult survivors reporting short stature (z score <1.96) increased with the geographic extent of their prior radiotherapy. Relative to nonirradiated leukemia survivors, those whose XRT was restricted to the head (CRT only) were nearly 3 times more likely to report being short. However, having undergone TBI raised that relative risk to 8-fold, and the cumulative effect of both modalities to 10.6-fold relative to nonirradiated survivors.[9]

Although growth hormone replacement under the direction of a pediatric endocrinologist can improve height velocity and body composition for those who are growth hormone deficient secondary to their cranial radiation, the radiated vertebrae are unlikely to respond to growth hormone as briskly as the native bones. In the experience of the author, it is common for young people to express disappointment with their height outcome even after years of growth hormone treatment, so practitioners should be cautious about predicting final adult height for these young people and reassuring them about their height growth.

Recommendation: Monitor height, weight, and body mass index (BMI) every 6 months until completion of growth. Refer to the pediatric endocrinology department for any decline in growth velocity or for failure to accelerate to a pubertal growth spurt. The COG Guidelines recommend referral to a pediatric endocrinologist for any child with open epiphyses who received >30 Gy XRT.[4] The author would urge evaluation by a pediatric endocrinologist for those who received TBI >10 Gy or CRT >18 Gy.[7,8] Be circumspect in discussing growth velocity, the pubertal growth spurt, and final adult height.

Table 1

Height (z score) and risk of short stature (z score <-1.96) among survivors of childhood leukemia, stratified by type of radiation exposure

Radiotherapy	n	Mean z-score (SD)	No. short stature (%)	Odds ratio*	95% Confidence interval
CRT/TBI					
None	983	0.02 (1.16)	37 (3.8)	1.0	Reference
CRT only	1872	-0.64 (1.12)	189 (10.1)	2.9	2.0, 4.2
TBI only	55	-1.00 (1.70)	13 (23.6)	8.0	3.7, 17.4†
CRT + TBI	35	-1.36 (1.30)	11 (31.4)	10.6	4.5, 25.3†
Spinal radiation therapy					
None	2672	-0.36 (1.18)	196 (7.3)	1.0	Reference
Any	273	-1.15 (1.15)	54 (19.8)	2.8	1.9-4.0

*Adjusted for sex, race/ethnicity, age at diagnosis/HCT and at follow-up, ALL vs AML, growth hormone supplementation, and all radiotherapy categories simultaneously.
†P <.05 compared with CRT-only group.
ALL, acute lymphoblastic leukemia; AML, acute myelogenous leukemia; CRT, cranial radiation therapy; HCT, hematopoietic cell transplant; TBI, total body irradiation.
Data from Chow et al.[9] Copyright © Wiley Periodicals, Inc. Used with permission.

ADRENOCORTICOTROPIC HORMONE AXIS

The adrenocorticotropic hormone (ACTH) axis is relatively radioresistant. Clinically apparent deficiency is rare for survivors of less than 50 Gy CRT and often is partial. In contrast, survivors of pituitary tumors are much more likely to have panhypopituitarism, including ACTH deficiency. This cohort is likely to already be under the care of an endocrinologist.

VASOPRESSIN

The posterior pituitary gland is resistant to damage from CRT. However, diabetes insipidus (DI) can represent the presenting symptom in craniopharyngioma and intracranial germinomas. Diabetes insipidus can also develop consequent to any neurosurgery in the suprasellar region. Patients may present with polyuria and polydipsia, often of abrupt onset. Very young children may refuse to eat solids and will be inconsolable unless provided with beverages constantly. Weight loss may be noted.

Recommendation: Prompt assessment (electrolytes, urinalysis) to differentiate DI from new-onset diabetes mellitus is indicated. Because of the specificity of treatment of DI and the high risk of additional hypothalamic-pituitary disorders, urgent referral to a pediatric endocrinologist is the standard of care.

REPRODUCTIVE AXIS

Increased risk of primary gonadal failure consequent to treatment for malignancies in childhood has been identified for many years. Gonads may be removed because of primary tumors or during en bloc pelvic resection.

Alkylating chemotherapeutic agents (Table 2), which have direct toxic effects on the germ cells, represent a major risk factor for delayed or absent pubertal development and for later infertility. Cumulative doses of the various chemotherapeutic agents can be determined by the treating oncology center and a risk profile developed.[4] Young women may experience primary ovarian failure. Young men exposed to sufficient doses of alkylating agent(s) are likely to be azoospermic and to have relatively smaller testes on physical examination relative to the sexual maturity rating of their other secondary sexual characteristics, because sperm and spermatic cords generally represent the bulk of testicular mass. Even low doses of alkylating agent(s) will cause gonadal failure when administered in combination with direct pelvic radiation or TBI.[4] Smoking will compound the risk of azoospermia. Testosterone production may be relatively spared unless there is concomitant gonadotropin deficiency.

In a CCSS study of self-reported fertility in 5149 female CCSS participants (ages 15-44 years) and 1441 female siblings,[10] those at highest risk for infertility were

Table 2
Alkylating chemotherapeutic agents

Cyclophosphamide
Procarbazine
Nitrogen mustard
Chlorambucil
Mechlorethamine
Melphalan
Ifosfamide
Carmustine
Lomustine
Busulfan
Thiotepa

survivors with direct XRT to the uterus and ovaries of even 5 Gy or more. Prepubertal ovaries are slightly more resistant to damage (see Figure 1). Germ cell retrieval and storage, and other assisted reproductive technologies, will not be discussed in this review.

The spectrum of gonadotropin deficiency following CRT is broad but in general can be appreciated as early as 12 months after XRT ≥40 Gy (see Figure 1). In the report by Green et al,[10] patients with cumulative radiation exposure of the hypothalamic-pituitary axis ≥30 Gy had gonadotropin deficiency. In the study by Chow et al,[9] self-reported pregnancies 5 or more years after completion of antineoplastic treatment were dramatically decreased in survivors who had undergone TBI for leukemia (Table 3). If additional CRT beyond the TBI conditioning was administered, fertility was a dramatic 97% lower relative to leukemia survivors who had received no radiotherapy.[9]

It has been noted that younger children undergoing high-dose CRT may be at risk for precocious puberty. For the adolescent patient presenting to a primary care office, this adverse effect will likely be reflected in short stature. Growth velocity will reflect postmenstrual age, and final adult height may be achieved quite early in adolescence.

Recommendation: Refer any child with bilateral gonadectomy to a pediatric endocrinologist to initiate hormone replacement therapy at age 11 years or as soon as gonadectomy is performed, whichever is later.[4] Perform sexual maturity rating of all patients at least annually. Monitor young men annually beginning at age 14 years with a first-morning testosterone concentration and consider referral if testosterone is not rising with age.[4] Take a careful menstrual history in young women and refer if there are signs of estrogen deficiency. Luteinizing hormone, follicular-stimulating hormone, and estradiol concentrations may be measured annually beginning at age 13.[4] Offer counseling promptly to those just learning of potential subfertility.

Table 3

Prevalence and odds of reproductive outcomes among survivors of childhood leukemia, stratified by type of radiation exposure

Radio-therapy	n	Ever Pregnant No. affected (%)	Odds ratio*	95% Confidence interval	Live Birth No. affected (%)‡	Odds ratio*	95% Confidence interval
CRT/TBI							
None	1200	527 (43.9)	1.0	Reference	451 (37.6)	1.0	Reference
CRT only	2143	773 (36.1)	0.5	0.5-0.6	666 (31.1)	0.6	0.5-0.7
TBI only	73	8 (11.0)	0.1	0.04-0.2†	5 (6.9)	0.07	0.03-0.18†
CRT + TBI	51	2 (3.9)	0.03	0.01-0.14†§	0	0	-
Spinal radiation therapy							
None	3160	1222 (38.7)	1.0	Reference	1048 (33.2)	1.0	Reference
Any	307	88 (28.7)	0.5	0.3-0.6	74 (24.1)	0.5	0.3-0.6

*Adjusted for sex, race/ethnicity, age at diagnosis/HCT and at follow-up, ALL vs AML, and all radiotherapy categories simultaneously.
†$P < .05$ compared with CRT-only group.
‡Same number analyzed as "ever pregnant."
§$P < .05$ compared with TBI-only group.
ALL, acute lymphoblastic leukemia; AML, acute myelogenous leukemia; CRT, cranial radiation therapy; HCT, hematopoietic cell transplant; TBI, total body irradiation.
Data from Chow et al.[9] Copyright © Wiley Periodicals, Inc. Used with permission.

BREAST HEALTH

The risk of developing breast cancer relative to the general population is increased after XRT to the chest for each age cohort.[11] A family history of breast cancer or a known breast cancer gene mutation will augment this risk.[4]

Recommendation: For young women who had TBI or with a cumulative radiation dose >10 Gy to the chest, counsel the patient on self breast examination monthly beginning at puberty. Perform a clinical breast examination yearly beginning at puberty.[4]

THYROID

Thyroid disorders consequent to antineoplastic therapy are generally attributable to direct radiation damage (see Figure 1) or to thyroid-stimulating hormone (TSH) deficiency[6] and may develop many years after treatment. The thyroid lies within the radiation fields for head and neck primary tumors and for craniospinal and TBI protocols. Radiation exposure may occur in those with Hodgkin lymphoma, mediastinal germinoma, or primary lung tumors. Of note, parathyroid function is generally spared.

In a CCSS study restricted to survivors of acute leukemia,[9] the relative risk of developing hypothyroidism was highest (10.9-fold) for those receiving both CRT and TBI (Table 4). Any spinal radiation therapy also resulted in a substantially increased risk of hypothyroidism relative to the reference population.[9] It is important to note that the study relied on self-report of thyroid conditions and did not attempt to delineate those whose hypothyroidism was attributable to TSH deficiency from those with primary thyroid failure.

Females have a higher risk for development of primary hypothyroidism, as do those with a younger age at cancer treatment and those with XRT ≥10 Gy or TBI. Hyperthyroidism is less common and is thought to be restricted to those with cumulative XRT ≥40 Gy (see Figure 1).[4] Thyroid nodules may develop after XRT, with similar high risk factors (female, young age at XRT; total XRT ≥25 Gy).[4]

Recommendation: For all of the potential thyroid problems, the history and physical examination, including vital signs, height, and weight, plus a careful thyroid examination and thyroid function tests (free T4, TSH) should be performed annually. Be mindful of the possibility that TSH may be inappropriately low in those who had CRT. Order a thyroid ultrasound for evaluation of any palpable nodules and consider referral for subspecialty care.

Table 4

Prevalence and odds of hypothyroidism among survivors of childhood leukemia, stratified by type of radiation exposure

Radiotherapy	No. analyzed*	No. affected (%)	Odds ratio†	95% Confidence interval
CRT/TBI				
None	1198	48 (4.0)	1.0	Reference
CRT only	2127	145 (6.8)	1.6	1.1, 2.3
TBI only	70	16 (22.9)	6.8	3.4, 13.5‡
CRT + TBI	47	14 (29.8)	10.9	5.3, 22.3‡
Spinal radiation therapy				
None	3148	180 (5.7)	1.0	Reference
Any	294	43 (14.6)	2.6	1.7-3.8

*Excludes individuals who underwent thyroidectomy before reporting hypothyroidism.
†Adjusted for sex, race/ethnicity, age at diagnosis/HCT and at follow-up, ALL vs AML, and all radiotherapy categories simultaneously.
‡P <.05 compared with CRT-only group.
ALL, acute lymphoblastic leukemia; AML, acute myelogenous leukemia; CRT, cranial radiation therapy; HCT, hematopoietic cell transplant; TBI, total body irradiation.
Data from Chow et al.[9] Copyright © Wiley Periodicals, Inc. Used with permission.

OBESITY, DIABETES MELLITUS, AND METABOLIC SYNDROME

In a report by Taskinen et al,[12] 52% of BMT survivors (median age 20 years) had hyperinsulinemia, either fasting or during a 2-hour oral glucose tolerance test. The combination of hyperinsulinemia plus hypertriglyceridemia indicative of the metabolic syndrome was noted in 39% of the BMT patients, compared with only 8% of the leukemia survivors and none of the healthy age and sex-matched controls. The number of subjects was small in this study, and the conditioning regimens before transplant varied. There was a trend toward greater risk of abdominal obesity, but the COG Survivorship Guidelines caution that survivors of TBI be considered at risk for metabolic syndrome even if they remain lean.[4] Neville et al[13] reported that 23% of Australian teen cancer survivors in their study had hyperinsulinemia, impaired glucose tolerance, or frank diabetes mellitus compared to a single control subject. Among pubertal and young adult BMT subjects who had undergone TBI, 64% exhibited 1 of the disorders of glucose homeostasis compared with 17% of those whose conditioning regimen before transplant did not include TBI. In a multivariate analysis, TBI, untreated hypogonadism, and abdominal adiposity represented independent risk factors, but a family history of type 2 diabetes mellitus did not.[13] Green et al[14] identified independent risk factors for obesity in CCSS participants, including age of cancer diagnosis between ages 5 to 9 years, low physical functioning, and CRT to the hypothalamic-pituitary axis of 20 to 30 Gy.

Self-report of diabetes mellitus was also studied in the CCSS, with n = 8599, compared to 2936 siblings.[15] Survivors had a statistically significant increased risk for reporting diabetes mellitus in each 5-year age cohort relative to their siblings. Furthermore, survivors who had XRT were at higher risk for developing diabetes mellitus than other survivors (Table 5; Figure 2). The authors state that the risk was independent of obesity or physical activity. There was a striking 23.8-fold increase in relative risk of diabetes for survivors of acute myelogenous

Table 5

Adjusted odds ratio estimates of diabetes mellitus in survivors of childhood cancer, by diagnosis and therapy, compared with siblings

	Not Adjusted for BMI		Adjusted for BMI	
Radiation therapy	OR (95% CI)	P value	OR (95% CI)	P value
Cranial irradiation	1.6 (1.1-2.4)	.02	1.6 (1.0-2.3)	.03
Abdominal irradiation	2.6 (1.8-3.8)	<.001	3.4 (2.3-5.0)	<.001
Total body irradiation	9.7 (4.9-19.1)	<.001	12.6 (6.2-25.3)	<.001

BMI, body mass index; CI, confidence interval; OR, odds ratio.
From Meacham LR, Sklar CA, Li S, et al. Diabetes mellitus in long-term survivors of childhood cancer. Arch Intern Med. 2009;169:1381-1388. Copyright © 2009 American Medical Association. All rights reserved. Used with permission.

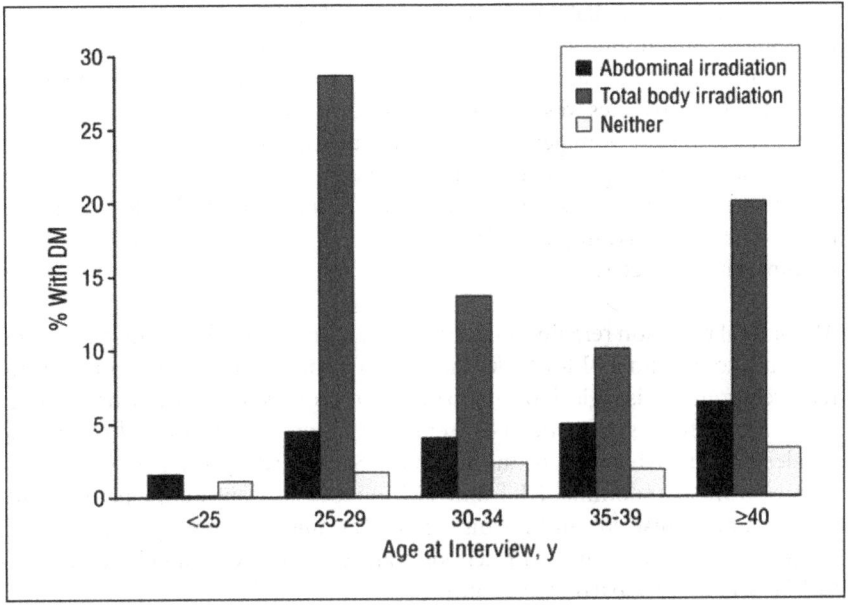

Fig 2. Risk of self-reported diabetes mellitus in survivors of childhood cancer, stratified by type of radiation exposure. (From Meacham LR, Sklar CA, Li S, et al. Diabetes mellitus in long-term survivors of childhood cancer. *Arch Intern Med.* 2009;169:1381-1388. Copyright © 2009 American Medical Association. All rights reserved. Used with permission.)

leukemia who had been treated with TBI. Within the cancer survivor cohort, the risk of diabetes in adulthood was increased 2.4-fold for those whose cancer diagnosis was made before age 5 years relative to those diagnosed at age 15 to 20 years. After adjustment for BMI, age, sex, race/ethnicity, household income, and health insurance, survivors were overall 1.8 times more likely than their siblings to report diabetes, but the odds ratio for those after XRT was higher. The authors suggest that there would be a greater likelihood of *undiagnosed diabetes* rather than a *false report* of having diabetes. At least 80% of diabetes cases across all groups were reported to be type 2 diabetes, and the risk factors for type 2 diabetes in the general population (non-Northern European background, lower household income, increased BMI) continued to be associated with increased risk of diabetes in this study as well.

In 2012, de Vathaire et al[16] published a striking study addressing the increased risk of diabetes in survivors of XRT. These researchers developed a software application to estimate radiation dose to 185 separate anatomic sites. They determined radiation exposure from detailed XRT records for 2520 survivors of childhood solid tumors or lymphoma (studied at least 20 years from their childhood cancer, at an average age of 28 years). Survivors of leukemia, the most common pediatric malignancy, were not included in the study. Sixty-five subjects (2.6%) were confirmed by their physicians to have diabetes. Although the absolute number of diabetes patients was rather low, the results showed a remarkable dose-response relationship of diabetes mellitus relative to prior XRT to the tail of the pancreas. If the tail of the pancreas received ≥10 Gy XRT, the relative risk for diabetes was 11.5-fold higher compared with those without XRT. Survivors who were younger than 2 years at the time of XRT were at increased risk for developing type 2 diabetes, but no increased risk of type 1 diabetes was reported. The study suggests intriguing areas for future research into the mechanism of diabetes risk, in particular why type 2 diabetes is more common than insulinopenic diabetes.

Abdominal radiation remains an integral part of treatment for Wilms tumor and neuroblastoma, and TBI for leukemias. Because many cancer survivors are still relatively young, it is logical to anticipate a "wave" of disorders of glucose homeostasis or metabolic syndrome in cancer survivors over time. Given the alarming incidence of diabetes in teens in the United States already, it would be prudent for survivors of abdominal XRT and TBI to receive detailed anticipatory guidance and be counseled carefully on lifestyle modification. Young people whose cancer was diagnosed in the preschool years and those with an elevated waist-to-hip ratio deserve particular scrutiny.

Recommendation: Monitor BMI and blood pressure at every visit. Record family history of type 2 diabetes mellitus and/or metabolic syndrome. Draw fasting blood glucose or hemoglobin A_{1c}, plus fasting lipid profile, every 2 years. More frequent testing may be warranted based on patient and family history factors.

MENTAL HEALTH

It is perhaps intuitive that young people who have chronic health conditions consequent to their cancer treatment may be at increased risk for depression, anxiety about their physical appearance, concern over future fertility, fatalistic outlook, and suicidal ideation. Survivors of central nervous system tumors and their treatment, and those who had therapy directed at the central nervous system for hematopoietic malignancies, are at the highest risk for mental health conditions within the survivor cohort. As is true for these mental health conditions in the population at large, female sex and lower socioeconomic status represent additive risk factors.[4]

Survivors of childhood cancer are more likely to engage in risky behaviors during adolescence. This risk is increased in those who were already teens at the time of diagnosis of the malignancy, those with lower household socioeconomic status, and those with lower educational achievement.[4] Anticipatory guidance may need to be reiterated and reinforced, for instance, regarding healthy eating, regular exercise, sun exposure, bone health, substance use, and unprotected sexual behavior.

References

1. Childhood cancer survivorship. American Society of Clinical Oncology. Available at: www.cancer.net/navigating-cancer-care/children/childhood-cancer-survivorship. Accessed May 26, 2015
2. Nathan PC, Daugherty CK, Wroblewski KE, et al. Family physician preferences and knowledge gaps regarding the care of adolescent and young adult survivors of childhood cancer. *J Cancer Surviv.* 2013;7:275-282
3. Kadan-Lottick NS, Robison LL, Gurney JG, et al. Childhood cancer survivors' knowledge about their past diagnosis and treatment: CCSS study. *JAMA.* 2002:287:1832-1839
4. Children's Oncology Group. Long-term follow-up guidelines for survivors of childhood, adolescent, and young adult cancers. October 2013. Available at: www.survivorshipguidelines.org. Accessed December 12, 2014
5. Armenian SH, Sun CL, Kawashima T. Long-term health-related outcomes in survivors of childhood cancer treated with HSCT versus conventional therapy: a report from the Bone Marrow Transplant Survivor Study (BMTSS) and Childhood Cancer Survivor Study (CCSS). *Blood.* 2011;118:1413-1420
6. Darzy KH, Shalet SM. Hypopituitarism following radiotherapy revisited. In: Wallace WHB, Kelnar CJH, eds. *Endocrinopathy after Childhood Cancer Treatment.* Basel, Switzerland: Karger; 2009:1-24
7. Costin G. Effect of low-dose cranial radiation on growth hormone secretory dynamics and hypothalamic-pituitary function. *Am J Dis Child.* 1988;142:847-852
8. Melin AE, Adan L, Levenger G, et al. Growth hormone secretion, puberty and adult height after cranial irradiation with 18 Gy for leukemia. *Eur J Pediatr.* 1998;157:703-707
9. Chow EJ, Liu W, Srivastava K, et al. Differential effects of radiotherapy on growth and endocrine function among acute leukemia survivors: a CCSS report. *Pediatr Blood Cancer.* 2013;60:110-115
10. Green DM, Kawashima T, Stovall M, et al. Fertility of female survivors of childhood cancer: A report from the CCSS. *J Clin Oncol.* 2009;27:2677-2685
11. Kenney LB, Yasui Y, Inskip PD, et al. Breast cancer after childhood cancer: a report from the CCSS. *Ann Int Med.* 2004;141:590-597
12. Taskinen M, Saarinen-Pihkala UM, Hovi L, Lipsanen-Nyman M. Impaired glucose tolerance and dyslipidaemia as late effects after bone-marrow transplantation in childhood. *Lancet.* 2000;356: 993-997
13. Neville KA, Cohn RJ, Steinbeck KS, Johnston K, Walker JL. Hyperinsulinemia, impaired glucose tolerance, and diabetes mellitus in survivors of childhood cancer: prevalence and risk factors. *J Clin Endocrinol Metab.* 2006;91:4401-4407
14. Green DM, Cox CL, Zhu L, et al. Risk factors for obesity in adult survivors of childhood cancer: a report from the CCSS. *J Clin Oncol.* 2012;30:246-255
15. Meacham LR, Sklar CA, Li S, et al. Diabetes mellitus in long-term survivors of childhood cancer. *Arch Intern Med.* 2009;169:1381-1388
16. de Vathaire F, El-Fayech C, Ben Ayed FF, et al. Radiation dose to the pancreas and risk of diabetes in childhood cancer survivors: a retrospective cohort study. *Lancet Oncol.* 2012;13:1002-1010

Note: Page numbers of articles are in **boldface** type. Page references followed by "*f*" and "*t*" denote figures and tables, respectively.

2,5-dichlorophenol (2,5-DCP), 271
3β-hydroxysteroid dehydrogenase deficiency, 346*t*, 347
5α-reductase-2 deficiency (5a-RD-2), 431–434
17-beta estradiol, 285
17β-hydroxysteroid dehydrogenase-3 deficiency (17b-HSD-3), 431–433
21-hydroxylase congenital adrenal hyperplasia, 431, 437
21-hydroxylase deficiency, 346*t*, 347, 348
25-hydroxyvitamin D (25OHD), 308, 309, 311

A

AAAS gene, 352
AAM. *See* Age at menarche (AAM)
Abdominal adiposity, 278
aBMD. *See* Areal BMD (aBMD)
Acne vulgaris, 329–330
ACTH. *See* Adrenocorticotropic hormone (ACTH)
ACTH axis. *See* Adrenocorticotropic hormone (ACTH) axis
ACTH deficiency. *See* Adrenocorticotropic hormone (ACTH) deficiency
Acute lymphocytic leukemia (ALL), 304, 306
Addison disease, 350, 354
Adipokines, 404. *See also* Adiponectin; Leptin
Adiponectin, 400, 405
Adolescent pregnancy, **382–392**
　contraception, 383–384
　diabetes mellitus, 385–386, 388
　folic acid supplementation, 385
　PCOS, 386–388, 388–389
　prepregnancy planning, 384–388
　thyroid dysfunction, 388, 389
　unintended pregnancies, 383
Adrenal androgen excess, 355
Adrenal carcinoma, 358
Adrenal dysfunction, **343–363**
　adrenal medullary diseases, 359–360
　adrenocortical hyperfunction, 355–357
　anatomy and physiology, 343–344
　causes of adrenal cortical insufficiency, 346–347*t*
　congenital adrenal hyperplasia (CAH), 345–349
　critically ill patients, 353
　Cushing syndrome, 357–358

　neuroblastoma, 359
　pheochromocytoma, 359–360
　premature adrenarche, 355–357
　primary adrenal insufficiency, 345, 346*t*, 349–351
　secondary adrenal insufficiency, 345, 346–347*t*, 351–352
　stress dosing, 354–355
Adrenal gland hyperplasia, 346*t*
Adrenal gland hypoplasia, 346*t*
Adrenal hypoplasia congenita, 346*t*
Adrenal medullary diseases, 359–360
Adrenal tumor, 358
Adrenalitis, 350
Adrenocortical hyperfunction, 355–357
Adrenocorticotropic hormone (ACTH)
　adrenal dysfunction, 345, 349, 350, 352, 354, 357, 358
　eating disorders, 402
Adrenocorticotropic hormone (ACTH) axis, 452
Adrenocorticotropic hormone (ACTH) deficiency, 452
Adrenoleukodystrophy, 346*t*
Age at menarche (AAM), 271–273
Agranulocytosis, 244
AIT. *See* Amiodarone-induced thyrotoxicosis (AIT)
Aldosterone, 343
Alendronate, 313, 314
Alkaline phosphatase, 297
Alkylating chemotherapeutic agents, 452, 453*t*
ALL. *See* Acute lymphocytic leukemia (ALL)
Alopecia, 330
Alpha-methyl-L-tyrosine, 360
Amenorrhea, 283–284, 286
AMG 785, 316
Amiodarone, 236, 237*t*
Amiodarone-induced thyrotoxicosis (AIT), 236
AN. *See* Anorexia nervosa (AN)
Anabolic steroids, 237*t*
ANCA-associated vasculitis. *See* Antineutrophil cytoplasmic antibody (ANCA)-associated vasculitis
Androgenic alopecia, 330
Androgens, 237*t*
Androstenedione, 332
Anorexia mirabilis, 394

Anorexia nervosa (AN)
 adiponectin, 405
 bone health, 294f, 301–302
 cortisol levels, 402
 defined, 394
 endocrine changes, 401
 estrogen replacement, 400
 ghrelin levels, 403
 GnRH pulsatility, 397
 irisin, 405
 peak bone mass, 294f
 puberty, 283–287
 recovery of normal reproductive function, 407
 resistin, 405
Antineutrophil cytoplasmic antibody (ANCA)-associated vasculitis, 243, 244
Antithyroperoxidase (anti-TPO), 239
APECED. See Autoimmune polyendocrine syndrome 1 (APECED)
Areal BMD (aBMD), 295
Aromatase inhibitors, 276
Artificial pancreas, 264, 266
Atypia of undetermined significance (AUS), 248
Atypical genital anatomy, 431. See also Disorders of sex development (DSD)
AUS. See Atypia of undetermined significance (AUS)
Autoimmune adrenalitis, 350
Autoimmune polyendocrine syndrome 1 (APECED), 350
Autoimmune polyendocrine syndrome 2, 350
Autoimmune thyroid disease, 233, 234, 240
Autonomously functioning nodules, 244–245
Avascular necrosis, 304

B

Ballet, 398
Bariatric surgery, 336
Basal-bolus therapy, 262–263
BED. See Binge eating disorder (BED)
Bilateral gonadectomy, 453
Bile acid sequestrants, 376, 377
Binge eating disorder (BED)
 defined, 394
 leptin levels, 405
Biochemical hyperandrogenism, 330
Bisphenol-A (BPA), 271
Bisphosphonates, 313–316
Block and replace method, 243–244
BMC. See Bone mineral content (BMC)
BMD. See Bone mineral density (BMD)
BMI. See Body mass index (BMI)
BMT. See Bone marrow transplant (BMT)
BN. See Bulimia nervosa (BN)
Body mass index (BMI)
 cardiovascular risk factors, 370

dyslipidemia, 370
 irisin, 405
 PCOS, 335
Body weight, 299
Bogalusa Heart Study, 371
Bone densitometry, 294–296
Bone development, 291–294
Bone health, **291–325**
 anorexia nervosa, 294f, 301–302
 assessment of, 294–298
 biochemical markers of bone metabolism, 297–298, 298t
 bisphosphonates, 313–316
 bone development, 291–294
 bone mass acquisition, 293–294
 bone remodeling cycle, 292f
 calcitonin, 316
 calcium, 307–308
 celiac disease, 304–305
 cerebral palsy (CP), 307
 childhood malignancy, 306
 contraceptives, 302–303, 399–400
 cystic fibrosis (CF), 305
 denosumab, 316
 DXA, 294–296
 eating disorders, 301–302, 399–401
 endocrine disorders, 306
 exercise and lifestyle, 309
 factors affecting bone mass, 298–300, 299t
 female athlete triad, 302
 gender, 299
 genetic factors, 298
 glucocorticoid-induced osteoporosis, 303–304
 hormonal status, 299
 hormone therapy, 312–313
 idiopathic juvenile osteoporosis (IJO), 301
 inflammatory bowel disease (IBD), 304
 main types of bones, 292
 osteogenesis imperfecta (OI), 300–301
 osteoporosis, 296, 310
 prevention, 307–310
 quantitative computed tomography (QCT), 296–297
 race, 299
 radiography, 297
 rheumatologic conditions, 305–306
 sclerostin antibody, 316
 teriparatide, 316
 treatment, 310–316
 vitamin D, 308–309, 310–312
Bone marrow transplant (BMT), 449, 456
Bone mass acquisition, 293–294
Bone mineral content (BMC), 295
Bone mineral density (BMD), 280, 286
Bone remodeling cycle, 292f
Bone-specific alkaline phosphatase, 297
Booster snack, 265
Boston and London twin/triplet studies, 258

Bounce at the Bell, 309
BPA. *See* Bisphenol-A (BPA)
Breast cancer, 421, 454
Browning of white fat, 405
Bulimia nervosa (BN)
    adiponectin, 405
    defined, 394
    dialectical behavior therapy (DBT), 406
    HPA axis, 403
    leptin levels, 405

C

CAH. *See* Congenital adrenal hyperplasia (CAH)
CAIS. *See* Complete androgen insensitivity syndrome (CAIS)
Calcitonin, 250, 293, 316
Calcium, 250, 307–308
Calcium channel-blocking drugs, 360
Canadian STOPP consortium, 305
Cancer survivors, Childhood cancer survivors
Carbamazepine, 237t
Carbamazepine/oxcarbamazepine, 237t
Carbimazole, 243
Carcinoembryonic antigen (CEA), 250
Cardiovascular disease, 364. *See also* Lipid disorders
Cardiovascular health integrated lifestyle diet-1 (CHILD-1), 372
Cardiovascular health integrated lifestyle diet-2 (CHILD-2), 372, 375, 376
Cardiovascular risk factors, 374t
Carney complex, 249
Casein milk proteins, 258
CBT. *See* Cognitive behavior therapy (CBT)
CCSS. *See* Childhood Cancer Survivor Study (CCSS)
CDGP. *See* Constitutional delay of growth and puberty (CDGP)
CEA. *See* Carcinoembryonic antigen (CEA)
Celiac disease, 304–305
Cerebral palsy (CP), 307
Cervical lymphadenopathy, 245, 246
CF. *See* Cystic fibrosis (CF)
CF-RBD. *See* CF-related bone disease (CF-RBD)
CF-related bone disease (CF-RBD), 305
CGMS. *See* Continuous glucose monitoring system (CGMS)
CGMS sensor-augmented insulin pump therapy, 263–264
CHARGE syndrome, 279
Chernobyl nuclear disaster, 249
CHILD-1 diet. *See* Cardiovascular health integrated lifestyle diet-1 (CHILD-1)
CHILD-2 diet. *See* Cardiovascular health integrated lifestyle diet-2 (CHILD-2)
Childhood Cancer Survivor Study (CCSS), 449

Childhood cancer survivors, **448–459**
    adrenocorticotropic hormone (ACTH) axis, 452
    alkylating chemotherapeutic agents, 452, 453t
    bilateral gonadectomy, 453
    bone marrow transplant (BMT), 449, 456
    breast cancer, 454
    Childhood Cancer Survivor Study (CCSS), 449
    COG guidelines, 448–449, 451, 456
    diabetes insipidus (DI), 452
    diabetes mellitus, 456–458
    gonadotropin deficiency, 453
    hypothalamic-pituitary axis, 449
    hypothyroidism, 455, 455t
    mental health, 458
    metabolic syndrome, 456, 458
    obesity, 456
    patient-specific recommendations, 448, 449
    reproductive axis, 452–453, 454t
    risk following radiation therapy, 450f
    risky behaviors, 458
    sexual maturity rating, 453
    short stature, 450–451, 451t
    thyroid disorders, 454–455
    total body irradiation (TBI) and graft-versus-host disease, 449
    vasopressin, 452
Cholecalciferol, 308
Cholesterol desmolase deficiency, 346t, 347
Chondrocyte, 292
Chronic lymphocytic thyroiditis, 245
Clinically significant fracture history, 296
Clomiphene citrate, 385, 386
Closed-loop insulin pump, 264, 266
Closed-loop pump automation, 267
Cognitive behavior therapy (CBT), 406
Colesevelam, 377, 378
Compartment dissection, 251
Complete androgen insensitivity syndrome (CAIS), 430, 431, 435
Congenital adrenal hyperplasia (CAH), 345–349, 431
Congenital Adrenal Hyperplasia Research Education & Support Foundation, 351
Congenital hypothyroidism, 241
Conjugated equine estrogens, 285
Consensus Statement on Management of Intersex Disorders, 429, 433, 437, 441
Constitutional delay of growth and puberty (CDGP), 274–277
Continuous glucose monitoring system (CGMS), 263
Contraception
    adolescent pregnancy, 383–384
    bone health, 302–303, 399–400
    Contraceptive CHOICE Project, 384
    hormonal contraceptives (HCs), 332

Contraception, *continued*
  LARC methods, 383, 384
  oral contraceptives, 286, 302, 303, 384, 385, 407
  US Medical Eligibility Criteria for Contraception (USMEC), 383, 384
Contraceptive CHOICE Project, 384
Copper IUD (ParaGard), 384
Corticosterone methyl oxidase deficiency, 346*t*
Corticotropin-releasing hormone (CRH), 396, 397, 402
Cortisol, 344, 349*t*, 400, 402
Cortisol deficiency, 344
Cortisone, 349*t*
Cosyntropin (ACTH 1-24) challenge test, 352
CP. *See* Cerebral palsy (CP)
Creatine kinase, 377
CRH. *See* Corticotropin-releasing hormone (CRH)
Cryptorchidism, 418–419
Cushing disease, 357
Cushing syndrome, 306, 357–358
Cyclical progesterone, 285
CYP21A2, 348
Cypionate, 280
Cystic fibrosis (CF), 305
Cytokine storm, 315

D

DAISY study, 258
DBT. *See* Dialectical behavior therapy (DBT)
DCCT. *See* Diabetes Control and Complications Trial (DCCT)
Dehydroepiandrosterone (DHEA), 344, 354, 356
Delayed puberty, 273–287
Demser, 360
Denosumab, 316
Depo-Provera, 302–303
Detemir, 262
DEXA. *See* Dual-energy X-ray absorptiometry (DXA)
Dexamethasone, 349*t*, 353
DHEA. *See* Dehydroepiandrosterone (DHEA)
DHEAS, 332
DI. *See* Diabetes insipidus (DI)
Diabetes Control and Complications Trial (DCCT), 261
Diabetes education, 264
Diabetes insipidus (DI), 452
Diabetes mellitus, **256–268**
  artificial pancreas, 264, 266
  booster snack, 265
  cancer survivors, 456–458
  categories, 256
  closed-loop pump automation, 267
  exercise, 265
  future directions, 266

glycemic goals, 264–265
MODY syndrome, 256
NIH-sponsored T1DM diabetes registries, 257
pregnancy, 385–386, 388
prevalence, 257*t*
SEARCH study, 257
T1DM. *See* Type 1 diabetes (T1DM)
T2DM, 256, 266
TODAY study, 266
Dialectical behavior therapy (DBT), 406
Diaphysis, 292
Diazepam binding inhibitor *(DBI)* gene, 271
DICER1PPB familial tumor predisposition syndrome, 249
Dietary cholesterol restriction, 372–376
Dietary (exogenous) fat pathway, 365*f*
Differentiated thyroid cancer (DTC), 249–250
Disorders of sex development (DSD), **428–447**
  adolescent medicine specialists, 441–442
  complaints/grievances of former patients, 438
  Consensus Statement, 429, 433, 437, 441
  consent, 438
  definitions and categories, 429–431
  DSD, defined, 429
  DSD nomenclature, 430*t*
  educating the patient, 441
  fertility, 436
  gender assignment, 433–434
  genital surgery, 434–435
  hypospadias, 429
  "lost to follow up," 440
  optimal gender policy, 438
  parents, 439–440, 439*f*
  patient centeredness, 437
  patient support organizations, 441
  poorly informed decisions, 440
  psychosocial adaptation, 436–437
  sex hormone replacement therapy, 435
  sexuality, 435–436
  shared decision-making, 438–440
  timing of diagnosis, 431
  transgender, distinguished, 431–432
  transition to adult health care, 440–441
DMPA, 302–303
Dopamine, 398
Dopamine agonists, 237*t*
Down syndrome, 233
DPD. *See* Lysyl Pyridinoline (DPD)
Drospirenone, 333, 333*t*, 334
DSD. *See* Disorders of sex development (DSD)
DTC. *See* Differentiated thyroid cancer (DTC)
Dual-energy X-ray absorptiometry (DXA), 294–296, 407
DXA. *See* Dual-energy X-ray absorptiometry (DXA)
Dyslipidemia. *See* Lipid disorders
Dyslipidemia of obesity, 371–372, 379

E

E$_2$, 285
Eating disorders, **393–410**
  adiponectin, 405
  AN. *See* Anorexia nervosa (AN)
  BED. *See* Binge eating disorder (BED)
  BN. *See* Bulimia nervosa (BN)
  bone health, 301–302, 399–401
  cardiac complications, 395
  clinical implications, 407
  endocrine complications, 393, 395
  gastrointestinal complications, 394–395
  ghrelin, 403–404
  growth hormone (GH), 401–402
  HPA axis, 402–403
  HPT axis, 406
  hypothalamic amenorrhea, 395–399
  IGF-1, 401–402
  irisin, 405
  leptin, 404–405
  peptide YY, 404
  refeeding syndrome, 407
  resistin, 405
  treatment, 406
  weight gain, 407
Ectopic thyroid tissue, 241
Enanthate, 280
Enteroviral (EV) illness, 260
Epiphyses, 292
Ergocalciferol, 308
Estrogen replacement therapy, 283, 284–285, 286, 312, 400, 413–414
Estrogens, 237*t*
Ethinyl estradiol, 285
Ethynodiol diacetate, 333*t*
Euglycemia, 404
Euthyroid autoimmune thyroiditis, 388
Euthyroid goiter, 248
EV illness. *See* Enteroviral (EV) illness

F

Familial adenomatous polyposis, 249
Familial combined hyperlipidemia (FCHL), 371
Familial glucocorticoid deficiency, 346*t*
Familial hypercholesterolemia (FH), 364, 369–370
Familial medullary thyroid carcinoma (FMTC), 250–251
Family-based therapy (FBT), 406
Fasciculata, 343
FBT. *See* Family-based therapy (FBT)
FCHL. *See* Familial combined hyperlipidemia (FCHL)
Female athlete triad, 302, 398
Fertility concerns, 334
FH. *See* Familial hypercholesterolemia (FH)

FHA. *See* Functional hypothalamic amenorrhea (FHA)
Fibrates, 378
Figure skating, 398
Fine needle aspiration (FNA), 247–249
Flat bones, 292
Fludrocortisone, 348, 354
Fluorouracil, 237*t*
FLUS. *See* Follicular lesion of undetermined significance (FLUS)
FMTC. *See* Familial medullary thyroid carcinoma (FMTC)
FNA. *See* Fine needle aspiration (FNA)
Folic acid supplementation, 385
Follicle-stimulating hormone (FSH), 270
Follicular lesion of undetermined significance (FLUS), 248
Follicular neoplasm, 248
Follicular thyroid cancer (FTC), 249
Fractures, 291. *See also* Bone health
Fragility fractures, 291
FSH. *See* Follicle-stimulating hormone (FSH)
FTC. *See* Follicular thyroid cancer (FTC)
Functional hyperandrogenism, 396
Functional hypothalamic amenorrhea (FHA), 283
Furosemide, 237*t*

G

GABA. *See* Gamma-amino butyric acid (GABA)
Gamma-amino butyric acid (GABA), 271
GEC. *See* Gene expression classifier (GEC)
Genant score, 297
Gender assignment, 433–434
Gender dysphoria, 431. *See also* Disorders of sex development (DSD)
Gene expression classifier (GEC), 248
Genital surgery, 434–435
Genomewide association studies (GWAS), 258
GH. *See* Growth hormone (GH)
Ghrelin, 275, 401, 403–404
Glargine, 262
Glomerulosa, 343
Glucocorticoid-induced osteoporosis, 303–304
Glucocorticoids
  adrenal dysfunction, 354
  bone fractures, 303
  GH and TSH suppression, 398
  hashitoxicosis, 245
  potencies, 349*t*
  protein synthesis, 303
  TSH secretion, 237*t*
Glutamate, 271
Glycemic goals, 264–265
GnRH. *See* Gonadotropin-releasing hormone (GnRH)

GnRH agonists. *See* Gonadotropin-releasing (GnRH) agonists
Goitrogens, 234
Gonadotropin deficiency, 453
Gonadotropin-releasing (GnRH) agonists, 240
Gonadotropin-releasing hormone (GnRH), 270, 396–398
Graves disease, 240, 242–244
Graves ophthalmopathy, 243
Growth hormone (GH), 270, 401–402, 413, 449, 450
Growth hormone deficiency, 306
Gut neuropeptides, 403. *See also* Ghrelin; Peptide YY
GWAS. *See* Genomewide association studies (GWAS)
Gymnastics, 398

H

HAIR-AN syndrome. *See* Hyperandrogenism-insulin resistance-acanthosis nigricans (HAIR-AN) syndrome
Hashimoto thyroiditis, 239–240
Hashitoxicosis, 245
HbA$_{1c}$ test, 260
HCG. *See* Human chorionic gonadotropin (HCG)
HCs. *See* Hormonal contraceptives (HCs)
HDL. *See* High-density lipoprotein (HDL)
Heparin, 237*t*
Hepatic cholesterol, 366
Hepatic (endogenous) fat pathway, 366*f*
Hepatic transaminase, 377
Hermaphrodite, 429. *See also* Disorders of sex development (DSD)
Heroin, 237*t*
Heterozygous familial hypercholesterolemia (FH), 370
High-density lipoprotein (HDL), 367
High-resolution pQCT (HR-pQCT), 296–297
Hirsutism, 329, 334
HLA haplotyping, 260
HMG co-A reductase, 366
Homozygous familial hypercholesterolemia (FH), 369–370
Hormonal contraceptives (HCs), 332
Hormone replacement therapy, 312
HPA axis. *See* Hypothalamic-pituitary-adrenal (HPA) axis
HPO axis. *See* Hypothalamic-pituitary-ovarian (HPO) axis
HPT axis. *See* Hypothalamic-pituitary-thyroid (HPT) axis
HR-pQCT. *See* High-resolution pQCT (HR-pQCT)
Human chorionic gonadotropin (HCG), 276, 281
Hydrocortisone, 348, 349*t*, 353

Hydroxylysyl-pyridinoline (PYD), 298
Hyperandrogenism, 333–334, 398
Hyperandrogenism-insulin resistance-acanthosis nigricans (HAIR-AN) syndrome, 328
Hypercortisolemia, 402
Hypergonadotropic hypogonadism
  characteristics, 277
  females, 281–283
  males, 277–278
  treatment, 280–282, 284–287
Hyperinsulinemia, 456
Hyperkalemia, 334
Hyperlipidemia, 239. *See also* Lipid disorders
Hyperpigmentation, 345
Hyperthyroidism, 235*f*, 242–245, 243*t*
Hypertrichosis, 334
Hypertriglyceridemia, 370–371, 378
Hypocalcemia, 244
Hypogonadism, 277–287. *See also* Hypergonadotropic hypogonadism; Hypogonadotropic hypogonadism
Hypogonadotropic hypogonadism
  characteristics, 277
  females, 281–282
  males, 279–280
  treatment, 280–282, 284–287
Hypoleptinemia, 406
Hypospadias, 429
Hypothalamic amenorrhea, 395–399
Hypothalamic-pituitary axis, 449
Hypothalamic-pituitary-adrenal (HPA) axis, 395, 397, 402–403, 404
Hypothalamic-pituitary-ovarian (HPO) axis, 395, 396, 398
Hypothalamic-pituitary-thyroid (HPT) axis, 395, 398, 404, 406
Hypothalamic suppression, 396, 398
Hypothyroidism, 234*f*, 238–241, 238*t*, 455, 455*t*

I

IBD. *See* Inflammatory bowel disease (IBD)
Idiopathic juvenile osteoporosis (IJO), 301
IDL. *See* Intermediate-density lipoprotein (IDL)
IGF-1. *See* Insulin like growth factor-1 (IGF-1)
IJO. *See* Idiopathic juvenile osteoporosis (IJO)
IMAGe syndrome, 346*t*
Incidentaloma, 245
Infertility, 420–421
Inflammatory bowel disease (IBD), 304
INHB. *See* Inhibin B (INHB)
Inherited medullary thyroid cancer syndromes, 250
Inhibin B (INHB), 275, 420

Insulin-induced hypoglycemia, 352
Insulin like growth factor-1 (IGF-1), 270, 328, 400, 401–402
Insulin pump therapy, 262
Insulin resistance, 334, 335, 337
Insulin therapy, 263
Insulin-to-carb ratio, 262
Intermediate-density lipoprotein (IDL), 366
Intersex, 428. *See also* Disorders of sex development (DSD)
Intrauterine device (IUD), 384
Iodide, 237*t*
Iodine, 236
Iodine-123 (^{123}I), 245
Iodine deficiency, 238
Irisin, 405
Irregular menses, 328–329, 332–333
Islet cell antibody testing, 260
Isolated ACTH deficiency, 347*t*
Isolated aldosterone deficiency, 346*t*
IUD. *See* Intrauterine device (IUD)

J

JIA. *See* Juvenile idiopathic arthritis (JIA)
Jöd-Basedow phenomenon, 236
Juvenile idiopathic arthritis (JIA), 305

K

Kallmann syndrome, 279–280
Kearns-Sayre syndrome, 346*t*
Ketoacidosis, 260
Kisspeptin, 271, 284, 287
Klinefelter syndrome (KS), 233, **417–423**, 430*t*. *See also* Disorders of sex development (DSD)
  autoimmune disorders, 422
  breast cancer, 421
  clinical features, 418*t*
  endocrinopathies, 421–422
  hypergonadotropic hypogonadism, 278–279, 419
  importance of early intervention, 422–423
  infertility, 420–421
  inhibin B levels, 420
  life expectancy, 422
  medical management and monitoring, 423*t*
  minipuberty, 419
  osteopenia and osteoporosis, 422
  SHOX gene, 419
  speech development and learning problems, 280, 421
  tall stature, 418–419
  testosterone replacement therapy (TRT), 280–281, 420
  underdeveloped male genitalia, 419–420
KS. *See* Klinefelter syndrome (KS)
Kussmaul respiration, 259

L

Labetalol, 360
LARC method of contraception. *See* Long-acting reversible contraceptive (LARC) methods
LC/MS/MS. *See* Liquid chromatography tandem mass spectrometry (LC/MS/MS)
LDL. *See* Low-density lipoprotein (LDL)
Leptin, 275, 284, 396–397, 400, 404–405, 406
Leptin replacement, 286
Letrozole, 276, 280, 388
Levonorgestrel, 333*t*
Levothyroxine, 236, 249
LH. *See* Luteinizing hormone (LH)
Lingual thyroid, 241
Lipid disorders, **364–381**
  2011 NHLBI guidelines for screening, 372, 373*t*
  cardiovascular risk factors, 374*t*
  causes of dyslipidemia, 368*t*, 369*t*
  controversy, 379
  dietary cholesterol restriction, 372–376
  dietary (exogenous) fat pathway, 365*f*
  dyslipidemia of obesity, 371–372, 379
  elevated LDL cholesterol, 376–378
  elevated triglycerides, 378
  familial combined hyperlipidemia (FCHL), 371
  familial hypercholesterolemia (FH), 369–370
  hepatic (endogenous) fat pathway, 366*f*
  hypertriglyceridemia, 370–371
  lipid profiles, 367–368
  NHLBI cholesterol cutpoints, 374*t*
  overview of lipid metabolism, 365–367
  pharmacologic therapy, 376–379
  reverse cholesterol transport, 367, 367*f*
  treatment, 372–379
Lipid profiles, 367–368
Lipoid hyperplasia, 346*t*
Liquid chromatography tandem mass spectrometry (LC/MS/MS), 356
Lithium, 234–235, 237*t*
Lithium-induced hyperthyroidism, 235
Long-acting reversible contraceptive (LARC) methods, 383, 384
Long bones, 292
Lovaza, 378
Low BMD for chronologic age, 296
Low-density lipoprotein (LDL), 366, 367, 370, 372
Luteinizing hormone (LH), 270, 284, 328
Lymphadenopathy, 245
Lysyl Pyridinoline (DPD), 298

M

Macrocytic anemia, 239
Marfanoid habitus, 250

Maturity-onset diabetes of youth (MODY) syndrome, 256
Mayer-Rokitansky-Küster-Hauser syndrome, 435
McCune-Albright syndrome, 249
MC2R, 352
MD-Logic, 264
Medullary thyroid carcinoma, 250–251
MEN2A. *See* Multiple endocrine neoplasia type 2A (MEN2A)
MEN2B. *See* Multiple endocrine neoplasia type 2B (MEN2B)
Menarche, 271, 395
Menstrual irregularity, 328–329, 332–333, 395
Metabolic diseases, 346*t*
Metabolic syndrome, 278, 456, 458
Metaiodobenzylguanidine (mIBG), 359
Metaphyses, 292
Metformin, 237*t*, 335, 336, 385, 386
Methadone, 237*t*
Methimazole (MMI), 237*t*, 243
Methylprednisolone, 349*t*
Metyrapone, 237*t*
mIBG. *See* Metaiodobenzylguanidine (mIBG)
mIBG scan, 360
Microdissection TESE, 420
Micronized 17-beta estradiol (E$_2$), 285
Micronized progesterone, 285
Microphallus, 420
Milk, 307, 308
Mineralocorticoids, 343
Minipuberty, 419
Mipomersen, 377
Mirena, 384
Mitotane, 237*t*
MMI. *See* Methimazole (MMI)
MODY syndrome. *See* Maturity-onset diabetes of youth (MODY) syndrome
Multiple endocrine neoplasia type 2A (MEN2A), 250
Multiple endocrine neoplasia type 2B (MEN2B), 250
Mutation analysis panel, 248

N

NAFLD. *See* Nonalcoholic fatty liver disease (NAFLD)
National Adrenal Diseases Foundation (NADF), 351
National Institutes of Health (NIH)-sponsored T1DM diabetes registries, 257
National Survey of Family Growth (NSFG), 384
NCAH. *See* Nonclassic CAH (NCAH)
Neo-osseous osteoporosis, 301
Neuroblastoma, 359, 458
Neurofibromatosis type 1, 360
Neurokinin B, 271
Nexplanon, 384

NHLBI cholesterol cutpoints, 374*t*
Niacin, 378
Nifedipine, 360
NIH-sponsored T1DM diabetes registries, 257
Nodule hypoechogenicity, 248
Nonalcoholic fatty liver disease (NAFLD), 336
Nonclassic CAH (NCAH), 347, 356
Nonsteroidal anti-inflammatory drugs, 237*t*
Noonan syndrome, 277
Norethindrone, 333*t*
Norgestimate, 333*t*
Norgestrel, 333*t*
Normocytic anemia, 239
Normosmic hypogonadotropic hypogonadism, 279
NSFG. *See* National Survey of Family Growth (NSFG)

O

Obesity
 adrenocortical hyperfunction, 356
 cancer survivors, 456
 dyslipidemia of obesity, 371–372, 379
 infertility, 387
 PCOS, 335, 337, 387
 secondary dyslipidemia, 364
 thyroid disorders, 233
Obstructive sleep apnea, 337
OGTT. *See* Oral glucose tolerance test (OGTT)
1,25(OH)$_2$D, 308
OI. *See* Osteogenesis imperfecta (OI)
Oliguria, 260
Omega-3 fatty acids, 378
OMIM. *See* Online Mendelian Inheritance of Man (OMIM)
Online Mendelian Inheritance of Man (OMIM), 345, 346*t*, 347*t*
OPG. *See* Osteoprotegerin (OPG)
Opioid peptides, 271
Optimal gender policy, 438
"Optimizing Bone Health in Children and Adolescents," 307
Oral contraceptives, 285, 286, 302, 303, 384, 385, 407. *See also* Contraception
Oral estrogen preparations, 285
Oral glucose tolerance test (OGTT), 260, 261
Orange juice, 308
Orthostatic hypotension, 344
Osteoblast, 292, 297
Osteocalcin, 298
Osteocyte, 293
Osteogenesis imperfecta (OI), 300–301
Osteomalacia, 310
Osteonecrosis, 304
Osteopenia, 278, 296, 422
Osteoporosis, 296, 310, 422. *See also* Bone health

Osteoporosis genes, 298
Osteoprotegerin (OPG), 293
Ovotesticular DSD, 430t
Oxandrolone, 276, 413

P

Pamidronate, 313, 314, 316
Pancreatitis, 370
Panhypopituitarism, 352, 452
Papillary thyroid carcinoma (PTC), 249
PAR1. *See* Pseudoautosomal region 1 (PAR1)
Paraganglioma, 360
ParaGard, 384
Partial androgen insensitivity syndrome, 433
Patient-Centered Outcomes Research Institute (PCORI), 440
PCOM. *See* Polycystic ovarian morphology (PCOM)
PCORI. *See* Patient-Centered Outcomes Research Institute (PCORI)
PCOS. *See* Polycystic ovarian syndrome (PCOS)
PCSK9. *See* Proprotein convertase subtilisin kexin type 9 (PCSK9)
Peak bone mass, 293
Peptide YY, 400, 404
Peripheral QCT (pQCT), 296
PG. *See* Plasma glucose (PG)
Phenobarbital, 237t
Phenoxybenzamine, 360
Phenytoin, 237t
Pheochromocytoma, 359–360
Phthalates, 272
Plasma glucose (PG), 259, 260, 262
Polycystic ovarian morphology (PCOM), 330–331
Polycystic ovarian syndrome (PCOS), **326–342**
 acne vulgaris, 329–330
 androgenic alopecia, 330
 bariatric surgery, 336
 biochemical hyperandrogenism, 330
 BMI, 335
 body weight, 335
 clinical features, 326
 clinical presentation, 328–331
 diagnosis, 331–332
 diagnostic criteria, 327t
 fertility concerns, 334
 genetics, 326
 hirsutism, 329
 hyperandrogenism, 333–334
 insulin resistance, 334, 335, 337
 irregular menses, 328–329, 332–333
 menstrual irregularity, 328–329, 332–333
 metabolic dysfunction, 334–336
 metformin, 335, 336
 multidisciplinary approach, 337
 NAFLD, 336
 obstructive sleep apnea, 337
 pathogenesis, 327–328
 PCOM, 330–331
 pregnancy, 386–388, 388–389
 psychosocial concerns, 336
 treatment, 332–337
Polydipsia, 345
Polygenic hypercholesterolemia, 370
Polyuria, 345
pQCT. *See* Peripheral QCT (pQCT)
Prednisolone, 349t
Prednisone, 349t, 353
Pregnancy. *See* Adolescent pregnancy
Premature adrenarche, 355–357
Preosteoclast, 292
Primary adrenal insufficiency, 345, 346t, 349–351
Progesterone, 285
Progestin-only subdermal implant (Nexplanon), 384
Progestins, 333t
Proopiomelanocortin deficiency, 347t
Proprotein convertase subtilisin kexin type 9 (PCSK9), 378
Propylthiouracil (PTU), 237t, 243
Prostaglandins, 270–271
Pseudoautosomal region 1 (PAR1), 419
Pseudohypoaldosteronism, 346t
PTC. *See* Papillary thyroid carcinoma (PTC)
PTEN hamartoma syndrome, 249
PTU. *See* Propylthiouracil (PTU)
Puberty and its disorders, **269–290**
 age at menarche (AAM), 271–273
 anorexia nervosa (AN), 283–287
 bone mineral density (BMD), 280, 286
 CHARGE syndrome, 280
 constitutional delay of growth and puberty (CDGP), 274–277
 delayed puberty, 273–287
 functional hypothalamic amenorrhea (FHA), 283
 growth charts, 274f, 278f
 hypogonadism (females), 281–287
 hypogonadism (males), 278–281
 Kallmann syndrome, 280
 Klinefelter syndrome (KS), 277, 278, 280
 physiology of puberty and pubertal growth, 270–271
 resumption of menses (ROM), 286
 testicular enlargement, 273
 timing of puberty, 271–273
 Turner syndrome (TS), 283–284
Pulmonary fibrosis, 250
PYD. *See* Hydroxylysyl-pyridinoline (PYD)

Q

Quantitative computed tomography (QCT), 296–297

R

Radioactive iodine ablation, 244, 249
Radioactive iodine uptake scan, 247
RANK-L, 293, 316
Recombinant human growth hormone (rhGH) therapy, 276
Recurrent pancreatitis, 370
Refeeding syndrome, 407
Remnant hypertrophy, 241
Resistin, 405
Resumption of menses (ROM), 286, 407
RET mutation analysis, 250
Reticularis, 343
Retropharyngeal mass, 241
Reverse cholesterol transport, 367, 367*f*
Rexinoids, 237*t*
Rhabdomyolysis, 377
Rheumatologic conditions, 305–306
rhGH therapy. *See* Recombinant human growth hormone (rhGH) therapy
Rickets, 309
Rifampin, 237*t*
Risedronate, 313
ROM. *See* Resumption of menses (ROM)
Runners, 398

S

Salicylates, 237*t*
Schmidt syndrome, 350
Sclerostin, 400
Sclerostin antibody, 316
SEARCH for Diabetes in Youth study, 257
Secondary adrenal insufficiency, 345, 346–347*t*, 351–352
Selective serotonin reuptake inhibitors (SSRIs), 406
Self-starvation, 393, 394. *See also* Eating disorders
Septo-optic dysplasia, 346*t*
Sertoli cells, 420
Serum E_2, 285
Sex chromosome DSD, 430
Sex determination, 429
Sex differentiation, 429
Sex hormone-binding globulin (SHBG), 328
Sex hormone replacement therapy, 435
Sexual maturity rating, 453
SHBG. *See* Sex hormone-binding globulin (SHBG)
Short stature, 411–412, 450–451, 451*t*
Short-stature-homeobox *(SHOX)* gene
  Klinefelter syndrome, 419
  Turner syndrome, 412
SHOX gene. *See* Short-stature-homeobox *(SHOX)* gene
Sick euthyroid syndrome, 406
Simple virilizers, 347
Sipple syndrome, 250
Skeleton, 291
Skyla, 384
Smith-Lemli-Opitz syndrome, 346*t*
Sodium chloride, 353
Somatostatin analogues, 237*t*
Spironolactone, 334
Sports, 398
SSRIs. *See* Selective serotonin reuptake inhibitors (SSRIs)
St. Catherine of Siena, 393
STAR 3 study, 263
Statins, 366, 376, 377, 379
StaTur Study, 414
Streak gonads, 435
Stress hyperglycemia, 260
Subclinical hypothyroidism, 240
Swimmers, 398
Swyer syndrome, 430

T

T1DM. *See* Type 1 diabetes (T1DM)
T2DM. *See* Type 2 diabetes (T2DM)
T3. *See* Triiodothyronine (T3)
T3 test. *See* Triiodothyronine (T3) test
T4. *See* Thyroxine (T4)
T4 test. *See* Thyroxine (T4) test
Tall stature, 418–419
TBII. *See* TSH-binding inhibitory immunoglobulin (TBII)
TBSRTC. *See* The Bethesda System for Reporting Thyroid Cytopathology (TBSRTC)
Teriparatide, 316
TESE. *See* Testicular sperm extraction (TESE)
Testicular enlargement, 272
Testicular sperm extraction (TESE), 420
Testosterone, 330, 331
Testosterone esters, 280
Testosterone replacement therapy (TRT), 277, 280, 312, 400
TG. *See* Triglyceride (TG)
TGF-α. *See* Transforming growth factor-α (TGF-α)
The Bethesda System for Reporting Thyroid Cytopathology (TBSRTC), 248
Thioamides, 237*t*, 243
Thyroglossal duct cyst, 241
Thyroid autoimmunity, 240
Thyroid cancer, 241
Thyroid disorders, **233–255**
  algorithm (hyperthyroidism), 235*f*
  algorithm (hypothyroidism), 234*f*
  algorithm (thyroid nodule), 246*f*, 247*f*
  autonomously functioning nodules, 244–245
  cancer survivors, 454–455

congenital hypothyroidism, 241
differentiated thyroid cancer, 249–250
drugs that cause thyroid dysfunction, 237t
evaluation of thyroid mass/nodule, 245–249
familial medullary thyroid cancer syndromes, 250–251
Graves disease, 242–244
Hashimoto thyroiditis, 239–240
hashitoxicosis, 245
hyperthyroidism, 235f, 242–245, 243t
hypothyroidism, 234f, 238–241, 238t
Jöd-Basedow phenomenon, 236
medullary thyroid carcinoma, 250–251
obesity, 233
physical examination, 238
pregnancy, 388, 389
subclinical hypothyroidism, 240
thyroid dysgenesis, 241
thyrotoxicosis, 242–245
Turner syndrome (TS), 415
Wolff-Chaikoff effect, 236
Thyroid dysgenesis, 241
Thyroid dyshormonogenesis, 241
Thyroid globulin antibodies, 242
Thyroid nodule, 245–249
Thyroid peroxidase antibodies, 242
Thyroid-stimulating hormone (TSH) test, 234
Thyroid-stimulating immunoglobulin (TSI), 242
Thyroid volume, 247
Thyroidectomy, 251
Thyrotoxicosis, 242–245, 306
Thyrotropin-releasing hormone (TRH), 397, 406
Thyroxine (T4), 239, 406
Thyroxine (T4) test, 234, 238
TODAY study, 266
Total thyroidectomy, 244, 251
Transforming growth factor-α (TGF-α), 270
Transient hypocalcemia, 315
Transient thyroiditis, 235
"Transition to Adult Health Care for Adolescents and Young Adults With Chronic Conditions," 441
TRH. *See* Thyrotropin-releasing hormone (TRH)
Triglyceride (TG), 365, 367, 372
Triiodothyronine (T3), 406
Triiodothyronine (T3) test, 234
Triple A syndrome, 346t, 352
TRT. *See* Testosterone replacement therapy (TRT)
True exophthalmos, 243
TS. *See* Turner syndrome (TS)
TSH-binding inhibitory immunoglobulin (TBII), 242
TSH receptor immunoglobulin (TSHrAb), 242
TSH test. *See* Thyroid-stimulating hormone (TSH) test

TSHrAb. *See* TSH receptor immunoglobulin (TSHrAb)
TSI. *See* Thyroid-stimulating immunoglobulin (TSI)
Tuberous sclerosis, 360
Turner syndrome (TS), **411–417**, 430t. *See also* Disorders of sex development (DSD)
autoimmune disease, 415
bone health, 306, 415
cardiac abnormalities, 414–415
clinical features, 412t
cognitive development and function, 416
congenital malformations, 416
estrogen therapy, 413–414
gonadal failure, 413
growth chart, 278f
growth failure shortly after birth, 413
growth hormone therapy, 413
hearing problems, 416
hypergonadotropic hypogonadism, 282–283
medical management and monitoring, 417t
oxandrolone, 413
pregnancy, 415
risk of mortality, 416
short stature, 411–412
SHOX gene, 412
streak gonads, 435
thyroid disorders, 415
Type 1 diabetes (T1DM), 256. *See also* Diabetes mellitus
advancements in management tools, 261
basal-bolus therapy, 262–263
booster snack, 265
Boston and London twin/triplet studies, 258
CGMS sensor-augmented insulin pump therapy, 263–264
continuous glucose monitoring system (CGMS), 263
DAISY study, 258
DCCT, 261
diabetes education, 264
diagnosis, 259–261
etiology, 258–259
exercise, 265
genomewide association studies (GWAS), 258
glycemic goals, 264–265
insulin pump therapy, 262
insulin therapy, 263
insulin-to-carb ratio, 262
management, 261–264
schools, 265–266
screening for T1DM, 259
STAR 3 study, 263
Type 2 diabetes (T2DM), 256, 266, 385. *See also* Diabetes mellitus
Type I collagen, 298

U

Undecanoate, 280
Urine ketones, 260
US Medical Eligibility Criteria for Contraception (USMEC), 383, 384
USMEC. See US Medical Eligibility Criteria for Contraception (USMEC)

V

Vaginoplasty, 349
Values clarification, 439
Vasopressin, 452
Vegan diet, 376
Vegetarian diet, 376
Vertebral radiography, 304, 317
Very-low-density lipoprotein (VLDL), 366
Vitamin D, 308–309, 310–312
Vitamin D deficiency, 308, 309
VLDL. See Very-low-density lipoprotein (VLDL)
von Hippel Lindau disease, 360

W

Welchol, 377, 378
Wilms tumor, 458
WNT signaling pathway, 293
Wolff-Chaikoff effect, 236
World Professional Association of Transgender Health (WPATH), 434
WPATH. See World Professional Association of Transgender Health (WPATH)

X

X-chromosome gene(s) haploinsufficiency, 306

Z

Zoledronate, 313